AI-Based Nutritional Intervention in Polycystic Ovary Syndrome (PCOS)

Rakesh Kumar • Meenu Gupta
Anand Nayyar
Editors

AI-Based Nutritional Intervention in Polycystic Ovary Syndrome (PCOS)

Springer

Editors
Rakesh Kumar
Department of Computer Science and Engineering
Chandigarh University
Chandigarh, Punjab, India

Meenu Gupta
Department of Computer Science and Engineering
Chandigarh University
Chandigarh, Punjab, India

Anand Nayyar
School of Computer Science
Duy Tan University
Da Nang, Vietnam

ISBN 978-981-96-2119-4 ISBN 978-981-96-2120-0 (eBook)
https://doi.org/10.1007/978-981-96-2120-0

This Springer imprint is published by the registered company Springer Nature Singapore Pte Ltd.
The registered company address is: 152 Beach Road, #21-01/04 Gateway East, Singapore 189721, Singapore

Preface

This book proposes a groundbreaking investigation into the synergy of Artificial Intelligence (AI) and nutritional interventions for Polycystic Ovary Syndrome (PCOS) management. Addressing the complexities of PCOS, this book explores AI applications in unraveling the genetic, metabolic, and lifestyle intricacies that influence the syndrome. PCOS is a prevalent endocrine disorder that affects countless women globally, often presenting complex challenges related to hormonal imbalances, insulin resistance, fertility issues, and overall well-being. Key focuses include AI-driven diagnostics for swift and accurate PCOS identification, personalized nutrition plans integrating genetic and hormonal data, and behavioral interventions promoting adherence. The book delves into real-time monitoring through wearable tech and ethical considerations surrounding AI implementation in healthcare. By bridging technological innovation and clinical practice, this book envisions a future where AI transforms PCOS management, ushering in a new era of precision medicine in women's health.

At the heart of this book lies a profound exploration of nutrient-based AI solutions. Readers will uncover how AI can tailor nutrition plans to suit individual PCOS profiles, offering insights into micronutrients, macronutrients, and dietary choices. With a spotlight on glycemic control, hormonal balance, and holistic wellness, this book sheds light on nutrition's vital role in PCOS management. It delves into the ethical dimensions of AI in healthcare while championing patient empowerment. Through real-life success stories, case studies, and practical guidance, "AI Solutions for PCOS" empowers women, healthcare professionals, and researchers to harness AI's potential in optimizing women's health and well-being.

The book comprises of 13 chapters contributed from diverse researchers across the world. Chapter 1 provides a comprehensive understanding of PCOS, including its pathophysiology, clinical manifestations, and diagnostic criteria, explores the intricate relationship between PCOS and nutritional status, detailing how the syndrome impacts nutritional status and metabolism and, conversely, how nutritional factors can influence the course of PCOS, presents evidence-based dietary management strategies tailored for patients with PCOS and highlights emerging research and potential future directions in the dietary management of PCOS. Chapter 2 highlights the shortcomings of traditional dietary guidelines which includes how well they work in controlling PCOS symptoms, examines the possible advantages of a more individualized and comprehensive approach to PCOS-affected women's nutrition, and suggests further investigations into the relationship between PCOS and nutrition. Chapter 3 summarizes current research and highlights the therapeutic potential of certain nutrients, such as minerals, vitamins, and substances that resemble vitamins, in treating pathways caused by PCOS. In addition, Artificial Intelligence (AI) and Deep Learning (DL) techniques are utilized to customize nutrient recommendations for women diagnosed with PCOS, aiding in personalized dietary plans aimed at managing symptoms and regulating metabolic imbalances. Chapter 4 proposes an AI-based precision nutrition model for providing customized dietary recommendations for PCOS by systematically assimilating multi-domain data, explores the use of explainable AI techniques for deciphering pathology and dissecting distinctive PCOS phenotypes, and outlines a methodology for mapping dietary components to outcomes via machine learning algorithms and continually updating recommendations. Chapter 5 highlights the gradual correction process and recommended practices for using gender-based data analytics to reduce prejudices and examines the revolutionary effects of large data sets on the identification of diseases, patient care, and the use of resources in the healthcare sector. Chapter 6 delves into the intersection of AI and nutrition, specifically focusing on the monitoring and optimization of nutrient intake and highlights the potential for AI-driven solutions to revolutionize how individuals track, analyze, and enhance their nutritional habits. In addition, the chapter enlightens prevalent challenges in conventional nutrient monitoring methods and their limitations and explores the integration of AI algorithms and machine learning techniques in processing vast amounts of dietary data. Chapter 7 highlights the potential of artificial intelligence (AI) in improving insulin management and glycemic control for diabetic patients, explores the use of AI systems to predict and reduce complications related to inadequate glycemic management, and provides insight into how AI might be used to develop intelligent insulin management systems. Chapter 8 illustrates the concept of AI-powered personalized nutrition for PCOS, enlightens critical considerations for AI in healthcare, and also highlights the future of PCOS care with AI. Chapter 9 streamlines the concept of comprehensive, personalized dietetics treatment strategy for PCOS, stresses to fallacy the conventional dietetics approach that results in non-unique, uniform dietary therapeutic plans and provides a better future treatment for PCOS and analysis of personal dietetics concept. Chapter 10 highlights nutritional supplements for PCOS, enlightens herbal remedies for PCOS, and discusses AI's role in Personalized Recommendations. Chapter 11 investigates the ethical implications of incorporating artificial intelligence into nutritional guidance systems by thoroughly examining current literature, case studies, and empirical analyses and illuminates the diverse challenges linked with AI-powered nutritional guidance. In addition, the chapter explores the use of LIME as a technical methodology for enhancing algorithm transparency, interpreting model decisions, and addressing potential biases and discusses robust privacy protocols and unbiased model development to ensure responsible deployment. Chapter 12 examines the role of mHealth solutions in PCOS nutrition, explores the integration of wearables for personalized health monitoring, and assesses the effectiveness of these technologies in improving PCOS outcomes. Chapter 13 presents how HAI enables users to monitor their eating patterns with precision and consistency, highlights how HAI-enabled algorithms can be utilized to provide individualized recommendations for nutritional intake, stresses on HAI-driven examination of eating behaviors that can offer useful behavioral insights, assisting individuals in identifying triggers for unhealthy eating habits or deficits to treat them effectively and enlightens how HAI systems can provide immediate feedback and coaching, assisting users in making improved food selections or proposing alternatives in cases where their diet lacks specific nutrients, future research trends, and lessons learned.

We hope this book empowers both healthcare professionals and patients on this journey of personalized dietary optimization through AI-driven insights. We invite you to delve deeper and explore the possibilities that AI-based interventions hold for PCOS treatment and overall well-being.

Chandigarh, India — Rakesh Kumar
Chandigarh, India — Meenu Gupta
Da Nang, Vietnam — Anand Nayyar

Contents

About the Editors

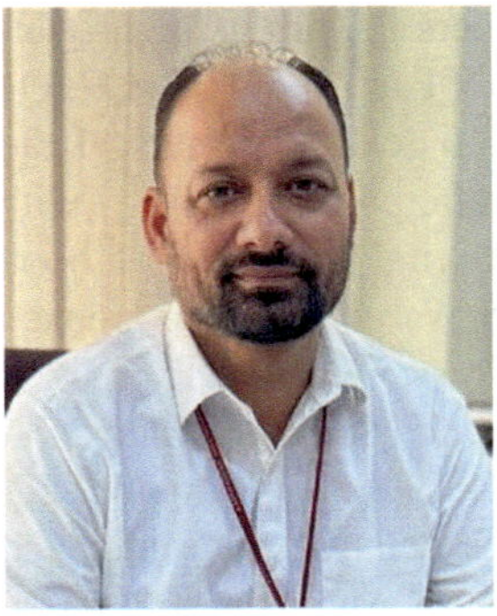

Rakesh Kumar is a Professor at the UIE-CSE Department, Chandigarh University, India. He completed his Ph.D. in Computer Science and Engineering from Punjab Technical University, Jalandhar 2017. He has more than 19 years of teaching experience. His research interests are IoT, Machine Learning, and Natural Language Processing. He has published many authored books with the reputed publisher. He works as a reviewer for several journals, including Big Data, CMC, Scientific Reports, and TSP. He has authored or co-authored more than 100 publications in various national and international conferences and journals. He also chaired many conferences and was the convener and organizer of IEEE and AIP conferences.

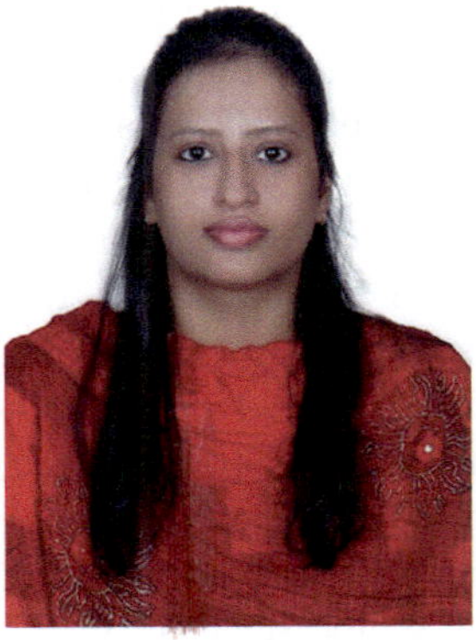

Meenu Gupta is an Associate Professor at the UIE-CSE Department, Chandigarh University, India. She completed her Ph.D. in Computer Science and Engineering with an emphasis on Traffic Accident Severity Problems from Ansal University, Gurgaon, India, in 2020. She has more than 15 years of teaching experience. Her research areas cover Computational Techniques, Intelligent Systems, and Data mining, with a specific interest in Artificial Intelligence, Image Processing and Analysis, Smart Cities, Data Analysis, and Human/Brain-Machine Interaction (BMI). She has five edited and four authored books. She has also written over 20 book chapters and 150+ papers in refereed international journals and conferences. She has five filled patents. She was awarded the Best Faculty of the Department and Best Researcher award in 2021 and 2022. She also chaired many conferences and was the convener and organizer of IEEE and AIP conferences.

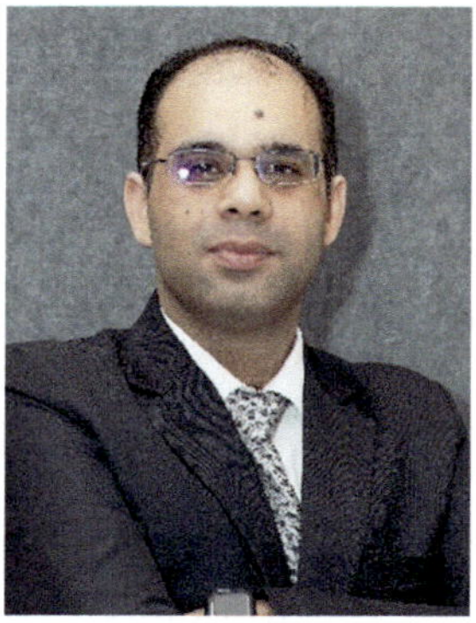

Anand Nayyar received Ph.D. (Computer Science) from Desh Bhagat University in 2017 in the area of Wireless Sensor Networks, Swarm Intelligence and Network Simulation. He is currently working in School of Computer Science-Duy Tan University, Da Nang, Vietnam as Professor, Scientist, Vice-Chairman (Research), and Director—IoT and Intelligent Systems Lab. A Certified Professional with 230+ professional certifications from CISCO, Microsoft, Amazon, Alibaba Cloud, Salesforce, Oracle, Google, Beingcert, EXIN, GAQM, Cyberoam, and many more. Published more than 250+ research papers in various high-quality ISI-SCI/SCIE/SSCI Impact Factor-Q1, Q2, Q3, Q4 Journals cum Scopus/ESCI Indexed Journals, 100+ papers in International Conferences indexed with Springer, IEEE, and ACM Digital Library, 70+ book chapters in various SCOPUS/Web of Science indexed books with Springer, CRC Press, Wiley, IET, Elsevier with citations: (Google Scholar): 18000+, H-Index: 70, and I-Index: 280; (Scopus): 9700+; H-Index: 52. Member of more than 60+ associations as senior and life member like: IEEE (Senior Member) and ACM (Senior Member). He has authored/co-authored cum edited 70+ books of Computer Science. Associated with more than 600+ International Conferences as Program Committee/Chair/Advisory Board/Review Board member. He has 18 Australian Patents, 16 German Patents, 4 Japanese Patents, 44 Indian Design cum Utility Patents, 13 UK Patents, 1 USA Patent, 3 Indian Copyrights and 2 Canadian Copyrights to his credit in the area of Wireless Communications, Artificial Intelligence, Cloud Computing, IoT, Healthcare, Drones, Robotics, and Image Processing. Awarded 54 Awards for Teaching and Research—Young Scientist, Best Scientist, Best Senior Scientist, Asia's Top 50 Academicians and Researchers, Young Researcher Award, Outstanding Researcher Award, Excellence in Teaching, Best Senior Scientist Award, DTU Best Professor and Researcher Award—2019, 2020–2021, 2021–2022 2022–2023, 2023–2024; Distinguished Scientist Award by the National University of Singapore, Obada Prize 2023, Lifetime Achievement Award 2023; Asian Admirable Achievers 2024; Distinguished Academic Leader 2024, and many more. He is listed in Top 2% Scientists as per Stanford

University (2019, 2020, 2021, 2022, 2023, 2024), Ad Index (Rank No: 1 Duy Tan University, Rank No: 1 Computer Science in Viet Nam), and Listed on *Research.com* (Top Scientist of Computer Science in Viet Nam-National Ranking: 2; D-Index: 42; World Ranking: 6968).

He is acting as Associate Editor for Computer Communications (Elsevier), International Journal of Sensor Networks (IJSNET) (Inderscience), Computers, Materials and Continua (CMC), Tech Science Press—IASC, Cogent Engineering, Human-Centric Computing and Information Sciences (HCIS), PeerJ Computer Science, IEEE Transactions on Artificial Intelligence (IEEE TAI), Indonesian Journal of Electrical Engineering and Computer Science, IJFC, IJISP, IJDST, IJCINI, IJGC, IJSIR, IJBDCN, IJNR, IJSI. He is acting as Managing Editor of IGI-Global Journal, USA, titled *International Journal of Knowledge and Systems Science (IJKSS)* and Editor-in-Chief of IGI-Global, USA Journal titled *International Journal of Smart Vehicles and Smart Transportation (IJSVST)*. He has reviewed more than 5100+ articles for diverse Web of Science and Scopus Indexed Journals. He is currently researching in the area of Wireless Sensor Networks, Internet of Things, Swarm Intelligence, Cloud Computing, Artificial Intelligence, Drones, Blockchain, Cyber Security, Healthcare Informatics, Big Data, and Wireless Communications.

Introduction to Polycystic Ovary Syndrome (PCOS) and Nutritional Challenges

1

Bancha Yingngam, Chakkrapong Chaiburi, and Abhiruj Navabhatra

Abbreviations

AI	Artificial intelligence
AMPK	AMP-activated protein kinase
ANNs	Artificial neural networks
BMI	Body mass index
CNNs	Convolutional neural networks
FSH	Follicle-stimulating hormone
GI	Glycemic food
HDL	High-density lipoprotein cholesterol
INH	The National Institute of Health
LDL	Low-density lipoprotein cholesterol
LH	Luteinizing hormone
PCOS	Polycystic ovary syndrome
SVM	Support vector machine

B. Yingngam (✉)
Faculty of Pharmaceutical Sciences, Ubon Ratchathani University, Ubon Ratchathani, Thailand
e-mail: bancha.y@ubu.ac.th

C. Chaiburi
Faculty of Science and Digital Innovation, Thaksin University (Phatthalung Campus), Pa Payom, Phatthalung, Thailand
e-mail: chakkrapong@tsu.ac.th

A. Navabhatra
College of Pharmacy, Rangsit University, Pathum Thani, Thailand
e-mail: abhiruj.c@rsu.ac.th

R. Kumar et al. (eds.), *AI-Based Nutritional Intervention in Polycystic Ovary Syndrome (PCOS)*, https://doi.org/10.1007/978-981-96-2120-0_1

1.1 Introduction

Women's health, particularly during their reproductive years, encompasses a broad spectrum of physiological and hormonal processes that are essential for overall well-being and the ability to conceive [1]. Among the myriad of conditions affecting women, hormonal disorders play a significant role, often impacting not only physical health but also emotional and psychological well-being [2, 3]. These disorders can range from common hormonal imbalances to more complex conditions, affecting a significant portion of the female population worldwide [4]. Understanding these conditions, their causes and symptoms, and management strategies is crucial for both healthcare professionals and patients to ensure effective treatment and improve quality of life [5].

Polycystic ovary syndrome (PCOS) is a complex endocrine disorder that affects approximately 2.2–26% of women of reproductive age and is one of the most common hormonal disorders in this population [2, 6, 7]. Nevertheless, the incidence of PCOS might be greater in some instances. For example, in worldwide studies that utilize population cohorts, the previously estimated incidence of PCOS varies widely, ranging from 0.9% to 41%, with significant variability across North America and Europe [8]. In addition, this syndrome represents the most common endocrine disorder among women in their premenopausal years [1]. PCOS is characterized by a combination of symptoms, such as irregular menstrual cycles, excessive hair growth, acne, and obesity, and is also a leading cause of infertility [9, 10]. This syndrome is associated with insulin resistance and hyperinsulinemia, which exacerbates symptoms and increases the risk of developing type 2 diabetes, cardiovascular diseases, and endometrial cancer [5, 11]. Epidemiological studies indicate that approximately 50–70% of individuals with PCOS exhibit insulin resistance [12]. Furthermore, women with PCOS often experience significant nutritional challenges [13]. Their altered hormonal and metabolic profiles make weight management particularly difficult, necessitating specialized dietary strategies [14]. The high prevalence of insulin resistance in patients with PCOS demands a tailored approach to diet, focusing on low-glycemic-index foods and balanced macronutrient intake to improve insulin sensitivity [15]. Additionally, the psychological burden of PCOS, including increased rates of anxiety and depression, can further complicate dietary adherence and overall management of the condition [16]. This interplay between PCOS and nutrition highlights the need for comprehensive management strategies that address both the physiological and the psychological aspects of the syndrome, highlighting the significant problems it poses to women's health globally [17]. Despite the common occurrence of PCOS, a significant number of women do not receive adequate treatment. This is often attributed to inconsistencies in clinical practices, a lack of adequate emphasis on lifestyle modifications and the prevention of long-term illnesses, and a primary focus on fertility treatments that usually involve expensive assisted reproductive technologies. While modern therapies for PCOS are available, they typically only target the symptoms of the disorder [18]. This approach is used predominantly owing to a limited understanding of the underlying causes of PCOS, which poses a challenge in developing treatments that effectively address the core underlying mechanisms of this syndrome.

Objectives of the Chapter

The objectives of the chapter are:

1. To provide a comprehensive understanding of PCOS, including its pathophysiology, clinical manifestations, and diagnostic criteria, thereby establishing a solid foundation for subsequent discussions on nutritional challenges and management strategies.
2. To explore the intricate relationship between PCOS and nutritional status and detail how the syndrome impacts nutritional status and metabolism and, conversely, how nutritional factors can influence the course of PCOS.
3. To present evidence-based dietary management strategies tailored for patients with PCOS, emphasizing the importance of individualized nutritional plans and lifestyle modifications that can alleviate symptoms and improve overall health outcomes.
4. To address the management of common comorbidities associated with PCOS through nutritional factors, such as insulin resistance, obesity, and cardiovascular risk, providing a holistic approach to treatment.
5. And, to highlight emerging research and potential future directions in the dietary management of PCOS, fostering an understanding of the evolving field of PCOS treatment and encouraging continuous learning and adaptation in clinical practice.

Organization of the Chapter

The rest of this chapter is organized as follows: Section 1.2 explores the detailed pathophysiology, clinical manifestations, and diagnostic criteria of PCOS, providing a comprehensive overview of the syndrome. Section 1.3 explains how PCOS affects nutritional status and metabolism and discusses the interplay between PCOS and various nutritional deficiencies or excesses. In Sect. 1.4, the authors examine specific dietary interventions and lifestyle modifications beneficial for managing PCOS symptoms, emphasizing evidence-based dietary guidelines and individualized nutritional plans. Section 1.5 focuses on the role of nutrition in managing common comorbid conditions associated with PCOS, such as insulin resistance, obesity, and cardiovascular risk factors. Section 1.6 highlights the latest related research in the field, exploring innovative dietary approaches and potential future therapies for PCOS. Finally, Sect. 1.7 summarizes the key points discussed in the chapter and proposes areas for future research, underscoring the evolving nature of understanding PCOS and its nutritional management.

1.2 Polycystic Ovary Syndrome

1.2.1 Definition

PCOS is a multifaceted endocrine disorder that predominantly affects women of reproductive age and impacts various aspects of their health [1]. The term "polycystic ovary syndrome" derives from the characteristic presence of numerous (poly)cysts—fluid-filled sacs—commonly found along the periphery of the ovaries [19]. Although not every individual with PCOS has these cysts, cysts containing undeveloped eggs are often not found [2]. Medically, PCOS is also known as hyperandrogenic anovulation or Stein–Leventhal syndrome [20]. It is characterized by the presence of numerous small cysts in one or both ovaries, which are typically approximately 2–9 mm in diameter [7]. A key diagnostic criterion is an ovarian volume greater than 10 mL in at least one ovary, a standard established by Stein and Leventhal's seminal work in 1935 [6]. Figure 1.1 presents a visual comparison between a normal ovary and a polycystic ovary, highlighting their anatomical differences. In the depiction of a normal ovary, one would expect to see an almond-shaped structure with a smooth exterior, typical of ovaries that measure approximately 3–5 cm in length. This ovary may show a single dominant follicle, which is representative of normal ovulation cycles. In contrast, polycystic ovaries are likely to appear enlarged and potentially two to three times larger than normal ovaries are, with a surface that may appear slightly bumpy or

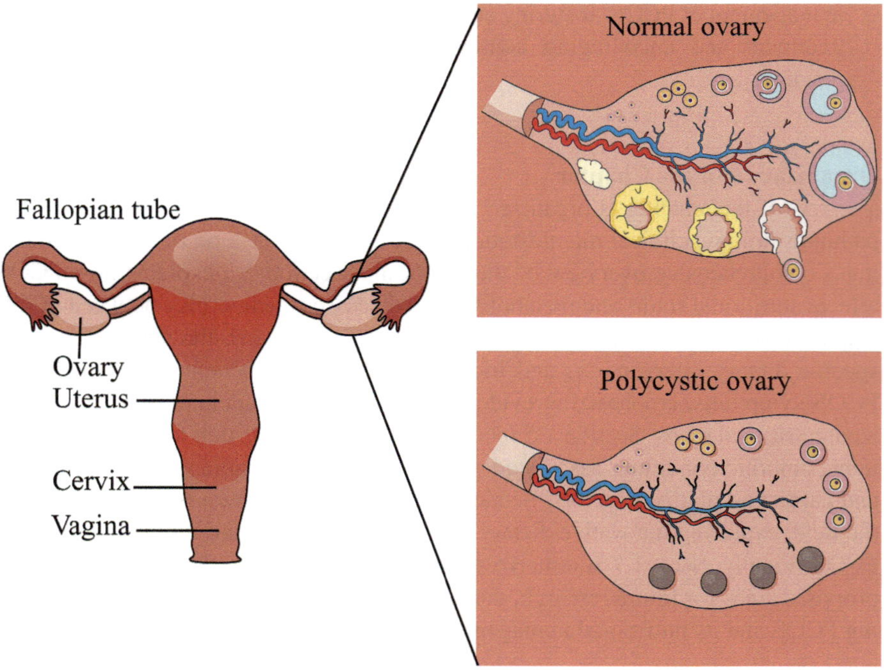

Fig. 1.1 Anatomical examples of a normal ovary compared with a polycystic ovary

smooth. This enlargement is due to the presence of multiple small follicles, often under 10 mm in size, which resemble a "string of pearls" around the periphery of the ovary [7]. These follicles represent immature eggs that have not progressed to full maturity or ovulation, illustrating the hallmark of irregular or absent ovulation associated with polycystic ovaries. This visual juxtaposition effectively illustrates the physical distinctions that underlie the differing reproductive functions and health implications of these two types of ovaries. Currently, PCOS is characterized by a range of symptoms and clinical signs, which include irregular or absent menstrual periods, hyperandrogenism (marked by excessive levels of male hormones leading to symptoms such as hirsutism, acne, and alopecia), and the presence of polycystic ovaries observable through ultrasound examination [21].

1.2.2 Prevalence

The prevalence of PCOS varies globally and is influenced by factors such as the diagnostic criteria used, the population studied, and methodology [22]. It is estimated that PCOS affects approximately 2.2–26.0% of women worldwide, making it one of the most common endocrine disorders among women of childbearing age [7, 23, 24]. However, this prevalence rate can vary; for example, some studies suggest that it could reach 15–20%, depending on the population and diagnostic criteria [25]. The prevalence of PCOS is also affected by factors such as race and ethnicity, with some groups showing higher or lower rates of PCOS [26]. The high prevalence of PCOS is significant not only because of its impact on reproductive health and fertility but also because of its association with long-term health risks, such as metabolic syndrome, type 2 diabetes, and cardiovascular diseases [27]. These findings underscore the importance of early diagnosis and effective management of this syndrome. The diverse manifestations of PCOS mean that it can affect various aspects of a woman's health and quality of life, making awareness and understanding of this condition crucial for healthcare providers and patients alike [28].

Table 1.1 presents a comprehensive overview of the incidence of PCOS in various populations globally using data from different studies and diagnostic criteria. For example, Chiaffarino et al. [30] conducted a systematic review and meta-analysis on the incidence of PCOS in Europe and the USA. The findings revealed that the incidence of PCOS varied according to the diagnostic criteria: 6.2% according to the NIH 1990 criteria, 19.5% according to the ESHRE/ASRM 2003 criteria, and 15.0% according to the AES-PCOS criteria. The study also revealed different PCOS phenotypes, with the most common being "complete PCOS" (phenotype A), followed by "nonhyperandrogenic PCOS" (phenotype D), "ovulatory PCOS" (phenotype C), and phenotype B, which resemble A but lack polycystic ovarian morphology. An increase in the prevalence of PCOS over time was noted, which was partially attributed to changes in diagnostic criteria. The study highlighted similar PCOS incidences in European countries and the USA, with some regional differences in phenotype frequencies, suggesting a need for further investigation into these variations for a better understanding of PCOS.

Table 1.1 Graph showing the prevalence of PCOS in different populations around the world

Region/ population	Incidence of PCOS	Notes	Reference
Global average	2.2–26.0%	Based on a synthesis of multiple studies	[7, 23, 24, 29]
USA and Europe	5.3–7.0% (average = 6.2%, NIH 1990), 17.3–21.6% (average = 19.5% ESHRE/ ASRM 2023), and 12.9–17.1% (average = 15.0%, AES-PCOS)	Variation based on diagnostic criteria	[30]
USA	5.2% (based on the international classification of diseases codes)	The prevalence of PCOS in the USA is shaped by genetic diversity, lifestyle, and environmental factors, as well as disparities in healthcare access and awareness. Different diagnostic criteria, including the international classification of disease codes, lead to varied prevalence rates. Ethnic and racial differences also influence the prevalence and presentation of PCOS across the country	[22]
Asia	5.6–14.3% (based on the Rotterdam criteria)	Higher prevalence in Southeast Asia	[31]
Southeast Asia	2.5–2.7%	Southeast Asia's lower PCOS prevalence compared to broader Asia may result from distinct genetic, dietary, and lifestyle factors. Variations in healthcare access and PCOS awareness, along with cultural and social influences, also affect its diagnosis and reporting in this subregion	[32]
Middle east	1.2–2.7%	Females aged between 15 and 45 years	[33, 34]
Australia	8.7–11.9%	Similar to north American trends	[35]

Note: The methodology used in this table is based on epidemiological studies that use varying diagnostic criteria, including the Rotterdam criteria and the NIH criteria. However, incidence rates can vary within regions due to ethnic, genetic, and lifestyle factors. The percentages are approximate and are subject to change as new research emerges

In Asian countries, studies using various diagnostic criteria, such as the Rotterdam, Japanese, and Chinese standards, have shown differing rates of PCOS occurrence. Specifically, in Chinese women, the occurrence of PCOS has been reported at rates of 6.1% (in the general population) and 13.7% (infertility patients) according to these criteria [36]. The frequency of PCOS in Asian regions shows significant variation: 5.6% among women in southern China, 5.7% among Thai women, and 6.3% among women from Sri Lanka, reaching 14.3% among Iranian women. These variations suggest that the incidence of PCOS is influenced by multiple factors, including ethnic diversity [31].

Like in North America, in Adelaide, Australia, the occurrence of PCOS shows notable differences when various diagnostic standards are used. According to the study referenced as number 31, the incidence rates in Adelaide were found to be 8.7% when the NIH criteria were used, 11.9% when the Rotterdam criteria were used, and 10.2% when the AES criteria were applied. These variations in prevalence rates highlight the impact of different diagnostic criteria on the reported incidence of PCOS in a given population [35].

The study of PCOS in the Middle East and North Africa, referencing data from the Global Burden of Disease 2019, provides significant insights into the prevalence and impact of PCOS across 21 countries. The data covering the period from 1990 to 2019 indicate a notable increase in both the point prevalence and incidence of PCOS, with age-standardized rates showing a substantial increase. In 2019, the age-standardized point prevalence rate was 2.079 per 100,000 people (approximately 2.1%), and the incidence rate was 77.2 per 100,000 people, indicating increases of 37.9% and 33.7%, respectively, since 1990. The percentage of years lived with disability also increased by 36.1% during this period. Notably, Kuwait reported the highest age-standardized years lived with disability rate, whereas Afghanistan had the lowest rate. Sudan experienced the most significant increase in years lived with disability. The prevalence of PCOS was found to be highest in women aged >20–14 years and to decline after age 45 [33]. Overall, the table highlights the significant variation in the incidence of PCOS across different regions and underscores the influence of diagnostic criteria and regional factors on these prevalence rates.

1.2.3 Symptoms

PCOS presents a spectrum of symptoms that can vary widely among individuals, contributing to the complexity of its diagnosis and management [13, 37]. One of the most common symptoms is menstrual irregularity, which may manifest as infrequent periods (oligomenorrhea), absent periods (amenorrhea), or irregular bleeding [7]. For example, in a study of Saudi women with PCOS, oligomenorrhea, characterized by extended intervals of at least 6 weeks between episodes of vaginal bleeding, was observed in 79.4% of the participants. Notably, increased menstrual irregularity is correlated with increased levels of luteinizing hormone/follicle-stimulating hormone (LH/FSH) and testosterone [38]. Another key symptom of this condition is hyperandrogenism, which causes excessive hair growth in areas typical for males (hirsutism), acne, and, in some cases, thinning of scalp hair (androgenic alopecia) [11, 39]. For example, in North America, the expenditure on PCOS and its associated comorbidities is estimated to be approximately 4 billion dollars. This condition represents the most frequently diagnosed endocrine disorder among women of reproductive age in this region. Dermatological issues, such as hirsutism, are present in 70% of these patients, whereas hair loss is reported in 38.5%. Additionally, 22.8% of patients with PCOS experience menstrual irregularities [8].

Additionally, many women with PCOS experience weight gain or difficulty losing weight, and obesity is commonly observed, although not universally [40]. As many as 80% of women diagnosed with PCOS are overweight or obese, with a body mass index (BMI) exceeding 25 kg/m^2. Particularly in Australia and the USA, the incidence of obesity (defined as a BMI greater than 30 kg/m^2) among women with PCOS ranges between 61% and 76%. Obesity is a significant concern for women with PCOS and is linked to a substantial decrease in quality-of-life scores [41].

Polycystic ovaries, as observed through ultrasound imaging, are typically characterized by the presence of numerous small cysts or follicles encircling the ovaries. These cysts are often described as resembling a string of pearls on ultrasound because of their arrangement around the periphery of the ovary. However, the presence of these cystic structures alone is insufficient for a PCOS diagnosis. Diagnosis requires a combination of symptoms and findings, as some women may have polycystic ovaries without experiencing the full spectrum of PCOS symptoms, whereas others may have PCOS without the characteristic cystic appearance of ultrasound [42].

Other symptoms can include infertility or subfertility, often due to irregular ovulation or anovulation [43]. For example, women with PCOS may experience longer or unpredictable menstrual cycles, making it difficult to predict ovulation. In some cases, they may not ovulate at all (anovulation), significantly reducing changes in natural conception. This irregularity in the reproductive cycle led to prolonged periods without pregnancy despite attempts to conceive, often necessitating medical intervention or fertility treatment [44].

Insulin resistance, a frequently undetected yet crucial characteristic of PCOS, can ultimately lead to symptoms related to high insulin and blood sugar levels. In their study, Chen et al. [45] reported that circulating insulin-like peptide 5 is significantly involved in metabolic activities both in laboratory settings and in living organisms. Their research revealed higher levels of this peptide in individuals with PCOS, and these levels were significantly correlated with the homeostasis model assessment of insulin resistance. Initially, individuals may not experience noticeable symptoms, but as insulin resistance progresses, it can lead to specific conditions [45]. For example, skin tags, which are small, soft, and skin-colored, may develop in various parts of the body. Additionally, one may observe darkened patches of skin, known as acanthosis nigricans, which typically appear in folds and creases such as the neck, groin, and under the breasts. These patches may initially seem to be mere dirt or discoloration but are a distinctive sign of certain underlying health issues. Often associated with insulin resistance, a key factor in conditions such as PCOS and type 2 diabetes, acanthosis nigricans can also indicate hormonal disorders. These symptoms are indicative of the body's impaired ability to use insulin effectively, a common issue in PCOS patients who can have broader metabolic implications if left unaddressed.

1.2.4 Pathophysiology and Causes

The pathophysiology of PCOS is multifaceted and not entirely understood; it involves a complex interplay of genetic, hormonal, and metabolic factors [1, 46,

47]. Central to the development of PCOS is the presence of hyperandrogenism, an elevated level of male hormones, particularly testosterone [48, 49]. This androgen excess often originates from the ovaries, although the adrenal glands may also contribute [21]. The adrenal glands can also contribute to increased androgen production. The adrenal glands, located above the kidneys, are responsible for producing a variety of hormones, including a small amount of androgen. The exact reason why the ovaries and sometimes the adrenal glands produce more androgens in PCOS patients is not entirely clear and is a subject of ongoing research. This hormonal imbalance underpins many of the clinical features of PCOS, making the management of androgen levels a key focus in the treatment of this syndrome.

Insulin resistance is another key aspect of PCOS pathophysiology and is present in a significant proportion of cases, especially those associated with obesity [50]. Insulin resistance leads to compensatory hyperinsulinemia (elevated insulin levels), which further exacerbates hyperandrogenism [17]. High insulin levels increase the production of androgens by the ovaries and reduce the hepatic synthesis of sex hormone-binding globulin (SHBG), which in turn increases the level of free testosterone [17]. This hormonal imbalance disrupts normal ovarian function, leading to anovulation (failure to ovulate) and menstrual irregularities [51]. Moreover, elevated androgens can lead to symptoms typical of PCOS, such as hirsutism, acne, and alopecia [11]. There is also the interplay between hyperandrogenism and dysregulation of the hypothalamic–pituitary–gonadal axis, further complicating ovulation and menstrual irregularities [52].

The exact causes of PCOS are not fully understood, but several factors likely contribute to its development. Genetics plays a significant role in this disease, as evidenced by the increased incidence of PCOS in women with a family history of this disease. Studies have identified various genetic markers associated with PCOS, although no single gene has been pinpointed as the definitive cause [53]. Environmental and lifestyle factors, such as diet, physical activity, and obesity, are also believed to contribute to the development of PCOS, particularly those that influence body weight and insulin resistance [54]. The onset of PCOS symptoms is often associated with weight gain, and obesity exacerbates insulin resistance and hyperandrogenism [50]. However, importantly, not all women with PCOS are overweight, and lean women can also be affected. Another proposed factor is fetal programming, where intrauterine exposures or conditions may predispose an individual to develop PCOS later in life [55]. This theory suggests that certain environmental exposures during fetal development could set the stage for hormonal and metabolic disturbances that manifest as PCOS in adulthood. Despite ongoing research, the exact etiology of PCOS remains a topic of investigation, with the current understanding pointing to a multifactorial origin involving complex interactions among genetic, hormonal, and environmental influences.

The pathophysiology of PCOS is complex and not completely understood, but it is known to involve hormonal imbalances, including increased levels of androgens (male hormones) and insulin resistance [45, 56]. These hormonal disturbances can lead to a variety of symptoms and increase the risk of other health problems, such as type 2 diabetes, cardiovascular diseases, and endometrial cancer [38]. There are several criteria for diagnosing PCOS, including the Rotterdam criteria, which require two of the following three criteria for a diagnosis: oligo- or anovulation, clinical or biochemical signs of hyperandrogenism, and polycystic ovaries [48]. PCOS has become the leading cause of female infertility, with estimates suggesting that it affects approximately 75% of women who suffer from infertility due to anovulation [6]. The variability in diagnostic criteria can sometimes lead to differences in the diagnosis and understanding of PCOS, making it a complex syndrome that requires careful and comprehensive evaluation [22].

1.2.5 Current Diagnostic Criteria

The diagnosis of PCOS typically involves a combination of clinical evaluation, laboratory tests, and imaging studies. It is based on the exclusion of other disorders that mimic similar symptoms [57]. The criteria for diagnosing PCOS have long been a topic of discussion and sometimes contention among gynecologists and endocrinologists. The core of this debate stems from the lack of a universally accepted, standardized definition for the syndrome. In regions such as Europe and Australia, the diagnosis of PCOS often hinges on ovarian ultrasound findings, particularly revealing the presence of chronic anovulation and hyperandrogenism. Currently, there are four established diagnostic criteria for PCOS: the National Institute of Health (NIH) (NIH 1990) criteria [58], the Rotterdam criteria [59], the criteria set by the Androgen Excess and PCOS Society (AE-PCOS Society) [60], and the International PCOS guidelines 2023 [61].

1. According to the 1990 NIH criteria, both clinical and biochemical hyperandrogenism and oligo-ovulation are needed for a diagnosis of PCOS, and other related disorders are excluded. This approach emphasizes androgen excess as a core feature of PCOS [58].
2. The Rotterdam criteria were expanded upon the NIH 1990 criteria by including two additional phenotypes. According to the Rotterdam criteria, PCOS can be diagnosed if two of the following three criteria are met: oligo- or anovulation, clinical and/or biochemical signs of hyperandrogenism, or polycystic ovaries. This expansion allows for the diagnosis of PCOS in women who have polycystic ovaries and either hyperandrogenism or ovulatory dysfunction, but not necessarily both [59].
3. The 2006 AE-PCOS Society criteria focus primarily on androgen excess in patients with PCOS. These conditions require the presence of clinical or biochemical hyperandrogenism, in addition to either polycystic ovaries or ovulatory dysfunction, for a PCOS diagnosis [60].
4. The International PCOS Guidelines 2023, the latest guidelines, emphasize a comprehensive and evidence-based approach to the assessment and management of PCOS. They incorporate the latest research and clinical practice insights to provide a more nuanced understanding of the condition. This includes refinements to diagnostic criteria, a recognition of the broader features of PCOS (such

as metabolic and psychological aspects), and an emphasis on personalized patient care.

To provide readers with a more understandable overview, Table 1.2 presents a side-by-side comparison of the four widely recognized diagnostic criteria for PCOS, highlighting the similarities and differences in their approaches. Notably, worldwide agreement on the diagnosis of PCOS was reached on the basis of the 1990 NIH criteria. Interestingly, this agreement did not support ovarian morphology as a key diagnostic factor, despite its role in the initial clinical description of the syndrome [58]. In May 2003, an international panel of experts convened during the Rotterdam proceedings to hold a consensus workshop on PCOS. The objective of these studies was to establish definitive diagnostic criteria for PCOS. A consensus was reached that a PCOS diagnosis should be considered when at least two out of the following three criteria are present: (1) oligo- or anovulation, (2) clinical or biochemical signs of hyperandrogenism, and (3) polycystic ovarian morphology confirmed by ultrasound scans. The relevance of detecting polycystic ovarian morphology via ultrasound scans, particularly in women without overt symptoms of PCOS, continues to be a topic of active discussion and research in the medical and scientific communities [59]. In 2006, the AE-PCOS established updated diagnostic criteria for PCOS. These criteria include the presence of (1) ovulation and menstrual irregularities, (2) hyperandrogenism, (3) clinical signs of elevated androgen levels, and (4) polycystic ovarian morphology. A significant number of individuals with PCOS present with menstrual irregularities, including infrequent menstruation or irregular uterine bleeding. In AE-PCOS, PCOS is a condition primarily characterized by excessive androgen [60]. The International PCOS Guidelines 2023 appear to continue emphasizing both oligo- or anovulation and hyperandrogenism as essential criteria, similar to earlier guidelines. However, specific details such as the primary features and any unique aspects of these latest guidelines are not provided in the information given. This evolution in diagnostic criteria reflects the ongoing research and understanding of PCOS, aiming to provide more accurate and inclusive diagnostic methods [61].

To enhance understanding, Fig. 1.2 presents a flowchart depicting the diagnostic criteria for PCOS according to the Rotterdam Consensus. According to these criteria, two out of three key features must be present for a diagnosis of PCOS: oligo-anovulation, clinical or biochemical signs of hyperandrogenism, and polycystic ovaries visible on ultrasound [21]. Oligo-anovulation refers to irregular menstrual cycles, which manifest as infrequent periods or prolonged cycles, typically more than 35 days apart [62]. This irregularity often points toward inconsistent ovulation or anovulation, where ovulation does not occur at all. Hyperandrogenism, the second criterion, can be identified through clinical signs such as hirsutism (excessive hair growth in areas where men typically grow hair), acne, and meal-pattern baldness or through elevated levels of androgens (male hormones) in blood tests [63]. The third criterion, polycystic ovaries, is determined via ultrasound. It is characterized by the presence of 12 or more follicles in each ovary or increased ovarian volume [21]. However, it is crucial to note that the presence of polycystic ovaries alone

Table 1.2 Comparison of different diagnostic criteria for PCOS

Criteria	National Institutes of Health (NIH) 1990 [58]	Rotterdam criteria 2003 [59]	Androgen excess society 2006 [60]	International PCOS guidelines 2023 [61]
Oligo- or anovulation	Required	At least of three criteria needed	Required	Required
Clinical and/or biochemical signs of hyperandrogenism	Required	At least one of three criteria needed	Required	Required
Polycystic ovaries on ultrasound	Not required	At least one of three criteria needed; presence of 12 or more follicles in each ovary measuring 2–9 mm in diameter and/or increased ovarian volume >10 cm^3	Not required	Not specified in the provided information
Exclusion of other etiologies	Required	Required	Required	Required
Primary feature	Oligo- or anovulation and hyperandrogenism	Two of the following three: oligo- or anovulation, hyperandrogenism, polycystic ovaries	Hyperandrogenism and ovarian dysfunction (oligo- or anovulation and/or polycystic ovaries)	Not specified in the provided information
Notes	Focuses on menstrual irregularity	More inclusive, considers PCO morphology	Emphasizers androgen excess as a central feature	Not specified in the provided information

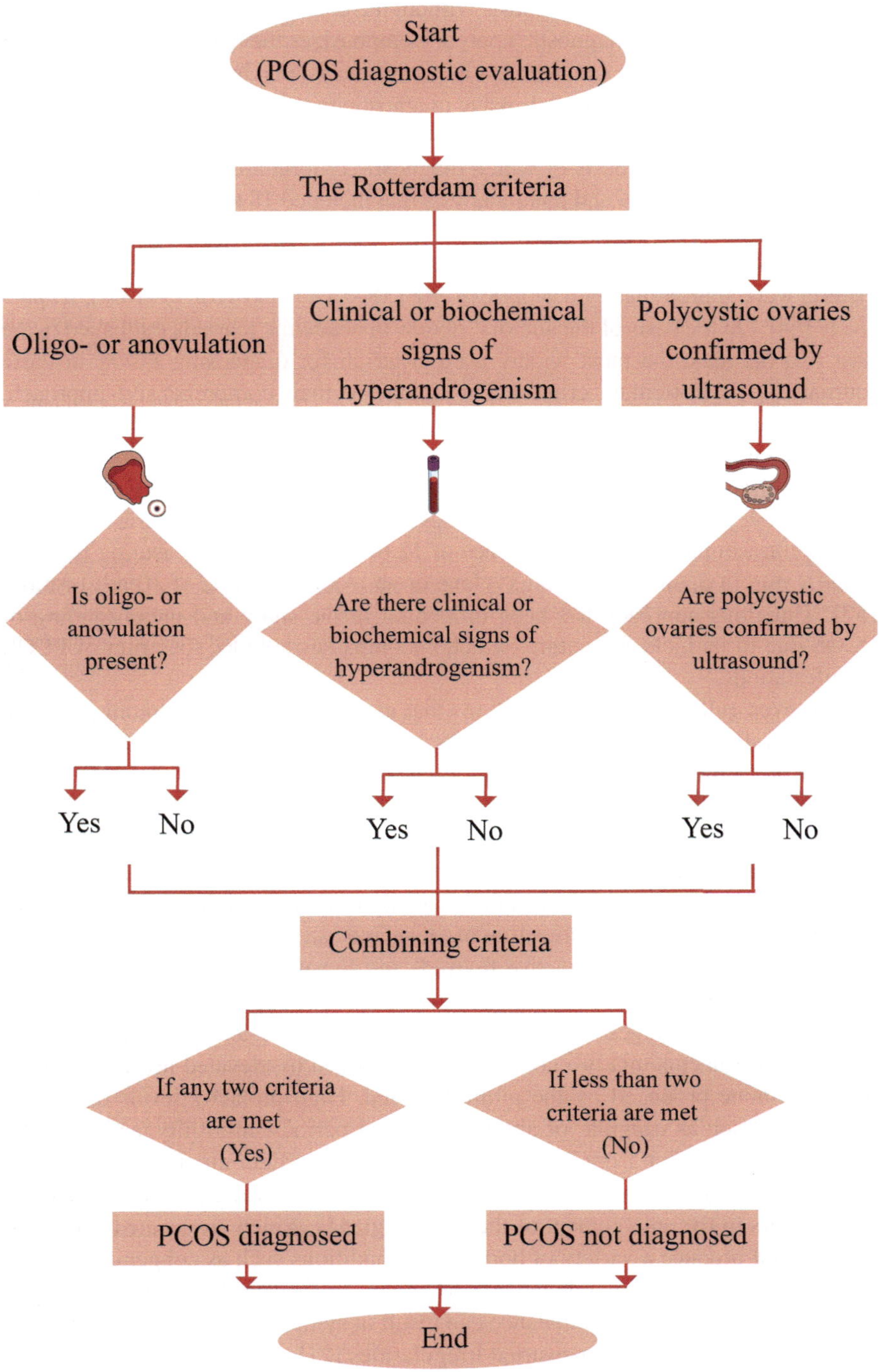

Fig. 1.2 A flowchart depicting the diagnostic criteria for PCOS according to the Rotterdam consensus scale

is not sufficient for a PCOS diagnosis without the concurrent presence of one of the other two criteria. This diagnostic approach emphasizes the heterogeneity of PCOS and acknowledges that it can manifest in various ways, making the Rotterdam criteria a more inclusive and comprehensive diagnostic tool.

Overall, each approach for the diagnosis of PCOS differs. The prevalence of PCOS can vary on the basis of which diagnostic criteria are used. For example, a recent systematic review and meta-analysis that included 18 trials for the NIH criteria, 15 trials for the Rotterdam criteria, and 10 trials for the AE-PCOS criteria revealed that the incidences (95% confidence intervals) of PCOS according to these criteria were approximately 6% (5–8%), 10% (8–13%), and 10% (7–13%), respectively [64]. On the basis of the authors' review of academic journals published in the past two decades, the most widely used criterion for diagnosing PCOS in these journals is the Rotterdam criteria. This is due to their comprehensive approach, which includes a broader range of symptoms than other criteria do. The Rotterdam criteria identify PCOS in women who present at least two of the following three features: oligo- or anovulation, clinical and/or biochemical signs of hyperandrogenism, or polycystic ovaries. Specifically, the criteria for polycystic ovaries to be visible on ultrasound include the presence of 12 or more follicles measuring between 2 and 9 mm in diameter in a single plane or an ovarian volume of 10 mL or more [57]. Thus, this approach has been influential in the study and understanding of PCOS due to its inclusive nature, which encompasses a wider spectrum of PCOS manifestations.

However, ruling out other conditions that can cause similar symptoms, such as thyroid dysfunction, hyperprolactinemia, and adrenal hyperplasia, is important [65]. In medicine, it is crucial to differentiate between similar symptoms to ensure accurate diagnosis and appropriate treatment. This process yields differential diagnosis. It involves considering various potential conditions (differential diagnoses) that could cause the patient's symptoms and systematically ruling out each one until the most likely diagnosis is determined. The thyroid gland produces hormones that regulate metabolism, and dysfunction of this gland can lead to a range of symptoms [66]. Hypothyroidism (underactive thyroid) and hyperthyroidism (overactive thyroid) can both present with symptoms that might overlap with other conditions, including weight changes, fatigue, menstrual irregularities, and mood disturbances [65]. Hyperprolactinemia is a condition characterized by elevated levels of prolactin, a hormone produced by the pituitary gland. High prolactin levels can cause symptoms, such as irregular or absent menstrual periods, infertility, and, in some cases, mild production from breasts unrelated to childbirth or nursing. These symptoms can be similar to those caused by other hormonal disorders [1]. Adrenal hyperplasia refers to the enlargement of the adrenal glands, which are located above the kidneys and produce a variety of hormones. Conditions such as congenital adrenal hyperplasia can lead to an imbalance in hormones such as cortisol, aldosterone, and androgens. This hormonal imbalance can result in symptoms such as early puberty, excessive hair growth, and menstrual irregularities [21].

In addition, a thorough medical history and physical examination are crucial, as they focus on menstrual patterns, signs of androgen excess, and weight changes

[21, 54]. Blood tests, including androgen, insulin, and glucose levels, are typically conducted to assess hormone levels and evaluate metabolic status and insulin resistance [67]. An ultrasound may be used to visualize the ovaries and assess the presence of polycystic morphology, although this alone does not confirm a diagnosis of PCOS [68]. The process of diagnosing PCOS can be challenging due to the overlap of symptoms with other conditions and the variability of symptoms among individuals with this syndrome [25]. Therefore, a careful and comprehensive approach is necessary to accurately diagnose PCOS and differentiate it from other similar disorders.

Table 1.3 provides a comprehensive overview of the various clinical signs and biochemical markers that are commonly associated with PCOS. Patients often present with irregular menstrual cycles, characterized by infrequent, irregular, or prolonged periods, a condition associated with hormonal imbalances [26]. Hirsutism, or excessive hair growth in areas typical for males, such as the face, chest, or back, is another common symptom, as is persistent or severe acne and alopecia, manifesting as thinning hair or male-pattern baldness [8, 11, 26, 37, 39]. Obesity or overweight, particularly fat accumulation around the waist, and acanthosis nigricans, characterized by dark, velvety patches of skin, especially in the neck and armpit areas, are also frequently observed [56, 74]. Biochemically, PCOS is characterized by elevated levels of androgens (male hormones); insulin resistance, indicated by elevated insulin levels and reduced sensitivity to insulin; dyslipidemia, characterized by abnormal cholesterol and triglyceride levels; and an imbalanced luteinizing

Table 1.3 Clinical and biochemical features commonly observed in PCOS patients

Feature type	Feature	Description	Reference
Clinical signs	Irregular menstrual cycles	Infrequent, irregular, or prolonged menstrual cycles	[26]
	Hirsutism	Excessive hair growth on the face, chest, and back	[26, 39]
	Acne	Persistent or severe acne, particularly on the face, chest, and upper back	[37]
	Alopecia	Thinning hair or male-pattern baldness	[8, 11]
	Obesity/overweight	Increased body weight or body mass index (BMI), often centered around the waist	[56]
	Acanthosis nigricans	Dark, velvety patches of skin, particularly in neck and armpit areas	[69]
Biochemical markers	Elevated androgens	Increased levels of male hormones, which may or may not be accompanied by clinical signs	[70]
	Insulin resistance	Elevated insulin levels in the blood and decreased sensitivity to insulin	[38]
	Dyslipidemia	Abnormal levels of cholesterol and triglyceride	[71]
	Elevated LH/FSH ratio	Imbalance in luteinizing hormone (LH) and follicle-stimulating hormone (FSH) levels	[72]
	Inflammation markers	Elevated levels of C-reactive protein (CRP) and other markers of systemic inflammation	[2, 73]

hormone (LH)/follicle-stimulating hormone (FSH) ratio, which refers to disproportionate levels of LH and FSH [38, 70–72].

In patients with PCOS, an elevated LH/FSH ratio is common. LH and FSH are hormones crucial for normal reproductive function. In a typical menstrual cycle, FSH promotes the growth of ovarian follicles, and LH triggers ovulation. However, in PCOs, the hormonal balance is often disrupted, leading to an increased LH/FSH ratio. For example, Xia et al. [72] reported that the LH/FSH ratio in patients with PCOS was significantly associated with factors, such as age, BMI, testosterone levels (both total and free), estradiol, and antihypertensive hormone levels. Women with PCOS and a higher LH/FSH ratio were found to have a poorer response to ovulation induction. This means that the changes in successful ovulation in response to treatment were lower than those in women with a lower LH/FSH ratio. Interestingly, while an elevated LH/FSH ratio negatively impacts ovulation, it is associated with more favorable outcomes in terms of clinical pregnancy and live birth rates, particularly for women with an LH/FSH ratio between 1 and 2. On the other hand, women with an LH/FSH ratio between 2 and 3 had a lower miscarriage rate. This study suggested that while an elevated LH/FSH ratio in women with PCOS can hinder ovulation, it does not necessarily preclude successful pregnancy outcomes. These findings indicate that LH and FSH levels in women with PCOS might play complex roles in achieving pregnancy, impacting ovulation but also influencing other aspects of reproductive function. This interesting finding contributes to our understanding of PCOS and its treatment, particularly in the context of fertility interventions.

Additionally, inflammatory markers, such as elevated levels of C-reactive protein and other indicators of systemic inflammation, are often present [2, 73]. One of the key underlying factors in PCOS is low-grade chronic inflammation, both at the local level (in the ovaries) and systemically throughout the body. This inflammation plays a significant role in the pathophysiology of PCOS and its various manifestations. Zhai and Pang [73] reported that, in PCOS patients, there is a notable increase in the number of circulating inflammatory cells. Compared with women without PCOS, women with PCOS have significantly greater concentrations of lymphocytes, neutrophils, eosinophilic granulocytes, monocytes, and T helper 17 (Th17) cells. Conversely, the percentage of regulatory T cells (Tregs), which are anti-inflammatory agents, is lower in patients with PCOS. This imbalance contributes to the chronic inflammatory state observed in PCOS patients. In contrast, the levels of anti-inflammatory cytokines are significantly lower in PCOS patients. These include interleukin (IL)-10, IL-17E, IL-27, IL-35, IL-37, transforming growth factor-beta (TGF-β), omemtin-1, and secreted frizzled-related protein 5 (SFRP5). The reduced presence of these cytokines further exacerbates the inflammatory state in PCOS patients. The inflammatory response in PCOS patients is not just systemic; it also occurs within the ovaries. Some inflammatory cells and cytokines may originate in the ovaries and subsequently enter the bloodstream, contributing to systemic inflammation. Systemic inflammation in PCOS patients is associated with other key features of the disorder, such as obesity, insulin resistance, and hyperandrogenism. This interaction creates a complex network of factors exacerbating PCOS symptoms. Alleviating inflammation is a critical aspect of managing PCOS. Strategies such as traditional Chinese medicine, multitargeted treatments, anti-inflammatory and antioxidant medications, and lifestyle modifications have been shown to help reduce inflammatory responses in patients with PCOS, thereby providing relief from various symptoms. These clinical signs and biochemical markers, as indicated in the referenced studies, collectively assist in the diagnosis and understanding of the complexities of PCOS.

1.2.6 Artificial Intelligence in PCOS Diagnosis

Artificial intelligence (AI) has revolutionized the field of medicine, offering innovative approaches to diagnosing complex conditions, including PCOS. AI, particularly machine learning and deep learning techniques, has shown promise in addressing these challenges. AI algorithms can identify patterns and correlations that may elude human clinicians. In this context, machine learning models trained with historical patient data have shown significant promise in improving the diagnosis of PCOS. Recent advancements in this field have demonstrated the use of various machine learning techniques combined with digital image processing to create automated systems for detecting PCOS. These systems are capable of classifying ovarian ultrasound images into PCOS or non-PCOS categories with high accuracy. For example, several researchers have employed techniques such as image enhancement, segmentation, feature extraction, and classification algorithms such as K-nearest neighbor (KNN), support vector machine (SVM), and artificial neural networks (ANNs) for this purpose [75].

Table 1.4 offers a detailed summary of recent developments in diagnosing PCOS via machine learning and image processing methods. Each entry in the table highlights a notable study in this area, providing information on the authors, year of publication, study focus, methodologies used, and key findings. For example, the study by Abouhawwash et al. [77] focused on the automatic diagnosis of PCOS via a wrapper methodology combined with deep learning techniques. Authors utilized deep learning models such as convolutional neural networks (CNNs), multilayer perceptron (MLPs), recurrent neural networks (RNNs), and bidirectional long short-term memory (Bi-LSTM), along with a tri-stage wrapper method for efficient feature selection, achieving high precision (97%), accuracy (98.67%), and recall (89%), particularly with CNNs, indicating effective feature extraction and classification. Sreejith et al. [78] developed a clinical decision support system for patients with PCOS via the red deer algorithm and random forest classifier. This innovative approach led to an accuracy of 89.81%, outperforming other methods in terms of accuracy, sensitivity, and specificity. Srinivas et al. [79] focused on enhancing the detection of polycystic ovarian follicles via an advanced Kalman filter (AKF) for ultrasound image segmentation, yielding efficient results in detecting dominant follicles. Suha and Islam [80] introduced an extended machine learning technique for PCOS detection using ultrasound images, combining a CNN with transfer learning and a stacking ensemble machine learning technique. Their methodology, which

Table 1.4 Overview of recent advances in diagnosing PCOS through machine learning and image processing techniques

Authors	Year	Study focus	Methodology	Key findings
Kavitha et al. [76]	2023	Detection of PCOS using machine learning algorithms with grid search CV optimization	Machine learning techniques like LightGBM boost, gradient boost, and XGBoost with grid search CV optimization	High accuracy in PCOS detection, evaluated in terms of accuracy, recall, f1_ score, and precision
Abouhawwash et al. [77]	2023	Automatic diagnosis of polycystic ovarian syndrome using wrapper methodology with deep learning techniques	Deep learning techniques like CNN, MLP, RNN, bi-LSTM with tri-stage wrapper method for feature selection	Highest precision (97%), accuracy (98.67%), and recall (89%) with CNN and effective feature extraction
Sreejith et al. [78]	2022	Clinical decision support system for PCOS using red deer algorithm and random forest classifier	Red deer algorithm and random Forest classifier for feature selection and optimization	Achieved an accuracy of 89.81%, superior to other methods in terms of accuracy, sensitivity, and specificity
Srinivas et al. [79]	2022	Improvised follicle polycystic ovarian detection using advanced Kalman filter (AKF)	AKF in ultrasound image segmentation for follicle detection	Efficient results in detecting dominant follicles, compared favorably with existing methods
Suha and Islam [80]	2022	Extended machine learning technique for PCOS detection using ultrasound images	CNN with transfer learning and stacking ensemble machine learning technique	Exceptional accuracy (99.89%) in classifying PCOS and non-PCOS ovaries using "VGGNet16" and "XGBoost"

employs "VGGNet16" for feature extraction and "XGBoost" for classification, achieved an exceptional accuracy of 99.89% in differentiating between PCOS ovaries and non-PCOS ovaries. Collectively, these studies represent significant advances in the application of advanced computational techniques for diagnosing and understanding PCOS, a complex and widespread endocrine disorder. These studies underscore the potential of machine learning and image processing to improve the accuracy, efficiency, and reliability of medical diagnostics.

Despite these advancements, challenges remain, such as the need for careful tuning of digital image processing techniques and the high computational power required for deep learning methods. However, the potential for ensemble machine learning techniques (which combine multiple models to improve prediction performance) has not been extensively explored in the context of PCOS detection. Some studies suggest combining the strengths of CNNs for feature extraction with traditional machine learning classifiers for categorizing medical images, but such hybrid approaches are still relatively rare in PCOS detection using ultrasound images [80].

Overall, the integration of AI and machine learning in the diagnosis of PCOS is highly effective. A study of 25 years of data was reported by the NIH, which revealed that AI- and machine learning-based programs were successful at detecting PCOS, with accuracy rates ranging from 80% to 90% in some studies [81, 82]. This research underscores the potential of AI and machine learning to increase the ability of healthcare systems to identify women with PCOS early, potentially leading to cost savings and a reduced burden of PCOS on patients and the health system. Moreover, the role of AI in PCOS diagnosis is not limited to clinical and imaging data analysis. It also extends to patient education and self-management. Mobile health applications powered by AI can assist patients in tracking their symptoms, understanding the implications of their lifestyle choices, and adhering to treatment plans. These applications can provide tailored advice and support, enhancing patient engagement and empowerment in managing their condition.

1.3 Nutritional Implications of PCOS

1.3.1 Link Between Diet and PCOS

The link between diet and PCOS is a critical aspect of managing this condition, given the significant role of nutritional factors in both the development and management of PCOS [83]. Diet directly influences several key features of PCOS, including insulin resistance, weight management, and hormonal balance [50]. Women with PCOS often exhibit insulin resistance, where the body becomes less effective at using lower blood sugar levels. Insulin resistance can lead to elevated insulin levels (hyperinsulinemia), which exacerbates the symptoms of PCOS by increasing insulin levels (hyperinsulinemia), which exacerbates the symptoms of PCOS by increasing the production of androgens (male hormones) and disrupting ovulation [17]. A diet rich in high-glycemic-index foods can worsen insulin resistance and hyperinsulinemia. Therefore, dietary recommendations for individuals with PCOS frequently emphasize a low glycemic index diet, which includes whole grains, legumes, fruits, and vegetables, to improve insulin sensitivity and reduce androgen levels [14].

Additionally, many women with PCOS struggle with overweight or obesity, which can further aggravate insulin resistance and hormonal imbalances [84]. Weight management through diet is thus a cornerstone in the treatment of PCOS [83]. Caloric restriction, balanced macronutrient distribution, and the incorporation of anti-inflammatory foods can aid in weight loss and reduce PCOS symptoms [85]. A diet that is balanced in carbohydrates, proteins, and healthy fats, with an emphasis on fiber-rich foods, lean protein, and omega-3 fatty acids, has been found to be beneficial [86]. The anti-inflammatory properties of certain foods, such as fatty fish, nuts, seeds, and leafy greens, may also help reduce the chronic low-grade inflammation observed in individuals with PCOS [87]. Moreover, specific micronutrient deficiencies, such as vitamin D, magnesium, and omega-3 fatty acids, are often noted in individuals with PCOS, and correcting these deficiencies through diet or supplementation can support overall hormonal balance and metabolic health [88, 89]. Thus, diet plays a pivotal role in the management of PCOS by influencing insulin resistance, weight, and hormonal regulation. Tailored nutritional interventions can significantly improve the symptoms and long-term health outcomes of women with PCOS.

1.3.2 Common Nutritional Deficiencies

Women with PCOS are often at risk for certain nutritional deficiencies, which can exacerbate their symptoms and contribute to their associated health risks [90]. Table 1.5 provides an overview of common nutritional deficiencies in patients with PCOS, their potential effects on PCOS, and their dietary sources. The list of nutrients included vitamin D, magnesium, omega-3 fatty acids, iron, B vitamins (including B6, B9, and B12), chromium, zinc, inositol, calcium, and vitamin B12. One of the most common deficiencies observed in women with PCOS is vitamin D deficiency. Vitamin D not only is crucial for bone health but also plays a role in insulin resistance and glucose metabolism. Low levels of vitamin D have been linked to worsened symptoms of PCOS, including insulin resistance, ovulatory dysfunction, and increased androgen levels. Ensuring adequate vitamin D intake through diet, supplementation, or sun exposure is therefore vital for women with PCOS [100].

Another nutrient of concern is magnesium. This mineral is essential for numerous biochemical reactions in the body, including glucose metabolism and insulin signaling. Many women with PCOS have been found to have lower levels of magnesium, which may contribute to insulin resistance and an increased risk of metabolic syndrome. The incorporation of magnesium-rich foods such as leafy greens, nuts, seeds, and whole grains or the use of supplements can help address this deficiency [101]. Additionally, women with PCOS may have lower levels of omega-3 fatty acids, which are important for reducing inflammation and improving lipid profiles [93]. Given that PCOS is often accompanied by low-grade chronic inflammation and dyslipidemia, increasing omega-3 intake through fish, flaxseeds, chia seeds, or supplements can be beneficial [102, 103].

There is also evidence suggesting that women with PCOS may have altered gut microbiota, leading to deficiencies in certain B vitamins produced by gut bacteria [93]. These vitamins play crucial roles in energy metabolism and maintaining proper hormonal balance [104]. Ensuring a balanced diet with enough whole grains, legumes, and leafy vegetables can help maintain healthy gut flora and prevent vitamin B deficiencies [105]. Furthermore, chromium, a trace mineral important for carbohydrate and lipid metabolism, is another nutrient that women with PCOS may lack [96]. Chromium supplementation has been suggested to improve insulin sensitivity in some individuals with PCOS. Importantly, nutritional needs can vary greatly among individuals with PCOS, and a tailored approach is often necessary [106].

Table 1.5 List of common nutritional deficiencies in PCOS patients and their dietary sources

Nutrient	Common deficiency in PCOS	Potential effects on PCOS	Dietary sources	Reference
Vitamin D	Often deficient	Linked to insulin resistance and inflammation	Fatty fish, fortified dairy products, egg yolks, sunlight exposure	[91]
Magnesium	Frequently low	Important for insulin metabolism and hormonal balance	Leafy greens, nuts, seeds, whole grains	[92]
Omega-3 fatty acids	Commonly inadequate	Reduce inflammation, may improve menstrual regularity and ovulatory function	Fatty fish (salmon, mackerel), flaxseeds, walnuts	[93]
Iron	Risk due to irregular menstruation	Anemia can exacerbate fatigue and weakness	Red meat, leafy greens, legumes, fortified cereals	[94]
B vitamins	Particularly B6, B9 (folate), B12	Involved in energy metabolism and may affect mood and stress levels	Whole grains, avocados, bananas, meats, dairy products	[95]
Chromium	Often low	Enhances insulin action and may improve blood sugar control	Broccoli, potatoes, meats, whole grains	[96]
Zinc	Deficiency observed in some cases	Important for immune function and skin health (acne management)	Shellfish, meat, nuts, dairy products	[37]
Inositol	Not typically a dietary deficiency, but supplementation can be beneficial	Used in cell signaling; shown to improve insulin sensitivity and ovary function	Cantaloupe, oranges, nuts, beans	[97]
Calcium	Risk due to vitamin D deficiency	Essential for bone health, may be involved in hormonal regulation	Dairy products, leafy greens, fortified plant-based milks	[98]
Vitamin B12	Risk in those on metformin or with dietary restrictions	Necessary for nerve function and red blood cell formation	Meats, dairy products, fortified plant-based milks	[99]

Consulting a healthcare provider or a dietitian for personalized dietary advice and potential supplementation is recommended for the optimal management of PCOS.

1.3.3 Impact of Obesity and Insulin Resistance

Obesity and insulin resistance are two interlinked factors that significantly impact the health and management of many conditions, including PCOS [84]. Obesity, characterized by an excessive accumulation of body fat, exacerbates the severity of PCOS symptoms and increases the risk of several comorbid conditions [84]. In the context of PCOS, obesity can worsen hormonal imbalances, particularly in terms of androgen (male hormone) and insulin levels [50]. Elevated androgen levels lead to more severe symptoms, such as hirsutism (excessive hair growth), acne, and menstrual irregularities [107]. Obesity is also associated with a greater risk of infertility in patients with PCOS due to anovulation (lack of ovulation) [108]. Furthermore, the accumulation of adipose tissue, especially abdominal fat, contributes to the development and worsening of insulin resistance [84].

Insulin resistance, a condition in which body cells do not respond effectively to insulin, is a key feature in many cases of PCOS and is closely linked to obesity [67]. Insulin resistance leads to increased circulating insulin levels (hyperinsulinemia), which can exacerbate the production of androgens by the ovaries, thereby worsening PCOS symptoms. Insulin resistance also increases the risk of developing type 2 diabetes, cardiovascular diseases, and metabolic syndrome. These conditions are particularly concerning for women with PCOS, as they already have an elevated risk for these metabolic disorders [109]. Moreover, insulin resistance can lead to weight gain and difficulty losing weight, creating a vicious cycle that further exacerbates PCOS symptoms and associated health risks [50, 67].

The combined impact of obesity and insulin resistance in PCOS patients is profound and affects not only reproductive health but also long-term metabolic and cardiovascular health [56, 84]. Effective management of weight and insulin sensitivity is therefore crucial in the treatment of PCOS. Lifestyle interventions, including diet and physical activity, are first-line approaches for managing these aspects of PCOS [63]. Weight loss, even a modest amount, can significantly improve insulin resistance, hormonal imbalances, and reproductive outcomes [17]. For some women, pharmacological treatments that improve insulin sensitivity, such as metformin, may also be beneficial [109]. The interplay between obesity and insulin resistance in PCOS patients underscores the importance of a comprehensive approach to treatment, targeting not only symptoms but also underlying metabolic disturbances.

1.4 Dietary Management Strategies

1.4.1 Macronutrient Composition

The macronutrient composition of the diet plays a crucial role in the dietary management of individuals with PCOS. A balanced intake of carbohydrates, proteins,

Table 1.6 Macronutrient composition recommendations for the dietary management of PCOS patients

Macronutrient	Recommended intake	Rationale for PCOS management	Examples of food sources	Reference
Carbohydrates	Approximately 45–65% of total daily calories	Focus on low glycemic index carbs to manage insulin sensitivity	Whole grains, legumes, fruits, vegetables	[111, 112]
Proteins	15–30% of total daily calories	Supports muscle mass, satiety, and stable blood sugar levels	Lean meats, fish, dairy, legumes, tofu	[113]
Fats	20–30% of total daily calories	Emphasize omega-3 and monounsaturated fats for anti-inflammatory benefits	Avocado, nuts, seeds, olive oil, fatty fish	[113, 114]
Fiber	At least 25–30 g/day	Aids in digestion, improves insulin sensitivity, and supports weight management	Fruits, vegetables, whole grains, legumes	[112]
Omega-3 fatty acids	No specific recommendation, but aim for 2–3 servings of fatty fish per week	Reduces inflammation and may help regulate menstrual cycles	Salmon, mackerel, sardines, flaxseeds, walnuts	[115, 116]

and fats is essential for managing symptoms and reducing the risk of associated metabolic complications [110]. Table 1.6 provides recommendations for the macronutrient composition of the diet for the management of PCOS. This section includes the rationale for each recommendation and examples of food sources. This information can assist in planning a balanced diet that addresses the specific nutritional needs and challenges associated with PCOS. Carbohydrates are a key component of nutrition, and their role is particularly significant in the dietary management of PCOS [117]. In patients with PCOS, the body often has difficulty effectively using insulin, a condition known as insulin resistance. This resistance leads to increased levels of insulin and glucose in the blood, which can exacerbate the symptoms of PCOS, including weight gain, hormonal imbalances, and an increased risk of type 2 diabetes. The type and quality of carbohydrates consumed can have a direct effect on these issues [118]. Low glycemic index (GI) carbohydrate levels are particularly beneficial for individuals with PCOS. The glycemic index is a measure that ranks foods on the basis of how quickly they increase their blood sugar levels after eating. Low-GI foods are digested and absorbed at a slower rate, resulting in a more gradual increase in blood sugar and insulin levels. This slower digestion and absorption process is crucial for managing insulin resistance in PCOS patients [14]. By preventing rapid spikes in blood sugar, low-GI foods help maintain better insulin sensitivity [17]. Examples of low-GI foods include whole grains (such as brown rice and whole grain bread), vegetables, most fruits, and legumes. These foods are rich in fiber, which further aids in the slow digestion process and adds to the feeling of fullness, thereby assisting in weight management. In contrast, high-GI carbohydrates, such as sugary snacks, refined grains (such as white rice and white bread), and processed foods, are digested and absorbed quickly, leading to rapid spikes in blood sugar and insulin levels. These spikes can worsen insulin resistance, a key issue in PCOS. High-GI foods are often low in fiber and can lead to a quick return of hunger, contributing to overeating and weight gain. For individuals with PCOS who are already at a greater risk for obesity and type 2 diabetes, consuming high-GI foods can therefore have particularly negative effects on their health [119]. The dietary approach for managing PCOS thus involves focusing on low-GI carbohydrates combined with a balanced intake of proteins and fats. This not only helps in stabilizing blood sugar levels but also plays a role in weight management, an important aspect of PCOS treatment. By choosing healthier carbohydrates and pairing them with adequate protein and fat, it is possible to create a diet that not only helps individuals manage PCOS symptoms but also contributes to overall health and well-being [120]. For individualized advice, consulting with a dietitian or a healthcare provider is always recommended to tailor dietary choices to personal health needs and preferences.

Protein is another important macronutrient for women with PCOS. Its importance lies in several key areas, such as weight management, muscle mass maintenance, and insulin resistance [117]. First, protein is highly effective for weight management, an area that is often challenging for individuals with PCOS. High-protein foods are known to increase feelings of fullness, which can help reduce overall caloric intake. This aspect is particularly important in PCOS, where weight management is a key part of managing the condition and reducing the risk of associated complications such as type 2 diabetes and cardiovascular diseases. Proteins play a crucial role in maintaining muscle mass. Muscle mass is essential not only for physical strength and endurance but also for metabolic health. Muscles are active tissues that burn calories, even at rest, thereby aiding in overall energy expenditure and weight management. For women with PCOS, maintaining healthy muscle mass is important, as it helps in the effective utilization of insulin and glucose, thereby improving insulin sensitivity. Combining protein intake with regular exercise, particularly strength training, can increase muscle mass and improve metabolic health [121]. The choice of source of protein is significant. Lean protein sources such as chicken, fish, tofu, legumes, and low-fat dairy products are recommended for treating PCOS. These sources provide essential amino acids (the building blocks of protein) without the added burden of saturated fats, which are found in relatively high quantities in red meat and full-fat dairy products. Saturated fats can contribute to weight gain and worsen insulin resistance, thus negating some of the benefits of protein intake. Lean proteins, on the other hand, support a healthy diet without these risks [122]. Furthermore, the inclusion of protein in meals can help reduce the glycemic load. This means that when combined with carbohydrates, protein can slow the absorption of sugar into the bloodstream, leading to more stable blood sugar levels. This approach is particularly beneficial for managing insulin resistance, a common issue in PCOS patients. Therefore, a balanced diet for individuals with PCOS should focus not only on low glycemic index carbohydrates but also on adequate protein intake at each meal to manage insulin sensitivity and support overall metabolic health.

Finally, dietary fat intake is an essential aspect of a balanced diet, even for individuals with PCOS [123]. However, the type of fat consumed is important. Monounsaturated and polyunsaturated fats are considered healthy fats. These compounds are found in foods such as avocados, nuts, seeds, olive oil, and fatty fish. These fats are beneficial for several reasons [124]. First, they can help improve insulin sensitivity. Insulin resistance is a core problem in PCOS patients and leads to elevated blood sugar and insulin levels, which can exacerbate the symptoms of PCOS and increase the risk of developing type 2 diabetes. By enhancing the body's response to insulin, these healthy fats can help mitigate this risk [125]. Additionally, monounsaturated and polyunsaturated fats are healthy for the heart. This is particularly important for those with PCOS, who are at increased risk for cardiovascular diseases. These fats can help lower low-density lipoprotein (LDL) cholesterol levels and increase high-density lipoprotein (HDL) cholesterol levels, thereby promoting a healthier lipid profile [126]. Conversely, saturated and trans fats, typically found in processed foods, fried foods, and certain types of meats, should be limited. These fats can worsen insulin resistance and negatively impact heart health. They are known to increase LDL cholesterol and decrease HDL cholesterol, contributing to the buildup of plaque in arteries, which can lead to heart disease. Given the increased cardiovascular risks associated with PCOS, it is particularly important for individuals with this condition to moderate their intake of these less healthy fats [123]. Omega-3 fatty acids, a type of polyunsaturated fat, deserve special mention for their role in managing PCOS. These compounds are abundantly found in fatty fish, such as salmon, mackerel, and sardines. Omega-3 fatty acids are known for their anti-inflammatory effects, which can be beneficial in managing PCOS, a condition often characterized by chronic low-grade inflammation. Additionally, they can improve the lipid profile by reducing triglycerides and potentially increasing HDL cholesterol. These benefits make omega-3 fatty acids a highly recommended component of the diet for individuals with PCOS [93].

1.4.2 Micronutrients and Supplements

The micronutrient composition plays a vital role in the dietary management of PCOS patients, as certain vitamins and minerals can significantly impact the metabolic and hormonal imbalances associated with this condition [117]. The key micronutrients that are often emphasized include vitamin D, vitamin B, magnesium, and chromium [117, 127]. Vitamin D is crucial for women with PCOS, as deficiencies are common and can exacerbate insulin resistance and hormonal imbalances [128]. Vitamin D exists in two main forms: vitamin D2 (ergocalciferol) and vitamin D3 (cholecalciferol) (Fig. 1.3). Vitamin D2 is found in some plants, mushrooms, and yeasts. It is also commonly used in vitamin D-fortified foods and supplements. When vitamin D2 is consumed, it is converted into 25-hydroxyvitamin D (25(OH)D) (Fig. 1.3) in the liver, which is measured in the blood to assess vitamin D status. On the other hand, vitamin D3 is synthesized in the skin when exposed to sunlight and is also found in animal products such as fatty fish, liver, and egg yolks. Like

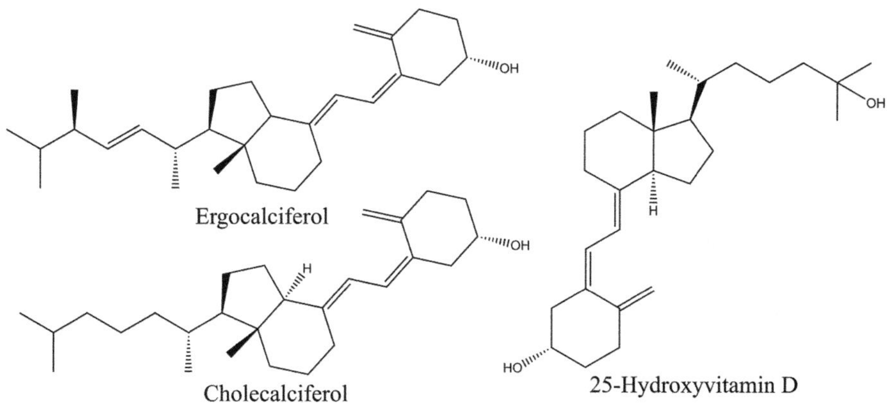

Fig. 1.3 Chemical structures of ergocalciferol, cholecalciferol, and 25-hydroxyvitamin D

vitamin D2, D3 is converted to 25(OH)D in the liver [129]. Several aspects of the role and effects of vitamin D in PCOS are considered significant.

- **Insulin resistance**: Women with PCOS often experience insulin resistance, which can lead to type 2 diabetes and other health issues. Vitamin D is thought to influence insulin secretion and sensitivity, and some studies suggest that vitamin D supplementation can improve insulin resistance in women with PCOS [89].
- **Hormonal balance**: Vitamin D may play a role in regulating the menstrual cycle by influencing the production of hormones such as estrogen and progesterone. Vitamin D deficiency is associated with menstrual irregularities, which are a key feature of PCOS [130].
- **Inflammation and immune function**: PCOS is associated with low-grade inflammation, and vitamin D has anti-inflammatory effects. It may help reduce inflammation and improve symptoms in patients with PCOS [131].
- **Ovary function**: There is some evidence suggesting that vitamin D can affect the function of the ovaries directly, potentially influencing the development of follicles and ovulation [132].

Despite these potential links, the relationship between vitamin D and PCOS is still an active area of research. While some studies have shown a correlation between vitamin D deficiency and the severity of PCOS symptoms, others have not shown significant effects of vitamin D supplementation on PCOS outcomes [133, 134].

B vitamins, particularly B2 (riboflavin), B6 (pyridoxine), B9 (folate), and B12 (cobalamin) (Fig. 1.4), play essential roles in energy metabolism and may support cardiovascular health. Women with PCOS may benefit from a diet rich in B vitamins, as these vitamins can aid in managing homocysteine levels, which are often elevated in patients with PCOS and are associated with an increased risk of cardiovascular diseases. Sources of B vitamins include whole grains, leafy greens, legumes, nuts, and lean meats [110].

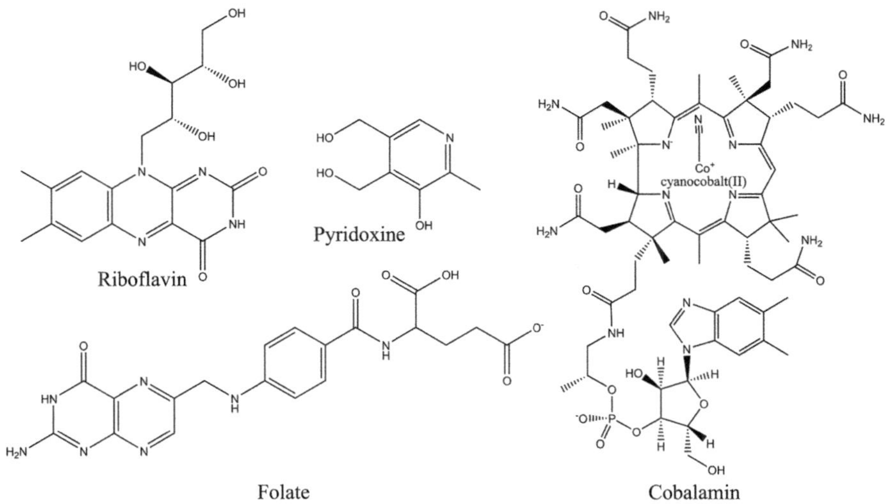

Fig. 1.4 Chemical structures of riboflavin, pyridoxine, folate, and cobalamin

Magnesium, a mineral involved in more than 300 enzymatic reactions in the body, is particularly important for glucose metabolism and insulin sensitivity [67]. Magnesium-rich foods, such as nuts, seeds, leafy greens, and whole grains, can help improve insulin resistance and reduce the risk of developing type 2 diabetes, a common concern in patients with PCOS [110]. Finally, chromium is another trace mineral that plays a role in carbohydrate and lipid metabolism. It enhances the action of insulin and may improve insulin sensitivity in women with PCOS. Whole grains, lean meats, fruits, and vegetables are good sources of chromium [135].

1.4.3 Specialized Diets (Anti-inflammatory and Low-Glycemic Diets)

Specialized diets play an integral role in managing PCOS and are tailored to address the unique metabolic and hormonal challenges associated with this syndrome [136]. Among the most effective and commonly recommended diets for treating PCOS are the low-GI diet, the Mediterranean diet, and the anti-inflammatory diet [50]. A low-GI diet focuses on foods that have a minimal impact on blood sugar levels [15]. This is crucial for PCOS management, as many women with this condition struggle with insulin resistance [137]. Foods with a low GI value, such as whole grains, legumes, nuts, seeds, most fruits, and nonstarchy vegetables, are emphasized [138]. These foods lead to a slower, more gradual increase in blood sugar and insulin levels, which can help individuals manage insulin resistance and reduce the risk of developing type 2 diabetes [137]. Additionally, this diet supports weight management, a key factor in PCOS, as it promotes satiety and reduces the likelihood of overeating [50].

The Mediterranean diet, which is rich in fruits, vegetables, whole grains, legumes, nuts, seeds, olive oil, and lean protein sources such as fish and poultry, is another excellent choice for PCOS management. This diet is high in anti-inflammatory foods and omega-3 fatty acids, which can help reduce the chronic inflammation often observed in patients with PCOS. It also promotes a healthy balance of macronutrients and is beneficial for cardiovascular health, an important consideration given the increased risk of heart disease in women with PCOS [14]. An anti-inflammatory diet is also highly recommended for PCOS management. This diet includes foods known for their anti-inflammatory properties, such as berries, fatty fish, leafy greens, nuts, and seeds, while limiting processed foods, refined carbohydrates, and high-sugar foods. Such a diet can help alleviate the low-grade inflammation associated with PCOS and improve symptoms such as acne and hirsutism [126]. In addition to these diets, some women with PCOS may benefit from specific dietary interventions, such as dairy-free or gluten-free diets, particularly if they are sensitive or intolerant [139]. However, these should be approached cautiously and ideally under the guidance of a nutritionist or healthcare professional to ensure that all nutritional needs are met.

1.5 Addressing Common Comorbidities Through Nutrition

1.5.1 Managing Insulin Resistance

Insulin resistance, where body cells become less responsive to insulin, is a key driver of many PCOS symptoms and associated health risks, including hyperandrogenism, menstrual irregularities, and an increased risk of developing type 2 diabetes [140]. Dietary strategies play a crucial role in improving insulin sensitivity and mitigating these risks. A diet rich in low-GI foods is foundational for managing insulin resistance [137]. Low-GI foods cause a slower, more gradual increase in blood glucose and insulin levels, which is beneficial for maintaining insulin sensitivity [14]. The incorporation of these foods into the diet can help stabilize blood sugar levels and prevent sharp spikes that exacerbate insulin resistance [109]. In addition to low-GI foods, high fiber intake is also beneficial, as fiber helps slow the digestion and absorption of carbohydrates, further aiding in blood sugar control [141].

In addition to focusing on carbohydrate quality, maintaining a balanced intake of macronutrients is important. Adequate protein intake from lean sources such as poultry, fish, legumes, and tofu can support muscle mass, which is important for glucose metabolism [142]. Moreover, regular meals and controlled portion sizes can help prevent large fluctuations in blood sugar and insulin levels, aiding in the management of insulin resistance [17].

In addition to macronutrients, certain micronutrients and dietary supplements may also improve insulin sensitivity in women with PCOS [117]. For example, zinc, chromium, selenium, magnesium, and vitamin D have been linked to improved insulin action and glucose metabolism. Adequate intake of these nutrients, either through diet or supplements, can be beneficial [143]. Authors suggested that it is important to approach supplementation with a certain degree of caution. Such practices should be undertaken under the careful supervision of a qualified healthcare professional. This ensures both safety and effectiveness in the use of supplements. Importantly, dietary management of insulin resistance in PCOS patients is not a one-size-fits-all approach. Individualized nutritional therapy, which considers personal dietary preferences, lifestyle, and overall health goals, is key to effectively managing insulin resistance in patients with PCOS. A registered dietician or nutrition specialist can provide personalized recommendations and support sustained dietary changes for optimal management of insulin resistance in patients with PCOS.

1.5.2 Weight Management Strategies

Effective weight management is pivotal, as a significant proportion of women with PCOS struggle with being overweight or obese, which exacerbates both the metabolic and reproductive manifestations of the syndrome [144]. Over half of the women suffering from PCOS were overweight, had a BMI ranging between 24.0 and 27.9 kg/m^2, or were obese, with a BMI of 28 kg/m^2 or more [145]. The cornerstone of weight management in individuals with PCOS involves creating a sustainable caloric deficit, typically through a combination of dietary modifications and increased physical activity. A balanced diet that emphasizes whole, minimally processed foods, including a variety of fruits, vegetables, whole grains, lean proteins, and healthy fats, is fundamental. This approach not only aids in reducing caloric intake but also ensures an adequate intake of essential nutrients. Portion control and mindful eating practices are also important strategies for preventing overeating and facilitating weight loss [146].

In addition to general caloric control, specific dietary patterns, such as the Mediterranean diet, low glycemic index diet, or anti-inflammatory diet, have shown benefits in managing PCOS-related weight issues. These diets focus on food quality, including high fiber content, which can improve satiety and reduce total caloric intake [147]. Regular physical activity, including both aerobic and resistance training, complements dietary efforts by increasing energy expenditure, preserving lean muscle mass, and improving insulin sensitivity [148]. It is also crucial to address any psychological factors that may contribute to weight issues, such as binge eating or emotional eating, as these can be common in patients with PCOS. Behavioral interventions, possibly with the support of a mental health professional, can be an important aspect of a comprehensive weight management strategy [16]. Personalized nutritional and lifestyle interventions, considering individual preferences, lifestyles, and metabolic needs, are key for effective and sustainable weight management in patients with PCOS [149]. Collaborating with healthcare providers, including dietitians and fitness professionals, can provide the necessary guidance and support for successfully implementing these strategies.

Table 1.7 offers a thorough comparison of various weight management strategies for patients with PCOS. It evaluates each strategy in terms of its effectiveness,

Table 1.7 Comparative analysis of weight management strategies in PCOS patients

Strategy	Approach	Effectiveness	Benefits	Challenges	Reference
Dietary intervention	Low glycemic index diet	High	Improves insulin sensitivity; reduces hyperinsulinemia	May require significant dietary changes	[150]
	High protein, low carbohydrate diet	Moderate to high	Aids in weight loss; improves satiety	Restrictive; may be hard to sustain long-term	[151]
	Mediterranean diet	Moderate	Heart-healthy; improves overall metabolic health	Requires consistent adherence; cost	[152]
Lifestyle modification	Regular exercise	High	Enhances weight loss; improves cardiovascular health	Requires time commitment; may be challenging for beginners	[121]
	Yoga and mindfulness	Moderate	Reduces stress; aids in weight management	Benefits may be more subtle and take time to manifest	[153]
Pharmacological intervention	Metformin	Moderate to high	Reduces insulin resistance; assists in weight management	Potential side effects; not a standalone solution	[154]
	Anti-obesity medications	Varies	Directly targets weight loss	Side effects; requires medical supervision	[155]
Surgical intervention	Bariatric surgery	High	Significant and rapid weight loss; improvement in metabolic syndrome	Invasive; potential risks and complications	[4]
Behavioral therapy	Cognitive behavioral therapy	Moderate	Addresses emotional eating; promotes sustainable lifestyle changes	Requires commitment; results may vary	[156]
Combined approaches	Diet + exercise + behavioral support	Very high	Holistic approach; sustainable weight loss	Requires multidisciplinary effort; time-intensive	[157]

benefits, and challenges and provides references for relevant studies. For dietary interventions, a low-glycemic-index diet is highly effective at improving insulin sensitivity and reducing hyperinsulinemia, although it may necessitate significant dietary changes [150]. A high-protein, low-carbohydrate diet shows moderate to high effectiveness, aiding in weight loss and improving satiety but can be restrictive and challenging to maintain long-term [151]. A Mediterranean diet is moderately effective and heart-healthy and enhances overall metabolic health but requires consistent adherence and can be costly [152]. In lifestyle modifications, regular exercise is highly effective at enhancing weight loss and cardiovascular health, but it demands time commitment and can be difficult for beginners [121]. Yoga and mindfulness, which are moderately effective, help reduce stress and aid in weight management, although their benefits may be subtler and more gradual [153]. Pharmacological interventions include metformin (Fig. 1.5), which is moderately to highly effective at reducing insulin resistance and aiding in weight management but has potential side effects and is not a standalone solution [154]. The primary action of metformin is to reduce the production of glucose by the liver. It inhibits gluconeogenesis, during which the liver synthesizes glucose from noncarbohydrate sources. This reduction in hepatic glucose output leads to a decrease in overall blood glucose levels [158]. Metformin also enhances the sensitivity of peripheral tissues, such as muscles, to insulin. By improving the response of these tissues to insulin, metformin helps the body utilize glucose more effectively, thus lowering blood glucose levels. This increased insulin sensitivity also contributes to improved

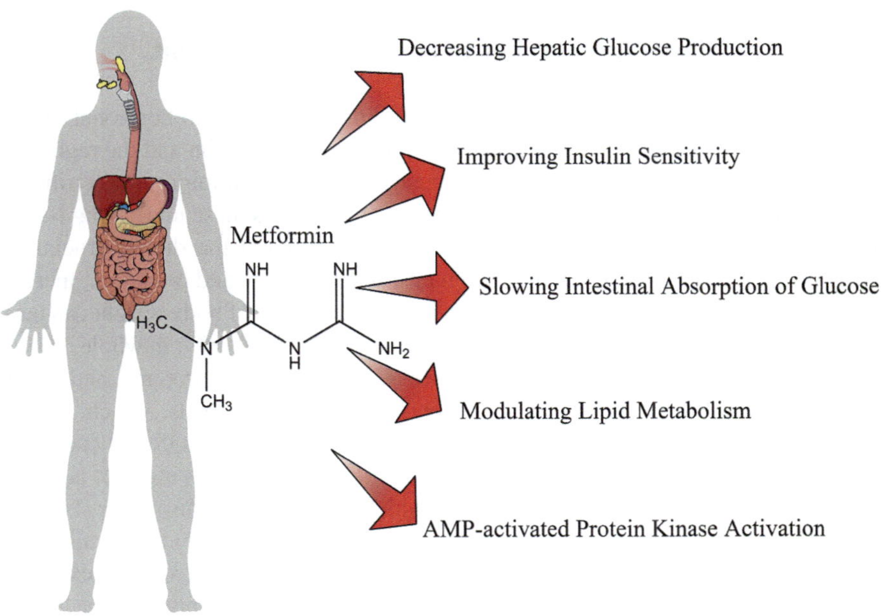

Fig. 1.5 Mechanisms of action of metformin in managing insulin resistance and metabolic disorders in patients with polycystic ovary syndrome

overall metabolic function, which can aid in weight management [159]. Another mechanism by which metformin works is by slowing the absorption of glucose in the intestine. This leads to a more gradual increase in blood sugar levels following meals, preventing sharp spikes that can be detrimental, especially in diabetic patients [50]. Metformin has been shown to affect lipid metabolism. It can lower the levels of LDL cholesterol and triglycerides, which are often elevated in individuals with conditions such as PCOS and type 2 diabetes. This modulation of lipid metabolism contributes to a reduction in cardiovascular risk [51]. In addition, metformin activates an enzyme called AMP-activated protein kinase (AMPK), a crucial regulator of the cellular energy balance. The activation of AMPK leads to a series of metabolic effects that increase insulin sensitivity, promote glucose uptake by cells, and reduce fat storage. This effect of metformin on AMPK is considered central to many of its beneficial actions in managing insulin resistance and metabolic syndrome [160]. The effectiveness of anti-obesity medications varies, as they target weight loss directly but require medical supervision due to side effects [155]. Surgical interventions, such as bariatric surgery, are highly effective at preventing significant and rapid weight loss and improving metabolic syndrome but are invasive and have potential risks and complications [4]. Behavioral therapy, such as cognitive behavioral therapy, is moderately effective at addressing emotional eating and promoting sustainable lifestyle changes, but commitment and results may vary [156]. Finally, combined approaches that integrate diet, exercise, and behavioral support are very effective, offering a holistic and sustainable method for weight loss, although they require a multidisciplinary effort and are time intensive [157].

1.5.3 Nutritional Approaches to Fertility Enhancement

Fertility challenges in patients with PCOS are linked primarily to hormonal imbalances, insulin resistance, and obesity, which can disrupt ovulation and the regularity of the menstrual cycle [69]. Nutritional management aimed at improving fertility in PCOS patients involves a multifaceted approach that targets these underlying issues. First, achieving and maintaining a healthy weight through the diet is crucial, as weight loss has been shown to improve menstrual regularity and ovulation, thereby increasing fertility [8]. Even a modest weight loss of 5–10% of body weight can have a significant positive impact on fertility outcomes [137]. A diet rich in whole, unprocessed foods that provide a balanced intake of carbohydrates, proteins, and fats is recommended. Emphasis is placed on low-glycemic-index foods, which help in managing insulin resistance, a common issue in patients with PCOS that can affect fertility [14]. The inclusion of whole grains, fruits, and vegetables in a diet is essential because of their high nutrient content, which includes vitamins, minerals, fiber, and antioxidants. These components play crucial roles in maintaining overall health and can specifically benefit reproductive health in several ways [137]. For example, whole grains are a great source of fiber that can help regulate blood sugar levels. Stable blood sugar levels are particularly important for individuals with reproductive health issues such as PCOS, where insulin resistance is a common problem [161].

In addition to macronutrients, specific micronutrients play pivotal roles in maintaining fertility. For example, adequate intake of folic acid is crucial for preventing birth defects and supporting healthy pregnancy, and omega-3 fatty acids are known for their anti-inflammatory properties and potential role in improving menstrual regularity and ovulatory function [74, 93]. Antioxidant-rich foods, such as berries, nuts, seeds, and leafy greens, can combat oxidative stress, which is thought to contribute to reproductive dysfunctions in individuals with PCOS [137]. Supplements such as inositol, particularly myoinositol, have also gained attention for their ability to improve ovarian function and insulin sensitivity, thereby aiding in enhancing fertility in patients with PCOS [162]. Importantly, while nutrition plays a significant role in enhancing fertility, it is only one component of a comprehensive management plan for individuals with PCOS. Individualized dietary planning is essential because of each woman's unique health profile, dietary preferences, and lifestyle factors. This tailored approach ensures that dietary interventions not only target fertility concerns but also address individuals' overall health and well-being.

1.6 Emerging Research and Future Directions

1.6.1 Recent Studies on Nutrition and PCOS

Recent research has expanded the body of knowledge on how specific dietary patterns and nutrients impact PCOS, offering new insights for more effective management strategies [163]. One area of recent focus has been the role of dietary patterns, such as Mediterranean and plant-based diets, in managing PCOS symptoms. Studies have shown that these diets, which are rich in fruits, vegetables, whole grains, and healthy fats and low in processed foods and red meat, can improve insulin sensitivity, reduce inflammation, and aid in weight management [141]. The Mediterranean diet, in particular, has a high content of monounsaturated fats, fiber, and antioxidants and has been associated with reduced insulin resistance and androgen levels in women with PCOS. Plant-based diets have also garnered attention, with research suggesting that such diets, when well-planned and nutritionally balanced, can improve PCOS symptoms. These diets are typically high in fiber, vitamins, and minerals but low in saturated fats and added sugars, which aligns well with the nutritional needs of PCOS patients [14].

Another key area of research is the impact of specific nutrients and supplements on PCOS. In PCOS, an altered metabolic process leads to increased transformation of myoinositol into D-chiro-inositol. Myoinositol and D-chiro-inositol are both forms of inositol (Fig. 1.6), a type of sugar crucial for cellular processes and hormone regulation. Myoinositol acts as a second messenger for follicle-stimulating hormone (FSH), whereas D-chiro-inositol functions as an aromatase inhibitor [164]. This shift toward more D-chiro-inositol and less myoinositol is significant because myoinositol is essential for healthy ovarian function [164]. A decrease in myoinositol levels in the ovaries disrupts normal ovulation, a process in which the ovaries release an egg each month and a key aspect of female fertility. Myoinositol

Fig. 1.6 Chemical structures of myoinositol and D-chiro-inositol

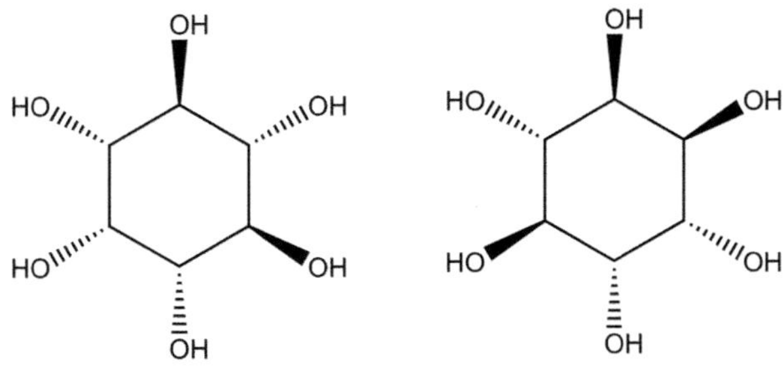

Myo-inositol D-Chiro-inositol

is involved in signaling pathways that influence the release of eggs from the ovaries [165]. Therefore, a reduced amount of myoinositol impairs this process, often leading to irregular or absent menstrual cycles, a common symptom of PCOS. Additionally, this imbalance in the myoinositol and D-chiro-inositol ratios contributes to other hormonal imbalances observed in PCOS patients. These can include increased levels of androgens (male hormones such as testosterone), which can cause symptoms such as acne, excess hair growth, and scalp hair loss [166]. The altered inositol conversion process plays a central role in the manifestation of PCOS symptoms by affecting hormone levels and ovarian function [167]. In addition, myoinositol has been extensively studied for its insulin-sensitizing effects and potential to improve ovulatory function and fertility in women with PCOS [168]. This is because, in PCOS, insulin resistance is a common concern, often leading to metabolic issues and affecting ovarian function [169]. Myoinositol works by improving insulin sensitivity (insulin-sensitizing compound), which helps in regulating blood sugar levels. This, in turn, can contribute to a better hormonal balance, reducing symptoms such as irregular menstrual cycles and facilitating ovulation [168]. Clinical studies have shown that supplementation with myoinositol can improve the metabolic and reproductive aspects of PCOS [170]. For example, a review by Joardar et al. [171] demonstrated that myoinositol significantly improved the metabolic profile and ovarian function in PCOS patients. Authors reported that myoinositol supplementation led to improved menstrual regularity and ovulation rates in women with PCOS. These findings suggested that myoinositol can be an effective adjunct therapy for managing PCOS, particularly for those with insulin resistance.

Omega-3 fatty acids, known for their anti-inflammatory properties, are another area of interest. Research indicates that omega-3 supplementation may help reduce androgen levels and improve menstrual regularity in patients with PCOS [126]. Additionally, interest in the role of the gut microbiota in PCOS is increasing, with studies suggesting that dietary modifications that favor a healthy gut microbiome could be beneficial [172, 173]. Probiotics and prebiotics, which support gut health, are being explored as potential therapeutic options to alleviate PCOS symptoms. For example, Zhang et al. [174] conducted a meta-analysis of randomized clinical trials examining the effect of probiotic supplementation on the management of type

II diabetes risk factors in adults with PCOS. They reported that probiotic supplementation may help control glucose homeostasis in adults with PCOS. Table 1.8 presents a curated overview of recent phase 4 clinical trials exploring dietary interventions for PCOS. These trials explored a range of dietary supplements and modifications, such as probiotic supplementation and its effects on hormonal levels, GLP-1 receptor agonists' impacts on body fat composition, and the combined influence of dietary advice with specific supplements such as myoinositol and folic acid. Additionally, comparisons between different types of dietary supplements, such as myoinositol and d-chiro-inositol, are made to assess their effectiveness on various clinical and metabolic factors associated with PCOS. These studies differ in their intervention methods and primary outcomes, offering valuable insights into the potential of diet-based treatments for PCOS.

The intersection of nutrition and genetics, known as nutrigenomics, is an emerging field that holds promise for personalized nutrition strategies in PCOS management. Recent studies have begun to explore how individual genetic variations can affect nutrient metabolism and the response to different dietary interventions in patients with PCOS. This research paves the way for personalized dietary recommendations on the basis of genetic profiles, offering a more targeted and effective approach to managing PCOS through nutrition. However, this area is still in its infancy, and additional research is needed to translate these findings into clinical practice [175]. Table 1.9 provides an insightful overview of the genetic variations linked to nutrient metabolism in patients with PCOS and their impacts on conditions, complemented by relevant literature references. For example, the FTO gene, known for its role in appetite regulation and energy expenditure, is associated with an increased risk of obesity and insulin resistance in patients with PCOS, as indicated in reference [176]. The INSIG2 gene, which affects insulin secretion and activity, influences insulin resistance and the risk of metabolic syndrome in patients with PCOS, as noted previously Irgam et al. [177]. CYP17A1, which is crucial for steroidogenesis and androgen metabolism, is associated with hyperandrogenism and menstrual irregularities in patients with PCOS [178]. The SHBG gene is involved in sex hormone binding and transport and is linked to variations in androgen levels and insulin sensitivity in patients with PCOS as highlighted by Raja et al. [179]. The VDR governs vitamin D metabolism and affects vitamin D status, which is related to insulin resistance in patients with PCOS [180]. TCF7L2, which is important for glucose homeostasis, is associated with an increased risk of type 2 diabetes in patients with PCOS [181]. The PPARG gene, which plays a role in lipid metabolism and adipogenesis, influences susceptibility to obesity and insulin sensitivity in patients with PCOS, as reported previously [182]. INSR, which is responsible for insulin receptor activity, affects insulin signaling, implicating insulin resistance in PCOS [184]. LHCGR, which is involved in luteinizing hormone receptor activity, impacts ovulatory dysfunction and infertility in patients with PCOS [183]. Finally, MC4R, which is crucial for appetite control and energy balance, is linked to obesity risk in patients with PCOS [176]. This comprehensive guide significantly enhances the understanding of genetic factors influencing the metabolic aspects of PCOS, providing valuable insights for further research and clinical applications. Overall, recent studies in the

Table 1.8 Overview of recently selected phase 4 clinical trials investigating dietary interventions in patients with PCOS

Study title	Intervention type	Primary outcome measures	Start and completion dates	Number of participants	Status	Phase
Probiotic intervention in PCOS (NCT04593459)	Probiotic supplementation	Change in free testosterone level (pg/mL) in serum	2020–ongoing	180 participants across three arms (probiotic, placebo, metformin)	Recruiting	4
GLP-1 RAs in patients with polycystic ovary syndrome (PCOS) (NCT04876027)	GLP-1 receptor agonist (a glucagon-like peptide 1 analog)	The change in visceral adipose tissue (pretreatment–posttreatment) after achievement of the weight loss target	2022–2022	68 participants (age 18–45 years) (12 weeks)	Completed	4
The gut microbiome in women with polycystic ovary syndrome (NCT03642600)	– Dietary supplement: dietary advice plus myoinositol and folic acid – Drug: dietary advice plus liraglutide pen injector	Weight loss	2019–2020	21 participants (32 weeks)	Completed	4
Myoinositol versus D-chiro-inositol in the treatment of polycystic ovary syndrome and insulin resistance: evaluation of clinical, metabolic, endocrine, and ultrasound parameters (NCT01514942)	Dietary supplement: containing myoinositol	Body mass index, menstrual cycle, acne scores (acne grading system by Cremoncini and colleagues), hirsutism scores (Ferriman-Gallwey score), alopecia, oral glucose tolerance test, glucagon levels, C-peptide test, myoinositol serum concentration, etc.	2019–2020	21 participants	Complete	4

Source: https://clinicaltrials.gov/, accessed 20 Jan 2024

Table 1.9 Summary of genetic variations associated with nutrient metabolism in PCOS patients

Gene	Nutrient/metabolism affected	Impact on PCOS	Reference
FTO	Appetite regulation and energy expenditure	Increased risk of obesity and insulin resistance in PCOS	[176]
INSIG2	Insulin secretion and action	Influences insulin resistance and risk of metabolic syndrome in PCOS	[177]
CYP17A1	Steroidogenesis and androgen metabolism	Associated with hyperandrogenism and menstrual irregularities in PCOS	[178]
SHBG	Sex hormone binding and transport	Linked to variations in androgen levels and insulin sensitivity in PCOS	[179]
VDR	Vitamin D metabolism	Impacts vitamin D status, which is related to insulin resistance in PCOS	[180]
TCF7L2	Glucose homeostasis	Associated with increased risk of type 2 diabetes in PCOS	[181]
PPARG	Lipid metabolism and adipogenesis	Influences susceptibility to obesity and insulin sensitivity in PCOS	[182]
INSR	Insulin receptor activity	Affects insulin signaling, with implications for insulin resistance in PCOS	[183]
LHCGR	Luteinizing hormone receptor activity	Impacts ovulatory dysfunction and infertility in PCOS	[184]
MC4R	Appetite control and energy balance	Linked to obesity risk in PCOS	[176]

field of nutrition and PCOS are expanding our understanding of how various dietary approaches and specific nutrients can impact this syndrome. This growing body of evidence underscores the importance of nutrition in managing PCOS and points toward more personalized and effective dietary strategies in the future. Continued research in this area is essential for developing refined nutritional guidelines that can better address the diverse needs of women with PCOS.

1.6.2 Potential Therapeutic Developments

This area of research is critical, as it offers hope for more effective and targeted interventions for women suffering from this complex syndrome. From our perspective, Fig. 1.7 represents the future of PCOS treatment and research that is poised for groundbreaking advancements across various domains. One such domain is innovative therapeutic approaches, which encompass a range of cutting-edge techniques, such as gene therapy, stem cell research, and personalized medicine. Gene therapy, for example, opens up possibilities for directly addressing the genetic roots of hormonal imbalances characteristic of PCOS, offering a more targeted and potentially curative approach [185]. Similarly, stem cell research holds promise for regenerative treatments, which have the potential to restore normal ovarian function and address infertility issues often associated with PCOS [186]. Personalized medicine represents a paradigm shift, moving away from a one-size-fits-all approach to

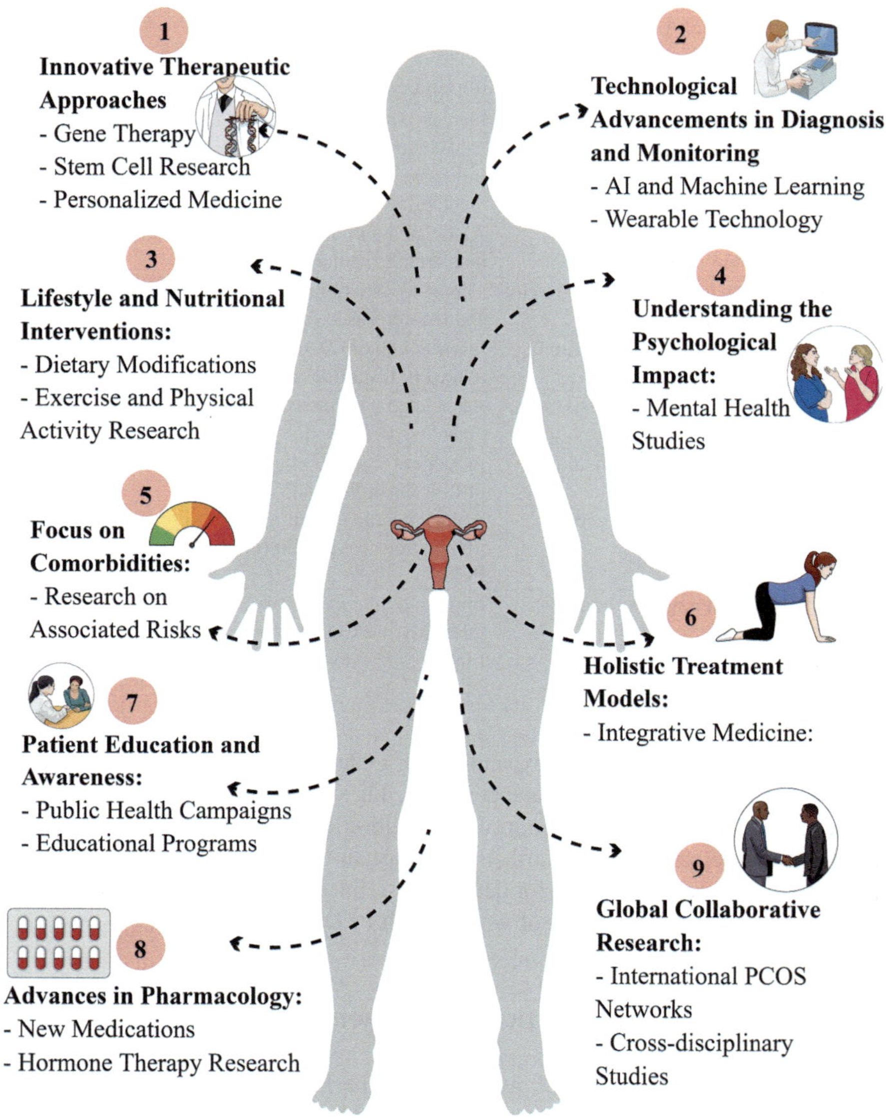

Fig. 1.7 Infographics summarizing potential future directions in PCOS research and treatment

tailoring treatments on the basis of individual genetic profiles, lifestyle choices, and specific symptomatology. This personalized approach ensures more effective and tailored treatment, reducing the trial-and-error aspect of current management strategies [187].

In parallel, substantial progress in technological advancements is significantly transforming the diagnosis and monitoring of PCOS. AI and machine learning offer tools for early detection and the development of personalized treatment plans. These technologies can analyze vast datasets to identify patterns and predict outcomes, potentially leading to earlier intervention and more effective management of the condition [188]. Wearable technology also plays a crucial role in enabling continuous monitoring of metabolic and hormonal parameters, thus providing real-time data that can inform treatment adjustments and lifestyle recommendations. This continuous monitoring approach is particularly beneficial for managing conditions as dynamic and individualized as PCOS [148]. In addition to direct treatment and monitoring, there is a growing focus on lifestyle and nutritional interventions, with research exploring how specific diets and exercise regimens can mitigate PCOS symptoms and improve quality of life [74]. Such interventions emphasize the importance of a holistic approach, addressing not only the physiological aspects of PCOS but also the lifestyle factors that can significantly impact the condition. This comprehensive approach extends to the field of mental health, with studies increasingly focused on the psychological impact of PCOS and the development of strategies to increase mental well-being among patients. This holistic perspective is further supported by research into the comorbidities associated with PCOS, such as diabetes, cardiovascular diseases, and infertility, providing a more integrated understanding of the condition and its wider health implications [189].

In addition, advances in pharmacology are poised to significantly impact the future of PCOS treatment, with a focus on developing more effective medications that minimize side effects [190]. This includes the creation of targeted insulin sensitizers and the evolution of hormone therapy for improved hormonal balance and symptom control, signifying a shift from the current limitations in treatment efficacy and tolerability [99, 109, 132, 191, 192]. Additionally, global collaborative efforts and cross-disciplinary studies are enhancing PCOS research. International networks facilitate extensive research across diverse populations to understand the various genetic, environmental, and lifestyle factors associated with PCOS [193]. These efforts, which integrate insights from multiple scientific fields, are essential for a comprehensive understanding of PCOS, addressing its hormonal, metabolic, reproductive, and psychological aspects. Such collaborative and interdisciplinary approaches are key in progressing PCOS treatment toward more effective and personalized care.

1.6.3 AI and Nutritional Interventions

Currently, studies directly linking AI applications in nutrition research to PCOS management are limited. Table 1.10 outlines three significant AI and machine learning studies in this area. Kaur et al. [194] used pretrained convolutional neural networks to analyze food images for nutrient identification, aiming to manage PCOS through dietary recommendations. Their work also included a review of image classification techniques useful for dieticians in PCOS management. Wang et al. [195] studied the effect of carnitine supplementation on body weight in PCOS patients. They reported that a specific dose of carnitine for a certain duration was needed for the optimal effect, with no significant dose–response relationship occurring within

Table 1.10 AI and machine learning studies have focused on nutritional interventions for PCOS

Artificial intelligence/machine learning method used	Focus of study	Key findings	Reference
Deep learning (convolutional neural network (CNN)	Analyzing food images to track nutrient intake for PCOS management	Utilized pretrained CNNs on food image datasets (Food-101, UEC-256, UEC-100, etc.) to identify nutrients in food. Aimed to overcome PCOS by recommending diets based on nutrient tracking. Proposed study also included a review of image classification and recommendation techniques for dieticians to manage PCOS	[194]
Machine learning (maximal effect model)	Predicting the effect of carnitine supplementation on body weight in PCOS	Explored carnitine's impact on body weight in PCOS patients. Found E_{max} of carnitine supplementation was −3.92% with E_{t50} at 3.6 weeks. Indicated that 250 mg/day of carnitine for at least 14.4 weeks is needed for optimal effect. No significant dose–response relationship within the used dosage range	[195]
Machine learning (various techniques: K-nearest neighbor, decision tree, random forest classifier, multilayer perceptron)	Prevention and diet recommendation for PCOS	Analyzed a PCOS dataset from Kaggle with 541 records and 43 attributes, selecting 21 key features for diet recommendation. Developed a system for recommending a PCOS diet based on clinical data using various machine learning techniques. Validated the performance of these algorithms through different evaluation indicators, aiding in early prevention and safe recovery of PCOS patients through nutrition diets	[196]

E_{max} = maximal effect
E_{t50} = the duration of treatment required to attain 50% of the maximum effect

the dosage range used. In addition, Selvaraj et al. [196] focused on dietary recommendations for preventing PCOS by analyzing a PCOS dataset from Kaggle with various machine learning techniques to select key dietary features, aiding in the early prevention and safe recovery of PCOS patients through nutritional diets. This research highlights the potential of AI in improving dietary management and understanding of PCOS.

The future of the use of AI in nutritional interventions for PCOS should include transformative changes in how this complex condition is managed. The potential of AI to analyze vast arrays of data—from genomics and metabolic responses to lifestyle and dietary habits—promises a new era of highly personalized nutritional therapy for PCOS [14]. In the future, AI systems are expected to provide individualized dietary recommendations on the basis of real-time health data and predict how changes in diet and lifestyle could influence the progression of PCOS [197]. These systems might be capable of integrating data from wearable health trackers, thus providing continuous feedback and enabling adjustments to dietary plans. Additionally, advancements in AI and machine learning could lead to the development of sophisticated models that understand the intricate relationships between different food components and their impact on PCOS symptoms and comorbidities. As nutrigenomics evolves, AI might become instrumental in uncovering the ways in which genetic variations among women with PCOS affect their responses to certain nutrients and dietary patterns. This advancement could lead to the development of increasingly customized nutritional strategies [197]. However, the success of these algorithms will hinge on addressing current challenges, such as ensuring data privacy, improving the accuracy of AI algorithms, and creating interoperable systems that can integrate diverse data types. Collaborative efforts between healthcare professionals, dietitians, computer scientists, and patients are crucial. These findings play a key role in revealing the full potential of AI for nutritional interventions in individuals with PCOS. This approach is instrumental in making AI a cornerstone of effective and personalized management for this condition.

This approach suggests a method for applying AI to personalize nutritional therapy for PCOS patients, as illustrated in Fig. 1.8. Flowcharts often begin with the AI system's data collection phase, where diverse and intricate data, such as genetic profiles, metabolic rates, individual lifestyle habits, and dietary preferences, are gathered from PCOS patients. This is followed by a crucial analysis stage, where AI algorithms, equipped with advanced pattern recognition capabilities, sift through the amassed data to discern unique PCOS-related patterns and correlations. For example, an AI may detect specific genetic markers that correlate with heightened PCOS symptoms or identify lifestyle factors that exacerbate the condition. On the basis of these insights, the AI subsequently formulated tailored dietary recommendations uniquely suited to each patient's physiological makeup and lifestyle considerations. This process may then depict a continuous feedback loop, highlighting the role of wearable health devices and regular health assessments in providing ongoing data to the AI system. This constant stream of data allows the AI to dynamically adjust its dietary recommendations, ensuring that they remain aligned with the patient's evolving health status and treatment response. This process involves not only personalized healthcare but also demonstrating how the analytical process of AI, when harnessed correctly, can lead to highly individualized, adaptive, and effective treatment strategies for complex health conditions such as PCOS.

It is believed that AI and machine learning methodologies, such as neural networks, decision trees, deep learning models, predictive analytics, and reinforcement learning, are highly promising in PCOS nutrition research. These advanced technologies are adept at identifying diet patterns that increase insulin sensitivity, predicting individual metabolic responses to dietary alterations, assessing nutritional deficiencies, and evaluating the influence of diet on PCOS symptoms. They also

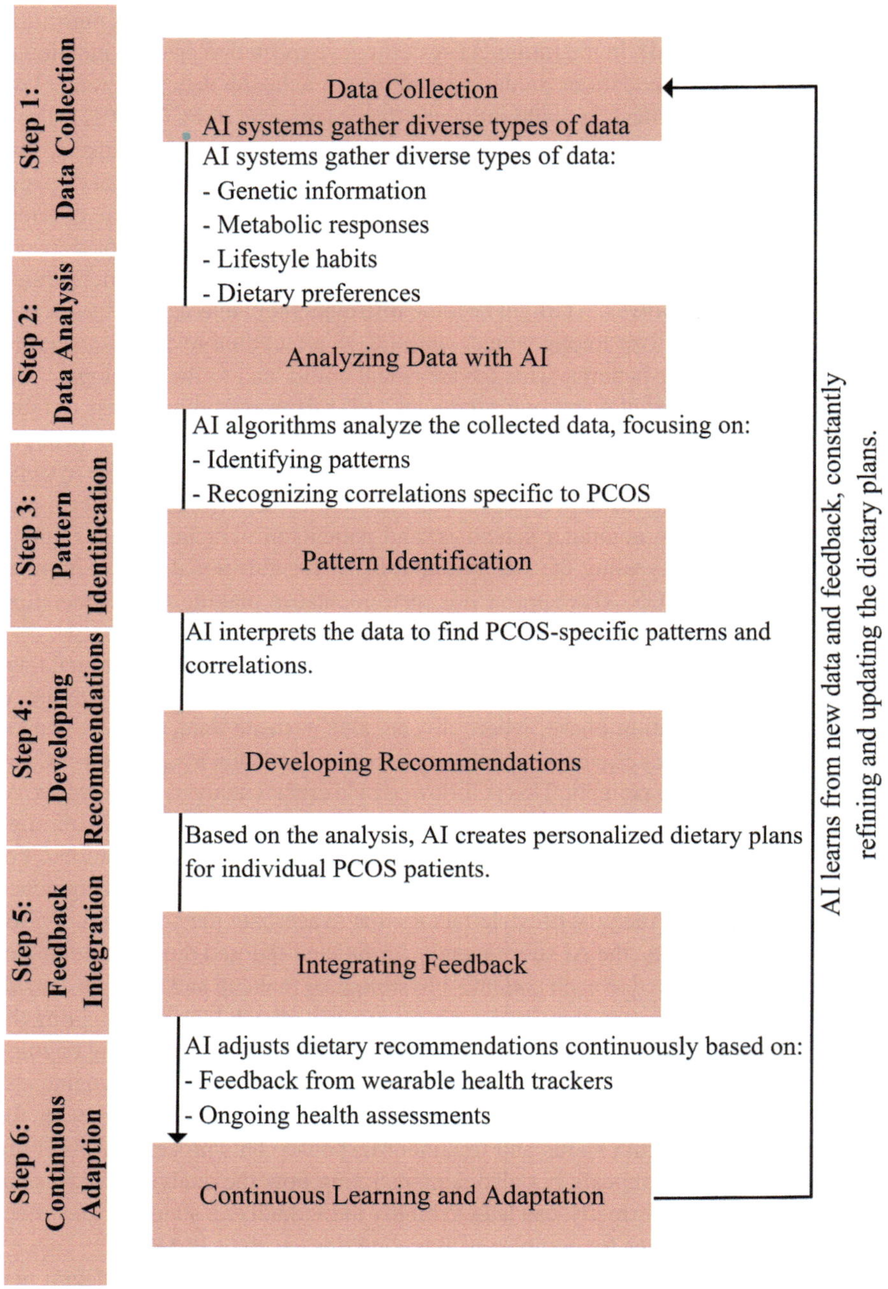

Fig. 1.8 Flow diagram showing the application of artificial intelligence in personalizing nutritional therapy for PCOS patients

excel in customizing dietary plans tailored to each individual's unique hormonal and metabolic profile, continually refining dietary interventions, and accurately predicting their success. This holistic strategy is poised to significantly advance the nutritional management of PCOS.

1.7 Conclusion and Future Scope

This chapter begins by elucidating the complexity of PCOS, a prevalent endocrine disorder characterized by symptoms such as menstrual irregularity, hyperandrogenism, and polycystic ovaries. The authors explored its multifaceted nature, highlighting how it intertwines with insulin resistance, obesity, and hormonal imbalances. The nutritional challenges associated with PCOS were then examined, underscoring the importance of dietary management strategies in alleviating symptoms and reducing the risk of comorbidities. The role of macronutrients and micronutrients in managing PCOS, including low glycemic indices, balanced macronutrient intake, and the importance of specific vitamins and minerals, was also described. Specialized diets, such as the Mediterranean and low-GI diets, were discussed for their ability to manage PCOS-related metabolic and reproductive issues. This chapter also reviews strategies for addressing common comorbidities through nutrition, with a focus on managing insulin resistance and obesity and increasing fertility. Emerging research and potential future directions are highlighted, particularly ongoing developments in pharmaceuticals and regenerative medicine and the utilization of advanced technologies such as AI in diagnosis and management. The potential of AI in revolutionizing nutritional therapy for PCOS has been particularly emphasized. The ability of AI to analyze extensive datasets for personalized diet recommendations and integrate this information into nutrigenomics opens new avenues for individualized treatment plans. In the future, significant advancements in the understanding and management of PCOS are anticipated. Continued research is essential to unravel the complex etiology and pathophysiology of PCOS. The role of AI and technology in advancing nutritional therapy is particularly promising. The potential of AI to provide tailored dietary recommendations on the basis of individual genetic, metabolic, and lifestyle factors could revolutionize the management of PCOS. This approach could lead to more effective, personalized treatments, improving the quality of life for women with PCOS. In conclusion, while the understanding of PCOS and its relationship with nutrition has increased, much still needs to be explored. Future research could uncover deeper insights into PCOS, paving the way for more effective and personalized management strategies. The integration of technological advancements such as AI in nutrition therapy is a particularly exciting prospect, offering the potential to significantly increase the precision and effectiveness of PCOS management.

References

1. Kamrul-Hasan ABM, Aalpona FTZ. Metabolic association of serum prolactin in polycystic ovary syndrome: a retrospective analysis of 840 patients in Bangladesh. Endocr Metab Sci. 2024;14:100153. https://doi.org/10.1016/j.endmts.2023.100153.
2. Zheng CY, Yu YX, Bai X. Polycystic ovary syndrome and related inflammation in radiomics; relationship with patient outcome. Semin Cell Dev Biol. 2024;154:328–33. https://doi.org/10.1016/j.semcdb.2023.02.013.
3. Hassan S, Thacharodi A, Priya A, Meenatchi R, Hegde TA, Thangamani R, et al. Endocrine disruptors: unraveling the link between chemical exposure and women's reproductive health. Environ Res. 2024;241:117385. https://doi.org/10.1016/j.envres.2023.117385.
4. Samarasinghe SNS, Woods C, Miras AD. Bariatric surgery in women with polycystic ovary syndrome. Metabolism. 2024;151:155745. https://doi.org/10.1016/j.metabol.2023.155745.
5. Wang M, Diao K, Richard M, Dai L, Hu T, Ding H. Discovering common pathogenetic processes between polycystic ovary syndrome and uterine corpus endometrial carcinoma by bioinformatics and experimental approach. Arab J Chem. 2024;17(2):105548. https://doi.org/10.1016/j.arabjc.2023.105548.
6. Chauhan N, Pareek S, Rosario W, Rawal R, Jain U. An insight into the state of nanotechnology-based electrochemical biosensors for PCOS detection. Anal Biochem. 2024;687:115412. https://doi.org/10.1016/j.ab.2023.115412.
7. Nazir S, Sadhu S. Effect of pilates on regulating menstrual cycle in females with polycystic ovarian syndrome. Eur J Obstet Gynecol Reprod Biol X. 2024;21:100271. https://doi.org/10.1016/j.eurox.2023.100271.
8. Shahid M, Wajid M. Chapter 30: Polycystic ovary syndrome in North America. In: Rehman R, Sheikh A, editors. Polycystic ovary syndrome. New Delhi: Elsevier; 2024. p. 229–36. https://doi.org/10.1016/B978-0-323-87932-3.00039-6.
9. Reka S, Suriya PT, Mohan K. Expeditious prognosis of PCOS with ultrasonography images—a convolutional neural network approach. Commun Comput Inf Sci. 2024;1929:367–76. https://doi.org/10.1007/978-3-031-48774-3_26.
10. Mazloomi S, Mousavi V, Aghadavod E, Mafi A. Circular RNAs: emerging modulators in the pathophysiology of polycystic ovary syndrome and their clinical implications. Curr Mol Med. 2024;24(2):153–66. https://doi.org/10.2174/1566524023666230110151155.
11. Ali SS, Jabeen S. Chapter 8: Clinical features and presentation of polycystic ovary syndrome. In: Rehman R, Sheikh A, editors. Polycystic ovary syndrome. New Delhi: Elsevier; 2024. p. 56–60. https://doi.org/10.1016/B978-0-323-87932-3.00017-7.
12. Bannigida DM, Nayak BS, Vijayaraghavan R. Insulin resistance and oxidative marker in women with PCOS. Arch Physiol Biochem. 2020;126(2):183–6. https://doi.org/10.1080/13813455.2018.1499120.
13. Francone NO, Ramirez T, Boots CE. Contemporary management of the patient with polycystic ovary syndrome. Obstet Gynecol Clin N Am. 2023;50(4):695–705. https://doi.org/10.1016/j.ogc.2023.08.003.
14. Dumesic D, Chazenbalk G, Heber D. Chapter 13: Precision nutrition in female reproductive health. In: Heber D, Li Z, Ordovas J, editors. Precision nutrition. Academic Press; 2024. p. 227–40. https://doi.org/10.1016/B978-0-443-15315-0.00002-X.
15. Butt AS, Devi J. Chapter 12: Polycystic ovary syndrome and nonalcoholic fatty liver disease. In: Rehman R, Sheikh A, editors. Polycystic ovary syndrome. New Delhi: Elsevier; 2024. p. 92–9. https://doi.org/10.1016/B978-0-323-87932-3.00021-9.
16. Asad N, Nadeem T, Noorullah A. Chapter 11: Polycystic ovary syndrome and mental health. In: Rehman R, Sheikh A, editors. Polycystic ovary syndrome. New Delhi: Elsevier; 2024. p. 87–91. https://doi.org/10.1016/B978-0-323-87932-3.00020-7.
17. Cherian KE, Paul TV. Chapter 33: Management of insulin resistance in PCOS. In: Mukhopadhyay S, Mondal S, editors. Metabolic syndrome. Academic Press; 2024. p. 407–13. https://doi.org/10.1016/B978-0-323-85732-1.00015-3.

18. Hu W, Xie N, Zhu H, Jiang Y, Ding S, Ye S, et al. The effective compounds and mechanisms of Cang-Fu-Dao-Tan formula in treating polycystic ovary syndrome based on UPLC/Q-TOF-MS/MS, network pharmacology and molecular experiments. J Pharm Biomed Anal. 2024;239:115867. https://doi.org/10.1016/j.jpba.2023.115867.
19. Das PK, Mukherjee J, Banerjee D. Female reproductive physiology. In: Das PK, Sejian V, Mukherjee J, Banerjee D, editors. Textbook of veterinary physiology. Singapore: Springer Nature; 2023. p. 513–68. https://doi.org/10.1007/978-981-19-9410-4_22.
20. Adashi EY, Cibula D, Peterson M, Azziz R. The polycystic ovary syndrome: the first 150 years of study. F S Rep. 2023;4(1):2–18. https://doi.org/10.1016/j.xfre.2022.12.002.
21. Kiran Z. Chapter 9: Diagnostic criteria for polycystic ovary syndrome. In: Rehman R, Sheikh A, editors. Polycystic ovary syndrome. New Delhi: Elsevier; 2024. p. 61–74. https://doi.org/10.1016/B978-0-323-87932-3.00018-9.
22. Yu O, Christ JP, Schulze-Rath R, Covey J, Kelley A, Grafton J, et al. Incidence, prevalence, and trends in polycystic ovary syndrome diagnosis: a United States population-based study from 2006 to 2019. Am J Obstet Gynecol. 2023;229(1):39.e1–39.e12. https://doi.org/10.1016/j.ajog.2023.04.010.
23. Mumusoglu S, Yildiz BO. Polycystic ovary syndrome phenotypes and prevalence: differential impact of diagnostic criteria and clinical versus unselected population. Curr Opin Endocr Metab Res. 2020;12:66–71. https://doi.org/10.1016/j.coemr.2020.03.004.
24. Rehman R, Alam F, Khan R. Chapter 25: Situation analysis of polycystic ovary syndrome in Central and East Asia. In: Rehman R, Sheikh A, editors. Polycystic ovary syndrome. New Delhi: Elsevier; 2024. p. 191–9. https://doi.org/10.1016/B978-0-323-87932-3.00034-7.
25. Hashmi MF. Chapter 1: Introduction to polycystic ovary syndrome. In: Rehman R, Sheikh A, editors. Polycystic ovary syndrome. New Delhi: Elsevier; 2024. p. 1–5. https://doi.org/10.1016/B978-0-323-87932-3.00010-4.
26. VanHise K, Wang ET, Norris K, Azziz R, Pisarska MD, Chan JL. Racial and ethnic disparities in polycystic ovary syndrome. Fertil Steril. 2023;119(3):348–54. https://doi.org/10.1016/j.fertnstert.2023.01.031.
27. Vidal-Cevallos P, Mijangos-Trejo A, Uribe M, Tapia NC. The interlink between metabolic-associated fatty liver disease and polycystic ovary syndrome. Endocrinol Metab Clin N Am. 2023;52(3):533–45. https://doi.org/10.1016/j.ecl.2023.01.005.
28. Barberis N, Calaresi D, Cannavò M, Verrastro V. Trait emotional intelligence and quality of life in women with polycystic ovary syndrome: dysmorphic concerns and general distress as mediators. Compr Psychiatry. 2023;122:152373. https://doi.org/10.1016/j.comppsych.2023.152373.
29. Deswal R, Narwal V, Dang A, Pundir CS. The prevalence of polycystic ovary syndrome: a brief systematic review. J Hum Reprod Sci. 2020;13(4):261–71 (in Eng). https://doi.org/10.4103/jhrs.JHRS_95_18.
30. Chiaffarino F, Cipriani S, Dalmartello M, Ricci E, Esposito G, Fedele F, et al. Prevalence of polycystic ovary syndrome in European countries and USA: a systematic review and meta-analysis. Eur J Obstet Gynecol Reprod Biol. 2022;279:159–70. https://doi.org/10.1016/j.ejogrb.2022.10.020.
31. Huang Z, Yong E-L. Ethnic differences: is there an Asian phenotype for polycystic ovarian syndrome? Best Pract Res Clin Obstet Gynecol. 2016;37:46–55. https://doi.org/10.1016/j.bpobgyn.2016.04.001.
32. Gao Y, Liu H, Qiao L, Liang J, Yao H, Lin X, Gao Y. Study of burden in polycystic ovary syndrome at global, regional, and national levels from 1990 to 2019. Healthcare. 2023;11(4):562. https://doi.org/10.3390/healthcare11040562.
33. Motlagh Asghari K, Nejadghaderi SA, Alizadeh M, Sanaie S, Sullman MJ, Kolahi AA, et al. Burden of polycystic ovary syndrome in the Middle East and North Africa region, 1990–2019. Sci Rep. 2022;12(1):7039. https://doi.org/10.1038/s41598-022-11006-0.
34. Mirza FG, Tahlak MA, Hazari K, Khamis AH, Atiomo W. Prevalence of polycystic ovary syndrome among females aged between 15 and 45 years at a major women: Hospital in Dubai, United Arab Emirates. Int J Environ Res Public Health. 2023;20(9):5717. https://doi.org/10.3390/ijerph20095717.

35. March WA, Moore VM, Willson KJ, Phillips DI, Norman RJ, Davies MJ. The prevalence of polycystic ovary syndrome in a community sample assessed under contrasting diagnostic criteria. Hum Reprod. 2010;25(2):544–51 (in Eng). https://doi.org/10.1093/humrep/dep399.
36. Wu Q, Gao J, Bai D, Yang Z, Liao Q. The prevalence of polycystic ovarian syndrome in Chinese women: a meta-analysis. Ann Palliat Med. 2021;10(1):74–87. https://doi.org/10.21037/apm-20-1893.
37. Masood S, Hashmani SR. Chapter 15: Pharmacologic management for polycystic ovary syndrome: hirsutism and acne. In: Rehman R, Sheikh A, editors. Polycystic ovary syndrome. New Delhi: Elsevier; 2024. p. 117–21. https://doi.org/10.1016/B978-0-323-87932-3.00024-4.
38. Hussein K, Karami M. Association between insulin resistance and abnormal menstrual cycle in Saudi females with polycystic ovary syndrome. Saudi Pharm J. 2023;31(6):1104–8. https://doi.org/10.1016/j.jsps.2023.03.021.
39. García-Sáenz MR, Lobaton-Ginsberg M, Ramírez-Rentería C, López-Juárez N, Saucedo R, Valencia-Ortega J, Ferreira-Hermosillo A. Hirsutism and polycystic ovarian morphology are the most frequent components of polycystic ovary syndrome in women with type 1 diabetes. Arch Med Res. 2023;54(7):102895. https://doi.org/10.1016/j.arcmed.2023.102895.
40. Bahri Khomami M, Moran LJ. Polycystic ovary syndrome and gestational weight gain. Curr Opin Endocr Metab Res. 2020;12:20–5. https://doi.org/10.1016/j.coemr.2020.02.009.
41. Siemienowicz K, et al. Insights into manipulating postprandial energy expenditure to manage weight gain in polycystic ovary syndrome. iScience. 2020;23(6):101164. https://doi.org/10.1016/j.isci.2020.101164.
42. Albogami SS, Albassam WB, Alghamdi EG, Alabdullatif A, Alajlan ZA, AlAwad SI, Hamd ZY. Prevalence of polycystic ovary syndrome by ultrasound and it is relation with endometrial hyperplasic and depression. J Radiat Res Appl Sci. 2023;16(3):100637. https://doi.org/10.1016/j.jrras.2023.100637.
43. Shan Y, Han X, Yang C, Li W, Zhou G, Han J, et al. The impact of metabolic surgery on natural conception rates in women with infertility, obesity and polycystic ovary syndrome: a retrospective study. Surg Obes Relat Dis. 2024;20(3):237–43. https://doi.org/10.1016/j.soard.2023.09.024.
44. Li M, Ruan X, Mueck AO. Management strategy of infertility in polycystic ovary syndrome. Glob Health J. 2022;6(2):70–4. https://doi.org/10.1016/j.glohj.2022.03.002.
45. Chen Y, Chen J, Li Y, Wu Y, Wu X, Zhang H, Zhang Z. Insulin-like peptide 5 is associated with insulin resistance in women with polycystic ovary syndrome. J Diabetes Complicat. 2023;37(7):108493. https://doi.org/10.1016/j.jdiacomp.2023.108493.
46. Ali RM, Lomteva SV, Aleksandrova AA, Gutnikova LV, Bugrimova ES, Sagamonova KY, et al. Effect of polymorphisms CYP17 (rs743572), SOD2 (rs4880) and CAT (rs1001179) on hormonal profile and redox status of blood serum and follicular fluid in patients with polycystic ovary syndrome. Gene Rep. 2023;33:101817. https://doi.org/10.1016/j.genrep.2023.101817.
47. Eivazi S, Kheirollahi A, Vatannejad A, Borumandnia N, Habibi B, Shapourizadeh S, et al. The hormone-sensitive lipase C-60G polymorphism is correlated with recurrent spontaneous abortion in women with polycystic ovary syndrome. Gene Rep. 2023;32:101788. https://doi.org/10.1016/j.genrep.2023.101788.
48. Appiah D, Hedderson MM, Kim C, Sidney S, Sternfeld B, Quesenberry CP Jr, et al. The prospective association of hyperandrogenism, oligomenorrhea and polycystic ovary syndrome with incident gestational diabetes: the coronary artery risk development in young adults women's study. Diabetes Res Clin Pract. 2023;198:110593. https://doi.org/10.1016/j.diabres.2023.110593.
49. Yi W, Zhang M, Yuan X, Shi L, Yuan X, Sun M, et al. model combining testosterone, androstenedione and free testosterone index improved the diagnostic efficiency of polycystic ovary syndrome. Endocr Pract. 2023;29(8):629–36. https://doi.org/10.1016/j.eprac.2023.05.007.
50. Lonardo MS, Cacciapuoti N, Guida B, Di Lorenzo M, Chiurazzi M, Damiano S, Menale C. Hypothalamic-ovarian axis and adiposity relationship in polycystic ovary Syndrome: physiopathology and therapeutic options for the management of metabolic and inflammatory aspects. Curr Obes Rep. 2024;13(1):51–70. https://doi.org/10.1007/s13679-023-00531-2.

51. Yousuf F, Rehman R. Chapter 14: Pharmacologic management of PCOS: menstrual irregularities. In: Rehman R, Sheikh A, editors. Polycystic ovary syndrome. New Delhi: Elsevier; 2024. p. 111–6. https://doi.org/10.1016/B978-0-323-87932-3.00023-2.
52. Aderemi Adelakun S, Babatunde O, Chidi Chinazo C, Abimbola Arowosegbe O, Obanijesu Adisa D. Histomorphological and histomorphometric evaluation of the therapeutic role of sulforaphane on the hypothalamic-pituitary-ovarian axis in polycystic ovary syndrome rats via its potential anti-inflammatory and antioxidant activities. Med Omics. 2024;10:100029. https://doi.org/10.1016/j.meomic.2023.100029.
53. Gao M, Liu X, Gu H, Xu H, Zhong W, Wei X, Zhong X. Association between single nucleotide polymorphisms, TGF-β1 promoter methylation, and polycystic ovary syndrome. BMC Pregnancy Childbirth. 2024;24(1):5. https://doi.org/10.1186/s12884-023-06210-3.
54. Eledath Kolasseri A, Eledath Kolasseri A, Sivaraman J, Ramasamy T. Assessment of factors related to poly cystic ovarian syndrome—a comparative and correlational study. J Psychosom Obstet Gynecol. 2024;45(1):2297166. https://doi.org/10.1080/0167482X.2023.2297166.
55. Urbanetz LAML, Soares JM Jr, Maciel GAR, Dos Santos Simões R, Baracat MCP, Baracat EC. Does bisphenol A (BPA) participates in the pathogenesis of polycystic ovary syndrome (PCOS)? Clinics. 2024;78:100310. https://doi.org/10.1016/j.clinsp.2023.100310.
56. Sheikh A. Chapter 10: Polycystic ovary syndrome and metabolic syndrome: risks in later life. In: Rehman R, Sheikh A, editors. Polycystic ovary syndrome. New Delhi: Elsevier; 2024. p. 75–86. https://doi.org/10.1016/B978-0-323-87932-3.00019-0.
57. Lim J, Li J, Feng X, Feng L, Xiao X, Xia Y, et al. Machine learning-based evaluation of application value of traditional Chinese medicine clinical index and pulse wave parameters in the diagnosis of polycystic ovary syndrome. Eur J Integr Med. 2023;64:102311. https://doi.org/10.1016/j.eujim.2023.102311.
58. Zawadzki JK, Dunaif A. Diagnostic criteria for polycystic ovary syndrome: toward a rational approach. In: Dunaif A, Givens JR, Haseltine FP, Merriam GE, editors. Polycystic ovary syndrome. Boston, MA: Blackwell Scientific Inc.; 1992. p. 377–84.
59. Carmina E. Diagnosis of polycystic ovary syndrome: from NIH criteria to ESHRE-ASRM guidelines. Minerva Ginecol. 2004;56(1):1–6 (in Eng).
60. Azziz R, Carmina E, Dewailly D, Diamanti-Kandarakis E, Escobar-Morreale HF, Futterweit W, et al. The Androgen Excess and PCOS Society criteria for the polycystic ovary syndrome: the complete task force report. Fertil Steril. 2009;91(2):456–88. https://doi.org/10.1016/j.fertnstert.2008.06.035.
61. Teede HJ, Tay CT, Laven JJ, Dokras A, Moran LJ, Piltonen TT, et al. Recommendations from the 2023 international evidence-based guideline for the assessment and management of polycystic ovary syndrome. Eur J Endocrinol. 2023;189(2):G43–G64. https://doi.org/10.1093/ejendo/lvad096.
62. Jarrett BY, Vanden Brink H, Oldfield AL, Lujan ME. Ultrasound characterization of disordered antral follicle development in women with polycystic ovary syndrome. J Clin Endocrinol Metabol. 2020;105(11):e3847–61. https://doi.org/10.1210/clinem/dgaa515.
63. Ganie MA, Rasool A, Sahar T, Geer MI. Chapter 40: Interrelationship between polycystic ovary syndrome and metabolic syndrome. In: Mukhopadhyay S, Mondal S, editors. Metabolic Syndrome. Academic Press; 2024. p. 479–91. https://doi.org/10.1016/B978-0-323-85732-1.00022-0.
64. Bozdag G, Mumusoglu S, Zengin D, Karabulut E, Yildiz BO. The prevalence and phenotypic features of polycystic ovary syndrome: a systematic review and meta-analysis. Hum Reprod Rev. 2016;31(12):2841–55. https://doi.org/10.1093/humrep/dew218.
65. Palomba S, Colombo C, Busnelli A, Caserta D, Vitale G. Polycystic ovary syndrome and thyroid disorder: a comprehensive narrative review of the literature. Front Endocrinol. 2023;14:1251866. https://doi.org/10.3389/fendo.2023.1251866.
66. You AS, Kalantar-Zadeh K, Brent GA, Narasaki Y, Daza A, Sim JJ, et al. Impact of thyroid status on incident kidney dysfunction and chronic kidney disease progression in a nationally representative cohort. Mayo Clin Proc. 2024;99(1):39–56. https://doi.org/10.1016/j.mayocp.2023.08.028.

67. Al-Kareem A, Ahmed T, Hassan SA, Abdalhadi SM. Polycystic ovary syndrome: pathogenesis, management, and treatment with metals and organic compounds. Cell Mol Biomed Rep. 2024;4(1):54–64. https://doi.org/10.55705/cmbr.2023.406103.1160.
68. Bedi P, Goyal SB, Rajawat AS, Kumar M. An integrated adaptive bilateral filter-based framework and attention residual U-net for detecting polycystic ovary syndrome. Decision Anal J. 2024;10:100366. https://doi.org/10.1016/j.dajour.2023.100366.
69. Chaudhuri A. Polycystic ovary syndrome: causes, symptoms, pathophysiology, and remedies. Obes Med. 2023;39:100480. https://doi.org/10.1016/j.obmed.2023.100480.
70. Ma C, Xu H, Zhang X, Feng G, Shi L, Su Y, et al. Association of classic and 11-oxygenated androgens with polycystic ovaries and menstrual cycle prolongation in infertile women with PCOS. Clin Chim Acta. 2023;547:117440. https://doi.org/10.1016/j.cca.2023.117440.
71. Huffman AM, Rezq S, Basnet J, Romero DG. Biomarkers in polycystic ovary syndrome. Curr Opin Physiol. 2023;36:100717. https://doi.org/10.1016/j.cophys.2023.100717.
72. Xia Q, Xie L, Wu Q, Cong J, Ma H, Li J, et al. Elevated baseline LH/FSH ratio is associated with poor ovulatory response but better clinical pregnancy and live birth in Chinese women with PCOS after ovulation induction. Heliyon. 2023;9(1):e13024. https://doi.org/10.1016/j.heliyon.2023.e13024.
73. Zhai Y, Pang Y. Systemic and ovarian inflammation in women with polycystic ovary syndrome. J Reprod Immunol. 2022;151:103628. https://doi.org/10.1016/j.jri.2022.103628.
74. Sheikh L, Islam ZS, Najmi N. Chapter 20: Management of associated risks of pregnancy in polycystic ovary syndrome. In: Rehman R, Sheikh A, editors. Polycystic ovary syndrome. New Delhi: Elsevier; 2024. p. 161–5. https://doi.org/10.1016/B978-0-323-87932-3.00029-3.
75. Subha R, Nayana BR, Rekha R, Sumalatha P. Computational intelligence for early detection of infertility in women. Eng Appl Artif Intell. 2024;127:107400. https://doi.org/10.1016/j.engappai.2023.107400.
76. Kavitha K, Tangudu N, Sahu SR, Narayana GVL, Anusha V. Detection of PCOS using machine learning algorithms with grid search CV optimization. Int J Eng Trends Technol. 2023;71(7):201–8. https://doi.org/10.14445/22315381/IJETT-V71I7P219.
77. Abouhawwash M, Sridevi S, Sundararajan S-C-M, Pachlor R, Karim F-K, Khafaga D-S. Automatic diagnosis of polycystic ovarian syndrome using wrapper methodology with deep learning techniques. Comput Syst Sci Eng. 2023;47(1):239–53. https://doi.org/10.32604/csse.2023.037812.
78. Sreejith S, Khanna Nehemiah H, Kannan A. A clinical decision support system for polycystic ovarian syndrome using red deer algorithm and random forest classifier. Healthc Anal. 2022;2:100102. https://doi.org/10.1016/j.health.2022.100102.
79. Srinivas K, Kumar P, Raghavendra C. An improvised follicle polycystic ovarian detection using AKF from a sequence of given ultrasound images. J Intell Fuzzy Syst. 2022;43(6):7717–32. https://doi.org/10.3233/JIFS-212857.
80. Suha SA, Islam MN. An extended machine learning technique for polycystic ovary syndrome detection using ovary ultrasound image. Sci Rep. 2022;12(1):17123. https://doi.org/10.1038/s41598-022-21724-0.
81. Barrera FJ, Brown ED, Rojo A, Obeso J, Plata H, Lincango EP, et al. Application of machine learning and artificial intelligence in the diagnosis and classification of polycystic ovarian syndrome: a systematic review. Front Endocrinol. 2023;14:1106625. https://doi.org/10.3389/fendo.2023.1106625.
82. The National Institutes of Health. NIH study reviews 25 years of data and finds AI/ML can detect common hormone disorder: AI and machine learning can successfully diagnose polycystic ovary syndrome. https://www.nih.gov/news-events/news-releases/ai-machine-learning-can-successfullydiagnose-polycystic-ovary-syndrome. Accessed 17 Jan 2024.
83. Butt MS, Saleem J, Zakar R, Aiman S, Bukhari GMJ, Fischer F. Comparison of physical activity levels and dietary habits between women with polycystic ovarian syndrome and healthy controls of reproductive age: a case–control study. BMC Womens Health. 2024;24(1):29. https://doi.org/10.1186/s12905-023-02866-3.

84. Bril F, Ezeh U, Amiri M, Hatoum S, Pace L, Chen YH, et al. Adipose tissue dysfunction in polycystic ovary syndrome. J Clin Endocrinol Metabol. 2024;109(1):10–24. https://doi.org/10.1210/clinem/dgad356.
85. Talebi S, Shab-Bidar S, Mohammadi H, Moini A, Djafarian K. The effects of intermittent fasting diet alone or in combination with probiotic supplementation in comparison with calorie-restricted diet on metabolic and hormonal profile in patients with polycystic ovary syndrome: study protocol for a randomized clinical trial. Trials. 2023;24(1):690. https://doi.org/10.1186/s13063-023-07691-5.
86. Angelico F, Baratta F, Coronati M, Ferro D, Del Ben M. Diet and metabolic syndrome: a narrative review. Intern Emerg Med. 2023;18(4):1007–17. https://doi.org/10.1007/s11739-023-03226-7.
87. Sharkesh EZ, Keshavarz SA, Nazari L, Abbasi B. Empirical dietary inflammatory pattern is positively associated with polycystic ovary syndrome: a case control study. Nutr Res. 2024;122:123–9. https://doi.org/10.1016/j.nutres.2023.12.009.
88. Shen JY, Xu L, Ding Y, Wu XY. Effect of vitamin supplementation on polycystic ovary syndrome and key pathways implicated in its development: a Mendelian randomization study. World J Clin Cases. 2023;11(23):5468–78 (in Eng). https://doi.org/10.12998/wjcc.v11.i23.5468.
89. Mohan A, Haider R, Fakhor H, Hina F, Kumar V, Jawed A, et al. Vitamin D and polycystic ovary syndrome (PCOS): a review. Ann Med Surg. 2023;85(7):3506–11. https://doi.org/10.1097/MS9.0000000000000879.
90. Sydora BC, Wilke MS, McPherson M, Chambers S, Ghosh M, Vine DF. Challenges in diagnosis and health care in polycystic ovary syndrome in Canada: a patient view to improve health care. BMC Womens Health. 2023;23(1):569. https://doi.org/10.1186/s12905-023-02732-2.
91. Amer W, Alnoury H. Vitamin D & E supplemental therapy could reduce insulin resistance and control PCOS-specific inflammatory and oxidative stresses. Evid Based Womens Health J. 2023;13(4):348–56. https://doi.org/10.21608/EBWHJ.2021.76595.1137.
92. Sharma P, Kapoor HS, Kaur B, Kamra P, Khetarpal P. Investigation of the association of serum trace elements concentrations and serum biochemical parameters with the risk of polycystic ovary syndrome: a case–control study. Biol Trace Elem Res. 2024;202(1):73–86. https://doi.org/10.1007/s12011-023-03664-6.
93. Zhang H, Zheng L, Li C, Jing J, Li Z, Sun S, et al. Effects of gut microbiota on omega-3-mediated ovary and metabolic benefits in polycystic ovary syndrome mice. J Ovarian Res. 2023;16(1):138. https://doi.org/10.1186/s13048-023-01227-w.
94. Al-Akabi DF, Hafth HA. Physiological effect of iron status on patients with polycystic ovary syndrome in Basrah city. J Med Biochem. 2023;42(3):530–5 (in Eng). https://doi.org/10.5937/jomb0-39091a.
95. Chatterjee S, Dutta M. Vitamins as nutraceuticals. In: Micronutrients and macronutrients as nutraceuticals. Apple Academic Press; 2024. p. 89–105.
96. Srnovršnik T, Virant-Klun I, Pinter B. Heavy metals and essential elements in association with oxidative stress in women with polycystic ovary syndrome: a systematic review. Antioxidants. 2023;12(7):1398. https://doi.org/10.3390/antiox12071398.
97. Greff D, Juhász AE, Váncsa S, Váradi A, Sipos Z, Szinte J, et al. Inositol is an effective and safe treatment in polycystic ovary syndrome: a systematic review and meta-analysis of randomized controlled trials. Reprod Biol Endocrinol. 2023;21(1):10. https://doi.org/10.1186/s12958-023-01055-z.
98. Sudhakaran G, Priya PS, Jagan K, Haridevamuthu B, Meenatchi R, Arockiaraj J. Osteoporosis in polycystic ovary syndrome (PCOS) and involved mechanisms. Life Sci. 2023;335:122280. https://doi.org/10.1016/j.lfs.2023.122280.
99. Kulkarni S, Gupta K, Ratre P, Mishra PK, Singh Y, Biharee A, Thareja S. Polycystic ovary syndrome: current scenario and future insights. Drug Discov Today. 2023;28(12):103821. https://doi.org/10.1016/j.drudis.2023.103821.

100. Yang M, Shen X, Lu D, Peng J, Zhou S, Xu L, Zhang J. Effects of vitamin D supplementation on ovulation and pregnancy in women with polycystic ovary syndrome: a systematic review and meta-analysis. Front Endocrinol (Lausanne). 2023;14:1148556 (in Eng). https://doi.org/10.3389/fendo.2023.1148556.
101. Abbasi S, Mohebbi M, Mousavi Vahed SH, Dadgar Moghaddam M, Afiat M, Nematy M, Jahanpak N. Comparison of magnesium status using 24-h urine magnesium content and magnesium fraction excretion in PCOS with non-PCOS control women: a cross-sectional study. Biol Trace Elem Res. 2023;201(12):5601–6. https://doi.org/10.1007/s12011-023-03626-y.
102. Sirotkin AV, Tarko A, Fabova Z, Valocky I, Alwasel S, Kotwica J, Harrath AH. Can flaxseed, chia or puncture vine affect mare ovarian cell functions and prevent the toxic effect of the environmental contaminant toluene? Theriogenology. 2023;208:178–84. https://doi.org/10.1016/j.theriogenology.2023.06.018.
103. FaragAllah EM, Algharib SA, Goda NI, El-Malkey NF, Mahboub HH, El-Fayoumi SH, et al. Protective effect of *Salvia hispanica* (chia seeds) against obesity induced ovarian disorders in rat model. Tissue Cell. 2023;83:102156. https://doi.org/10.1016/j.tice.2023.102156.
104. Corrie L, Awasthi A, Kaur J, Vishwas S, Gulati M, Kaur IP, et al. Interplay of gut microbiota in polycystic ovarian syndrome: role of gut microbiota, mechanistic pathways and potential treatment strategies. Pharmaceuticals. 2023;16(2):197. https://doi.org/10.3390/ph16020197.
105. Bykowska-Derda A, Kaluzna M, Ruchała M, Ziemnicka K, Czlapka-Matyasik M. The significance of plant-based foods and intense physical activity on the metabolic health of women with PCOS: a priori dietary-lifestyle patterns approach. Appl Sci. 2023;13(4):2118. https://doi.org/10.3390/app13042118.
106. Hu X, Wang W, Su X, Peng H, Tan Z, Li Y, Huang Y. Comparison of nutritional supplements in improving glycolipid metabolism and endocrine function in polycystic ovary syndrome: a systematic review and network meta-analysis. PeerJ. 2023;11:e16410. https://doi.org/10.7717/peerj.16410.
107. Sharma A, Bansal K, Bajpai M. The role of different medicinal herbs in treatment of polycystic ovary syndrome: a review. Nat Prod J. 2024;14(1):68–76. https://doi.org/10.2174/2210315513666230502104141.
108. Hu X, Yan E, Peng W, Zhou Y, Jin L, Qian K. Higher pre-pregnancy body mass index was associated with adverse pregnancy and perinatal outcomes in women with polycystic ovary syndrome after a freeze-all strategy: a historical cohort study. Acta Obstet Gynecol Scand. 2024;103(5):884–96. https://doi.org/10.1111/aogs.14771.
109. Rashid O, Fatima M. Chapter 17: Role of insulin sensitizers in the management of polycystic ovary syndrome. In: Rehman R, Sheikh A, editors. Polycystic ovary syndrome. New Delhi: Elsevier; 2024. p. 130–5. https://doi.org/10.1016/B978-0-323-87932-3.00026-8.
110. Guimarães TCM, Taranto DODL, Couto CA, Nardelli MJ, Cândido AL, Hott CDA, et al. Dietary pattern in women with polycystic ovary syndrome with and without associated nonalcoholic fatty liver disease: a cross-sectional study. Clinics. 2023;78:100288. https://doi.org/10.1016/j.clinsp.2023.100288.
111. Zhang X, Zheng Y, Guo Y, Lai Z. The effect of low carbohydrate diet on polycystic ovary syndrome: a meta-analysis of randomized controlled trials. Int J Endocrinol. 2019;2019:4386401. https://doi.org/10.1155/2019/4386401.
112. Krystock A. Role of lifestyle and diet in the management of polycystic ovarian syndrome. In: Pal L, editor. Polycystic ovary syndrome: current and emerging concepts. New York: Springer; 2014. p. 147–64. https://doi.org/10.1007/978-1-4614-8394-6_9.
113. Frary J, Bjerre K, Glintborg D, Ravn P. The effect of dietary carbohydrates in women with polycystic ovary syndrome. Minerva Endocrinol. 2014;10(10):57.
114. Farshchi H, Rane A, Love A, Kennedy RL. Diet and nutrition in polycystic ovary syndrome (PCOS): pointers for nutritional management. J Obstet Gynecol. 2007;27(8):762–73. https://doi.org/10.1080/01443610701667338.
115. Mínguez-Alarcón L, Williams PL, Souter I, Sacha C, Amarasiriwardena CJ, Ford JB, et al. Hair mercury levels, intake of omega-3 fatty acids and ovarian reserve among women attending a fertility center. Int J Hyg Environ Health. 2021;237:113825. https://doi.org/10.1016/j.ijheh.2021.113825.

116. Bahramian H, Sherafatmanesh S, Asadi N, Bakhshi A, Hassan Eftekhari M, Ekramzadeh Comma M. Effects of single-dose and cosupplementation of vitamin D and omega-3 on metabolic profile in women with polycystic ovary syndrome: an RCT. Int J Reprod Biomed. 2023;21(7):541–50 (in Eng). https://doi.org/10.18502/ijrm.v21i7.13889.
117. Naz MSG, Jahanfar S, Tehrani FR. An overview on effects of micronutrients and macronutrients interventions in management of polycystic ovary syndrome. Clin Nutr ESPEN. 2022;52:218–28. https://doi.org/10.1016/j.clnesp.2022.11.007.
118. Babu A, Devi Rajeswari V, Ganesh V, Das S, Dhanasekaran S, Usha Rani G, Ramanathan G. Gut microbiome and polycystic ovary syndrome: interplay of associated microbial-metabolite pathways and therapeutic strategies. Reprod Sci. 2024;31(6):1508–20. https://doi.org/10.1007/s43032-023-01450-2.
119. Begum RF, Singh A, Mohan S. Impact of junk food on obesity and polycystic ovarian syndrome: mechanisms and management strategies. Obes Med. 2023;40:100495. https://doi.org/10.1016/j.obmed.2023.100495.
120. Bykowska-Derda A, Kałużna M, Garbacz A, Ziemnicka K, Ruchała M, Czlapka-Matyasik M. Intake of low glycemic index foods but not probiotics is associated with atherosclerosis risk in women with polycystic ovary syndrome. Life. 2023;13(3):799. https://doi.org/10.3390/life13030799.
121. Cowan S, Lim S, Alycia C, Pirotta S, Thomson R, Gibson-Helm M, et al. Lifestyle management in polycystic ovary syndrome—beyond diet and physical activity. BMC Endocr Disord. 2023;23(1):14. https://doi.org/10.1186/s12902-022-01208-y.
122. Fighera TM, Dos Santos BR, Spritzer PM. Lean mass and associated factors in women with PCOS with different phenotypes. PLoS One. 2023;18(10):e0292623. https://doi.org/10.1371/journal.pone.0292623.
123. Han Y, Wu H, Sun S, Zhao R, Deng Y, Zeng S, Chen J. Effect of high fat diet on disease development of polycystic ovary syndrome and lifestyle intervention strategies. Nutrients. 2023;15(9):2230. https://doi.org/10.3390/nu15092230.
124. Emami N, Moini A, Bakhtiarizadeh MR, Yaghmaei P, Shahhoseini M, Alizadeh A. Fatty acids in subcutaneous adipose tissue of pregnant women with and without polycystic ovary syndrome are associated with genes related to steroidogenesis: a case–control study. Int J Fertil Steril. 2023;17(2):127–32 (in Eng). https://doi.org/10.22074/ijfs.2022.551310.1284.
125. Tian Y, Zhang J, Li M, Shang J, Bai X, Zhang H, et al. Serum fatty acid profiles associated with metabolic risk in women with polycystic ovary syndrome. Front Endocrinol. 2023;14:1077590. https://doi.org/10.3389/fendo.2023.1077590.
126. Siddique R, Mehmood MH. Chapter 22: Role of complementary and alternative medicine in polycystic ovary syndrome. In: Rehman R, Sheikh A, editors. Polycystic ovary syndrome. New Delhi: Elsevier; 2024. p. 171–80. https://doi.org/10.1016/B978-0-323-87932-3.00031-1.
127. Gholizadeh-Moghaddam M, Ghasemi-Tehrani H, Askari G, Jaripur M, Clark CC, Rouhani MH. Effect of magnesium supplementation in improving hyperandrogenism, hirsutism, and sleep quality in women with polycystic ovary syndrome: a randomized, placebo-controlled clinical trial. Health Sci Rep. 2023;6(1):e1013. https://doi.org/10.1002/hsr2.1013.
128. Lee W-L, Lee F-K, Wang P-H. Vitamin D and polycystic ovary syndrome. Taiwan J Obstet Gynecol. 2022;61(6):919–20. https://doi.org/10.1016/j.tjog.2022.06.010.
129. Seaward Brain HP, Georgiou C, Mason HD, Rice S. Mechanism of action of vitamin D (1,25-(OH) 2-D3) on ovarian follicle growth: implications for women with vitamin D deficiency and PCOS. bioRxiv. 2023; https://doi.org/10.1101/2023.06.16.545289.
130. Lejman-Larysz K, Golara A, Baranowska M, Kozłowski M, Guzik P, Szydłowska I, et al. Influence of vitamin D on the incidence of metabolic syndrome and hormonal balance in patients with polycystic ovary syndrome. Nutrients. 2023;15(13):2952. https://doi.org/10.3390/nu15132952.
131. Ersahin A, Celik O, Gungor ND, Celik N, Melil S, Yardim M, et al. Long pentraxin 3 and vitamin D receptor mRNA expression pattern of cumulus granulosa cells isolated from PCOS oocytes at different stages of nuclear maturation. Reprod Biol Endocrinol. 2024;22(1):6. https://doi.org/10.1186/s12958-023-01176-5.

132. Naz S, Amerjee A. Chapter 19: Management of subfertility in polycystic ovary syndrome. In: Rehman R, Sheikh A, editors. Polycystic ovary syndrome. New Delhi: Elsevier; 2024. p. 141–60. https://doi.org/10.1016/B978-0-323-87932-3.00028-1.
133. Zhang B, Yao X, Zhong X, Hu Y, Xu J. Vitamin D supplementation in the treatment of polycystic ovary syndrome: a meta-analysis of randomized controlled trials. Heliyon. 2023;9(3):e14291. https://doi.org/10.1016/j.heliyon.2023.e14291.
134. Tawfeek F. Study vitamin D3 effect on polycystic ovarian induction by letrozole of rat. Egypt J Vet Sci. 2024;55(2):473–86. https://doi.org/10.21608/ejvs.2023.233155.1594.
135. Zhao Y, Zhou M, Shang Y, Dou M, Gao S, Yang H, Zhang F. Effects of cosupplementation of chromium and magnesium on metabolic profiles, inflammation, and oxidative stress in impaired glucose tolerance. Diab Vasc Dis Res. 2024;21(1):14791641241228156. https://doi.org/10.1177/14791641241228156.
136. Hariri Z, Yari Z, Hoseini S, Abhari K, Sohrab G. Synbiotic as an ameliorating factor in the health-related quality of life in women with polycystic ovary syndrome. A randomized, triple-blind, placebo-controlled trial. BMC Womens Health. 2024;24(1):19. https://doi.org/10.1186/s12905-023-02868-1.
137. Sengupta P, Dutta S, Fallah Hassan M. Polycystic ovary syndrome (PCOS) and oxidative stress. J Integr Sci Technol. 2023;12(3):752. https://doi.org/10.62110/sciencein.jist.2024.v12.752.
138. Ahmed IA, Mikail MA. Diet and skin health: the good and the bad. Nutrition. 2024;119:112350. https://doi.org/10.1016/j.nut.2023.112350.
139. Kumar MM. Eating disorders in youth with chronic health conditions: clinical strategies for early recognition and prevention. Nutrients. 2023;15(17):3672. https://doi.org/10.3390/nu15173672.
140. Parveen S, Khan S, Ahsan H, Manger PT, Gupta B, Alam R. Fat mass and obesity associated (FTO) gene and polycystic ovary syndrome: insight into pathogenesis and association with insulin resistance. Hum Nutr Metab. 2022;30:200174. https://doi.org/10.1016/j.hnm.2022.200174.
141. Deepak Kumar K, Huntriss R, Green E, Bora S, Pettitt C. Development of a nutrition screening tool to identify need for dietetic intervention in female infertility. J Hum Nutr Diet. 2023;36(1):154–68. https://doi.org/10.1111/jhn.13055.
142. Ruan H, Zhang Y, Tang Q, Zhao X, Zhao X, Xiang Y, et al. Longitudinal changes in body weight of breastfeeding mothers in the first year after delivery and its relationship with human milk composition: a combined longitudinal and cross-sectional cohort study. Food Sci Human Wellness. 2024;13(1):254–64. https://doi.org/10.26599/FSHW.2022.9250021.
143. ElObeid T, Awad MO, Ganji V, Moawad J. The impact of mineral supplementation on polycystic ovarian syndrome. Metabolites. 2022;12(4):338. https://doi.org/10.3390/metabo12040338.
144. Muscogiuri G, Barrea L, Caprio M, Ceriani F, Chavez AO, El Ghoch M, et al. Nutritional guidelines for the management of insulin resistance. Crit Rev Food Sci Nutr. 2022;62(25):6947–60. https://doi.org/10.1080/10408398.2021.1908223.
145. Min M, Ruan X, Mueck AO. Advanced therapy of overweight or obese polycystic ovary syndrome: a prospective study. Glob Health J. 2022;6(2):75–9. https://doi.org/10.1016/j.glohj.2022.04.004.
146. Sangouni AA, Sasanfar B, Ghadiri-Anari A, Hosseinzadeh M. Effect of l-carnitine supplementation on liver fat content and cardiometabolic indices in overweight/obese women with polycystic ovary syndrome: a randomized controlled trial. Clin Nutr ESPEN. 2021;46:54–9. https://doi.org/10.1016/j.clnesp.2021.08.005.
147. Nadjarzadeh A, Ghadiri-Anari A, Ramezani-Jolfaie N, Mohammadi M, Salehi-Abargouei A, Namayande SM, et al. Effect of hypocaloric high-protein, low-carbohydrate diet supplemented with fennel on androgenic and anthropometric indices in overweight and obese women with polycystic ovary syndrome: a randomized placebo-controlled trial. Complement Ther Med. 2021;56:102633. https://doi.org/10.1016/j.ctim.2020.102633.

148. Wang A, Noel M, Christ JP, Corley J, Lenhart N, Cedars MI, Huddleston H. Vigorous versus moderate exercise to improve glucose metabolism in inactive women with polycystic ovary syndrome and insulin resistance: a pilot randomized controlled trial of two home-based exercise routines. F S Rep. 2024;5(1):80–6. https://doi.org/10.1016/j.xfre.2023.12.004.
149. Qureshi RN. Chapter 23: Evidence-based recommendations for clinical practice (future directions: research and practice). In: Rehman R, Sheikh A, editors. Polycystic ovary syndrome. New Delhi: Elsevier; 2024. p. 181–4. https://doi.org/10.1016/B978-0-323-87932-3.00032-3.
150. Faghfoori Z, Fazelian S, Shadnoush M, Goodarzi R. Nutritional management in women with polycystic ovary syndrome: a review study. Diabetes Metab Syndr Clin Res Rev. 2017;11:S429–32. https://doi.org/10.1016/j.dsx.2017.03.030.
151. Mehrabani HH, Salehpour S, Amiri Z, Farahani SJ, Meyer BJ, Tahbaz F. Beneficial effects of a high-protein, low-glycemic-load hypocaloric diet in overweight and obese women with polycystic ovary syndrome: a randomized controlled intervention study. J Am Coll Nutr. 2012;31(2):117–25. https://doi.org/10.1080/07315724.2012.10720017.
152. Mei S, Ding J, Wang K, Ni Z, Yu J. Mediterranean diet combined with a low-carbohydrate dietary pattern in the treatment of overweight polycystic ovary syndrome patients. Front Nutr. 2022;9:876620. https://doi.org/10.3389/fnut.2022.876620.
153. Young CC, Monge M, Minami H, Rew L, Conroy H, Peretz C, Tan L. Outcomes of a mindfulness-based healthy lifestyle intervention for adolescents and young adults with polycystic ovary syndrome. J Pediatr Adolesc Gynecol. 2022;35(3):305–13. https://doi.org/10.1016/j.jpag.2021.10.016.
154. Anbar HS, Vahora NY, Laghman Shah H, Azam MM, Islam T, Hersi F, et al. Promising drug candidates for the treatment of polycystic ovary syndrome (PCOS) as alternatives to the classical medication metformin. Eur J Pharmacol. 2023;960:176119. https://doi.org/10.1016/j.ejphar.2023.176119.
155. Wang FF, Wu YYHZ, Zhu YH, Ding T, Batterham RL, Qu F, Hardiman PJ. Pharmacologic therapy to induce weight loss in women who have obesity/overweight with polycystic ovary syndrome: a systematic review and network meta-analysis. Obes Rev. 2018;19(10):1424–45. https://doi.org/10.1111/obr.12720.
156. Cooney LG, Milman LW, Hantsoo L, Kornfield S, Sammel MD, Allison KC, et al. Cognitive–behavioral therapy improves weight loss and quality of life in women with polycystic ovary syndrome: a pilot randomized clinical trial. Fertil Steril. 2018;110(1):161–71. https://doi.org/10.1016/j.fertnstert.2018.03.028.
157. Kazemi M, McBreairty LE, Zello GA, Pierson RA, Gordon JJ, Serrao SB, et al. A pulse-based diet and the therapeutic lifestyle changes diet in combination with health counseling and exercise improve health-related quality of life in women with polycystic ovary syndrome: secondary analysis of a randomized controlled trial. J Psychosom Obstet Gynecol. 2020;41(2):144–53. https://doi.org/10.1080/0167482X.2019.1666820.
158. ul haq Shah MZ, Shrivastava V, Mir MA. Metformin treatment ameliorates endocrine-metabolic disturbances in letrozole-induced PCOS mice model by modulating adiponectin status. Obes Med. 2022;31:100392. https://doi.org/10.1016/j.obmed.2022.100392.
159. Sparić R, Andjić M, Rakić A, Bjekić-Macut J, Livadas S, Kontić-Vučinić O, et al. Insulin-sensitizing agents for infertility treatment in woman with polycystic ovary syndrome: a narrative review of current clinical practice. Hormones. 2024;23(1):49–58. https://doi.org/10.1007/s42000-023-00494-y.
160. Garcia-Beltran C, Malpique R, Andersen MS, Bas F, Bassols J, Darendeliler F, et al. SPIOMET4HEALTH—efficacy, tolerability and safety of lifestyle intervention plus a fixed dose combination of spironolactone, pioglitazone and metformin (SPIOMET) for adolescent girls and young women with polycystic ovary syndrome: study protocol for a multicenter, randomized, double-blind, placebo-controlled, four-arm, parallel-group, phase II clinical trial. Trials. 2023;24(1):589. https://doi.org/10.1186/s13063-023-07593-6.
161. Assaf-Balut C, de la Torre NG, del Valle L, Valerio J, Durán A, Bordiú E, et al. Gestational diabetes mellitus and Mediterranean diet principles. In: Preedy VR, Watson RR, editors. The Mediterranean diet. 2nd ed. Academic Press; 2020. p. 313–26.

162. Kamenov Z, Gateva A, Dinicola S, Unfer V. Comparing the efficacy of myo-inositol plus alpha-lactalbumin vs. myo-inositol alone on reproductive and metabolic disturbances of polycystic ovary syndrome. Metabolites. 2023;13(6):717. https://doi.org/10.3390/metabo13060717.
163. Xu Q, Zhang J, Lu Y, Wu L. Association of metabolic-dysfunction associated steatotic liver disease with polycystic ovary syndrome. iScience. 2024;27:108783. https://doi.org/10.1016/j.isci.2024.108783.
164. Facchinetti F, Unfer V, Dewailly D, Kamenov ZA, Diamanti-Kandarakis E, Laganà AS, et al. Inositols in polycystic ovary syndrome: an overview on the advances. Trends Endocrinol Metab. 2020;31(6):435–47. https://doi.org/10.1016/j.tem.2020.02.002.
165. Gambioli R, Forte G, Buzzaccarini G, Unfer V, Laganà AS. Myo-inositol as a key supporter of fertility and physiological gestation. Pharmaceuticals. 2021;14(6):504. https://doi.org/10.3390/ph14060504.
166. Wojciechowska A, Osowski A, Jóźwik M, Górecki R, Rynkiewicz A, Wojtkiewicz J. Inositols' importance in the improvement of the endocrine–metabolic profile in PCOS. Int J Mol Sci. 2019;20(22):5787. https://doi.org/10.3390/ijms20225787.
167. Almalki WH. A review on inositol's potential in cyclic disturbances of adipose-endocrinology-associated polycystic ovary syndrome. Mol Cell Biochem. 2021;476(8):2943–9. https://doi.org/10.1007/s11010-021-04123-3.
168. Bevilacqua A, Dinicola S, Bizzarri M. Chapter 4: Treating PCOS with inositols: choosing the most appropriate myo- to d-chiro-inositol ratio. In: Unfer V, Dewailly D, editors. A clinical guide to inositols. Academic Press; 2023. p. 53–64.
169. Rashid R, Mir SA, Kareem O, Ali T, Ara R, Malik A, et al. Polycystic ovarian syndrome-current pharmacotherapy and clinical implications. Taiwan J Obstet Gynecol. 2022;61(1):40–50. https://doi.org/10.1016/j.tjog.2021.11.009.
170. Etrusco A, Laganà AS, Chiantera V, Buzzaccarini G, Unfer V. Myo-inositol in assisted reproductive technology from bench to bedside. Trends Endocrinol Metab. 2024;35(1):74–83. https://doi.org/10.1016/j.tem.2023.09.005.
171. Joardar S, Duarah P, Purkait MK. Recent advances in myo-inositol recovery and purification from agricultural sources as potential dietary supplements: a review. Sustain Chem Pharm. 2023;36:101331. https://doi.org/10.1016/j.scp.2023.101331.
172. Wang R, Zhao Y, Fang X, Miao C, Ren N, Chen Y, et al. Effect of the ketogenic diet on gut microbiome composition and metabolomics in polycystic ovarian syndrome rats induced by letrozole and a high-fat diet. Nutrition. 2023;114:112127. https://doi.org/10.1016/j.nut.2023.112127.
173. Li JW, Chen YZ, Zhang Y, Zeng LH, Li KW, Xie BZ, et al. Gut microbiota and risk of polycystic ovary syndrome: insights from Mendelian randomization. Heliyon. 2023;9(12):e22155. https://doi.org/10.1016/j.heliyon.2023.e22155.
174. Zhang C, Sheng Y, Jiang J, Xue Y, Yu L, Tian F, et al. Probiotics supplementation for management of type II diabetes risk factors in adults with polycystic ovarian syndrome: a meta-analysis of randomized clinical trial. Food Sci Human Wellness. 2023;12(4):1053–63. https://doi.org/10.1016/j.fshw.2022.10.023.
175. Devi R, Sharma E, Thakur R, Lal P, Kumar A, Altaf MA, et al. Nondairy prebiotics: conceptual relevance with nutrigenomics and mechanistic understanding of the effects on human health. Food Res Int. 2023;170:112980. https://doi.org/10.1016/j.foodres.2023.112980.
176. Shewchuk BM. Chapter 15: Epigenetics and obesity. In: Peedicayil J, Grayson DR, Tollefsbol T, editors. Neuropsychiatric disorders and epigenetics. 2nd ed. Boston: Academic Press; 2024. p. 325–52.
177. Irgam K, Reddy BS, Hari SG, Banapuram S, Reddy BM. The genetic susceptibility profile of type 2 diabetes and reflection of its possible role related to reproductive dysfunctions in the southern Indian population of Hyderabad. BMC Med Genet. 2021;14(1):272. https://doi.org/10.1186/s12920-021-01129-0.

178. Rosato E, Sciarra F, Anastasiadou E, Lenzi A, Venneri MA. Revisiting the physiological role of androgens in women. Expert Rev Endocrinol Metab. 2022;17(6):547–61. https://doi.org/10.1080/17446651.2022.2144834.
179. Raja MHR, Javed MA, Rehman R. Chapter 4: Pathophysiology of polycystic ovary syndrome. In: Rehman R, Sheikh A, editors. Polycystic ovary syndrome. New Delhi: Elsevier; 2024. p. 23–32. https://doi.org/10.1016/B978-0-323-87932-3.00013-X.
180. Huynh K, Kempegowda P, Tamblyn J, O'Reilly MW, Mueller JW, Hewison M, Jenkinson C. Development of a LC–MS/MS method to measure serum 3-sulfate and 3-glucuronide 25-hydroxyvitamin D3 metabolites; comparisons to unconjugated 25OHD in pregnancy and polycystic ovary syndrome. Steroids. 2021;169:108812. https://doi.org/10.1016/j.steroids.2021.108812.
181. Rashid R, Shah IA, Asrar MM, Godha M, Ganai BA, Ganie MA. Family history of menstrual irregularity or diabetes mellitus enhances the susceptibility to polycystic ovary syndrome among subjects harboring rs7903146 genetic variant of TCF7L2. J Diabetes Metab Disord. 2022;21(1):769–76. https://doi.org/10.1007/s40200-022-01050-y.
182. Siemienowicz KJ, Coukan F, Franks S, Rae MT, Duncan WC. Aberrant subcutaneous adipogenesis precedes adult metabolic dysfunction in an ovine model of polycystic ovary syndrome (PCOS). Mol Cell Endocrinol. 2021;519:111042. https://doi.org/10.1016/j.mce.2020.111042.
183. Dakshinamoorthy J, Jain PR, Ramamoorthy T, Ayyappan R, Balasundaram U. Association of GWAS identified INSR variants (rs2059807 & rs1799817) with polycystic ovarian syndrome in Indian women. Int J Biol Macromol. 2020;144:663–70. https://doi.org/10.1016/j.ijbiomac.2019.10.235.
184. Singh R, Kaur S, Yadav S, Bhatia S. Gonadotropins as pharmacological agents in assisted reproductive technology and polycystic ovary syndrome. Trends Endocrinol Metab. 2023;34(4):194–215. https://doi.org/10.1016/j.tem.2023.02.002.
185. Chamanara S, Hozouri V, Irandoost E. Inhibition of NLRP3 inflammasome—a potential mechanistic therapeutic for treatment of polycystic ovary syndrome? J Biochem Mol Toxicol. 2023;38(1):e23592. https://doi.org/10.1002/jbt.23592.
186. Nejabati HR, Nikzad S, Roshangar L. Therapeutic potential of mesenchymal stem cells in PCOS. Curr Stem Cell Res Ther. 2024;19(2):134–44. https://doi.org/10.2174/1574888X18666230517123256.
187. Tay CT, Garrad R, Mousa A, Bahri M, Joham A, Teede H. Polycystic ovary syndrome (PCOS): international collaboration to translate evidence and guide future research. J Endocrinol. 2023;257(3):e220232. https://doi.org/10.1530/joe-22-0232.
188. Brown EDL, Hannah-Shmouni F, Shekhar S. Chapter 21: Artificial intelligence in endocrinology. In: Krittanawong C, editor. Artificial intelligence in clinical practice. Academic Press; 2024. p. 187–93.
189. Das B, Fatima T. Chapter 21: Importance of lifestyle modifications. In: Rehman R, Sheikh A, editors. Polycystic ovary syndrome. New Delhi: Elsevier; 2024. p. 166–70.
190. Jung W, Choi H, Kim J, Kim J, Kim W, Nurkolis F, Kim B. Effects of natural products on polycystic ovary syndrome: from traditional medicine to modern drug discovery. Heliyon. 2023;9(10):e20889. https://doi.org/10.1016/j.heliyon.2023.e20889.
191. Wang B, Li Z. Hypersecretion of basal luteinizing hormone and an increased risk of pregnancy loss among women with polycystic ovary syndrome undergoing controlled ovarian stimulation and intrauterine insemination. Heliyon. 2023;9(5):e16233. https://doi.org/10.1016/j.heliyon.2023.e16233.
192. Nadeem S, Merchant AAH. Chapter 16: Pharmacologic management for polycystic ovary syndrome: weight loss. In: Rehman R, Sheikh A, editors. Polycystic ovary syndrome. New Delhi: Elsevier; 2024. p. 122–9. https://doi.org/10.1016/B978-0-323-87932-3.00025-6.
193. Mohamed Rashid Sokwala SB, Dodia R. Chapter 29: Global approach to polycystic ovary syndrome in Africa. In: Rehman R, Sheikh A, editors. Polycystic ovary syndrome. New Delhi: Elsevier; 2024. p. 220–8. https://doi.org/10.1016/B978-0-323-87932-3.00038-4.

194. Kaur R, Kumar R, Gupta M. Food image-based nutritional management system to overcome polycystic ovary syndrome using deep learning: a systematic review. Int J Image Graph. 2023;23(5):2350043. https://doi.org/10.1142/S0219467823500432.
195. Wang D-D, Li Y-F, Mao Y-Z, He S-M, Zhu P, Wei Q-L. A machine-learning approach for predicting the effect of carnitine supplementation on body weight in patients with polycystic ovary syndrome. Front Nutr. 2022;9:851275 (in Eng). https://doi.org/10.3389/fnut.2022.851275.
196. Selvaraj S, Nidhyananthan SS, Vanmathi R, Ramya M. Diet recommendation for poly cystic ovarian syndrome of Indian patients using multiattribute and multilabeling classifier. J Pharm Negat Results. 2022;13:1660–72.
197. Kaur R, Kumar R, Gupta M. Lifestyle and dietary management associated with chronic diseases in women using deep learning. In: Combating women's health issues with machine learning. CRC Press; 2024. p. 59–73.

2 Traditional Dietary Approaches for PCOS: A Review of Conventional Dietary Recommendations for PCOS and Their Limitations

Virgina Varghese, Janitha Plackal Ayyappan, and Gopi Vankudre

2.1 Introduction

Polycystic ovary syndrome (PCOS) is a heterogeneous disorder of unknown etiology that manifests as hyperandrogenism and chronic anovulation. It is the one of the key causes of anovulation among the reproductive-aged women group having infertility. Polycystic ovaries have harmless follicles that measure up to 8 mm in diameter [1, 2]. These follicles are responsible for egg development; however, in PCOS, these sacs are incapable of developing eggs as they are underdeveloped [1].

Although PCOS cannot be cured, symptoms can be relieved through lifestyle modifications and managerial approaches [3]. Also, even if it has an unknown etiology, women having heredity of type II diabetes mellitus are at a higher risk of developing the condition [3]. It can be classified as the global public health burden among reproductive-aged women, having the condition prevalence ranging from 4% to 20% [3, 4]. The prevalence of this condition is higher in India than in other Asian countries [5]. Despite the higher prevalence of endocrinopathy, it has not yet received the needed attention and almost 70% of the affected women remain undiagnosed [3]. The condition is also susceptible to pose other risk factors. Adult women with PCOA have a ten times higher risk of developing type II diabetes mellitus [5]. In addition to diabetes mellitus type II, conditions such as hypertension, high cholesterol, heart disease, and endometrial cancer are also observed [3].

Along with the physiological aspects, the condition is also known to have a negative psychological impact [3, 6]. Anxiety, depression, and low self-esteem are commonly observed among affected individuals. Infertility, obesity, and unwanted hair growth could contribute to these psychological illnesses, affecting the familial and social domains of affected women [3].

V. Varghese · J. P. Ayyappan (✉) · G. Vankudre
College of Health Science, University of Buraimi, Al Buraimi, Oman

R. Kumar et al. (eds.), *AI-Based Nutritional Intervention in Polycystic Ovary Syndrome (PCOS)*, https://doi.org/10.1007/978-981-96-2120-0_2

Although heredity is a common factor for this condition, variations exist in relation to demography and ethnicity [3]. Also, variations exist in etiological factors and associated managerial protocols [4, 6]. This review focuses on the clinical features of this condition, associated risk factors, and their prevalence in India. This study presents current nutritional approaches for treating PCOS.

2.1.1 Key Terminologies

- **Polycystic ovarian syndrome (PCOS)**: It is a syndrome that causes the ovaries to overproduce androgens or male sex hormones, which are typically seen in modest amounts in women. Numerous tiny cysts or sacs packed with fluid develop in the ovaries and are referred to as polycystic ovarian syndrome [7].
- **World Health Organization (WHO)**: It is an agency of the United Nations that works mainly to promote health among the member countries.
- **Glycemic index (GI)**: It is a measure used to determine how much a food can affect your blood sugar levels [8].
- **In vitro fertilization (IVF)**: It is a procedure in which mature eggs are removed from ovaries and incubated with sperm in a laboratory. Next, one or more fertilized eggs, known as embryos, are placed into the uterus, where infants develop through a surgical operation [9].
- **Very-low-calorie ketogenic diet (VLCKD)**: It means low daily protein intake (1–2 g/kg of ideal body weight), low daily carbohydrate intake (<50 g), and low daily calorie intake (less than 800 kcal) [10].
- **Mediterranean diet (MD)**: It is mostly plant-based and calls for the daily consumption of whole grains, fruits, vegetables, nuts, olive oil, beans, and other legumes, herbs, and spices. Smaller amounts of other foods, such as animal proteins, are consumed, and fish and seafood are the most popular animal proteins [11].
- **Follicle-stimulating hormone (FSH)**: It is a hormone that plays a significant role in sexual development and reproduction by affecting the function of the ovaries and testes [12].
- **Luteinizing hormone (LH)**: It is a hormone produced by the pituitary. It affects female ovaries by causing follicles to release eggs and produce hormones that prepare the uterus for the implantation of a fertilized egg [13].

2.1.2 Background of the Study

Polycystic ovarian syndrome (PCOS) is a prevalent endocrine condition that affects women of reproductive age. Hyperandrogenism, polycystic ovaries, and irregular menstrual periods are the defining features. Although the precise origin of PCOS is still unknown, genetics, insulin resistance, and inflammation are thought to be the major contributing factors. Conventional dietary strategies for PCOS have focused on lowering insulin resistance and controlling weight with low-GI meals, calorie restriction, and consistent exercise. However, these traditional dietary guidelines have not been able to control PCOS symptoms or enhance long-term health outcomes. A growing amount of research indicates that controlling PCOS may benefit from a more individualized and comprehensive approach to nutrition.

There isn't, however, a thorough analysis of the drawbacks of conventional dietary methods for PCOS.

Objectives of the Chapter
The objectives of the chapter are:

- To examine the body of data on conventional dietary treatments for PCOS, such as calorie restriction, low-GI diets, and weight-loss techniques.
- To highlight the shortcomings of traditional dietary guidelines, which includes how well they work in controlling PCOS symptoms and enhancing health outcomes.
- To examine the possible advantages of a more individualized and comprehensive approach to PCOS-affected women's nutrition.
- And, to suggest further investigations into the relationship between PCOS and nutrition.

This study attempts to contribute to a more thorough understanding of the function of nutrition in controlling PCOS symptoms and improving health outcomes by highlighting the shortcomings of conventional dietary treatments for PCOS.

This study may also inform the development of more personalized and effective dietary interventions for women with PCOS. One of the most frequent reasons for infertility in women is PCOS, a complicated endocrine condition that affects 5–10% of women of reproductive age. Polycystic ovaries, hyperandrogenism, and irregular menstrual periods are the hallmarks of PCOS. Genetics, inflammation, and insulin resistance are thought to be the major factors in the development of PCOS. Conventional dietary strategies for PCOS have focused on lowering insulin resistance and controlling weight with low-GI meals, calorie restriction, and consistent exercise. These treatments have been somewhat successful in lowering weight and increasing insulin sensitivity; however, they have not been very effective in controlling PCOS symptoms or enhancing long-term health outcomes. According to recent research, a more individualized and comprehensive diet approach may be more successful in managing PCOS.

This strategy considers a person's genetic predisposition, lifestyle choices, and nutritional requirements. Nonetheless, there is a dearth of thorough research on the drawbacks of conventional dietary strategies for PCOS and the possible advantages of a more individualized approach. By examining existing studies on conventional dietary therapies for PCOS and their drawbacks, the proposed study seeks to close this knowledge gap. Additionally, a more individualized and comprehensive approach to diet for women with PCOS was investigated in this study. This study attempts to add to a more thorough understanding of the function of nutrition in controlling PCOS symptoms and improving health outcomes by offering a thorough overview of the existing state of knowledge in this area. Additionally, this research might help in the creation of more customized and effective dietary interventions for women with PCOS.

Organization of Chapter
The rest of the chapter is organized as: Section 2.2 enlightens methodology. Section 2.3 focuses on Bibliometric Analysis. Section 2.4 highlights discussion on Prevalence of PCOS, Clinical Features of PCOS, Associated factors of PCOS and Quality of Life in PCOS. Section 2.5 illustrates impact of Nutritional Approach in PCOS. Section 2.6 discusses traditional dietary approaches for managing PCOS. And, finally, Sect. 2.7 concludes the chapter with limitations, recommendations and future directions.

2.2 Methodology

A contemporary review of PCOS demonstrated an ongoing interest in traditional, complementary, and integrative medicinal management approaches related to the condition. However, there are limitations of such evidence on the nutritional or dietary impact on the condition and its integration into clinical practice. From these studies, it is observed that a specific nutritional or dietary pattern helps to improve condition-related outcomes that underscores the importance of considering the nutritional or dietary approach as a PCOS treatment strategy.

This comprehensive review of the traditional dietary approaches for polycystic ovary syndrome involves the following pivotal steps, ensuring rigorous methodology and reliable findings. It provides a structural approach while reviewing the literature on nutritional and traditional dietary approaches for PCOS to support the conclusions that are based on a critical analysis of the available evidence. For this purpose, the bibliometric data was extracted from the Scopus database as recommended by [14–16].

2.2.1 Literature Search

The literature review involved a systematic search of scholarly articles within databases, including PubMed, Scopus, and Web of Science. These articles focused on traditional dietary approaches for PCOS. The terms used and the literature findings are as follows.

"PCOS" or "polycystic ovary syndrome": For the year range of 2004–2024, using this term, a total of 29,227 articles were found of which 25,350 were in English. From 2019 to the present, there were 14,784 articles.

"Nutrition*" and "PCOS" or "polycystic ovary syndrome": There were a total of 645 articles from the year 2004, of which 588 were in English. A total of 294 articles were published between the years 2019 and 2024.

"PCOS" or "polycystic ovary syndrome" and "traditional diet*": There was only one study found with this keyword.

"Traditional diet*": Based on this keyword, a total of 1926 articles were found from the year 2004. From 2019 to 2024, there were 17,074 articles of which 996 were published in English.

2.2.2 Inclusion and Exclusion Criteria

Well-defined study inclusion and exclusion criteria were used in the literature review. The inclusion criteria were randomized control trials and observational studies focusing on the nutritional or dietary impact of PCOS. Studies including the female population within adolescent or reproductive age groups were included. Interventions specific to nutritional and dietary components were analyzed in this review. The study outcomes of interest were metabolic profiles, symptom relief, and fertility outcomes. This review provides implications of the findings in the context of the current knowledge related to nutritional and dietary approaches to PCOS and its impact on the condition for potential integration into patient counseling and clinical practice. The observed heterogeneity of the data provides recommendations for future research, preferably interventional studies involving larger sample sizes within the Indian context. Cohort studies that observe the long-term effects of interventions may also be useful.

2.3 Bibliometric Analysis

2.3.1 Analysis for the Keywords "PCOS" or "Polycystic Ovary Syndrome"

Figure 2.1 represents the associations observed terms within the literature such as "human," "insulin resistance," "ovary polycystic disease," and "female." The nodes observed within the diagram represent the term associations through the lines, with the thickness-dependent strength or frequency of the relationship. The colors (green and red, as observed in the diagram) represent the categories and types of relationships between them. From the picture, we can see that "human" is the key node.

There were three minimum occurrences, and six keywords were found in the literature (Table 2.1).

The graph shows the relationship between keywords in the articles. Human and ovarian polycystic disease" were observed to have the highest strength of 15, followed by the "female," "insulin resistance," and "review." The "premature ovarian failure" was observed to have the least strength.

The clustering mentioned in Table 2.2 highlights two primary areas of focus in the literature. The cluster reflects the key women's health issues, hormonal, and reproductive health issues. A general review of the literature related to PCOS is

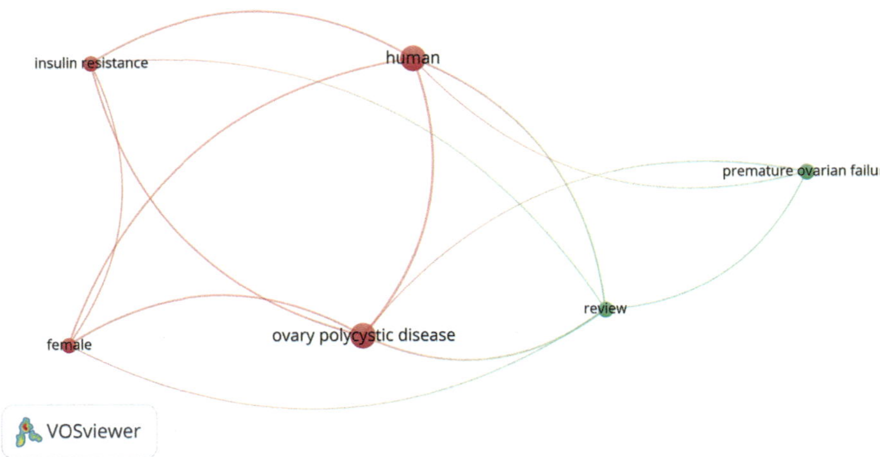

Fig. 2.1 Literature nodes and associations for "PCOS" or "polycystic ovary syndrome"

Table 2.1 Link strength of the keywords associated with "PCOS" or "polycystic ovary syndrome"

Sr. no.	Keyword	Occurrences	Total link strength
46	Human	5	15
98	Ovary polycystic disease	5	15
30	Female	3	9
57	Insulin resistance	3	9
112	Premature ovarian failure	3	3
115	Review	3	9

Table 2.2 Literature cluster analysis associated with "PCOS" or "polycystic ovary syndrome"

Cluster 1	Cluster 2
Female	Premature ovarian failure
Human	Review
Insulin resistance	
Ovary polycystic disease	

presented in cluster 1. The analysis shows that only two terms highlighted in the literature reflect the current evidence gap and scope for future research.

2.3.2 Citation Analysis for "PCOS" or "Polycystic Ovary Syndrome"

Surprisingly, very few articles were cited in the literature, and only in 2014. In addition, it was observed that there is no cross-citation in the literature. This suggests that attention should be paid to condition-related evidence in volatile, and collaborative research efforts need to be taken to address this issue (Fig. 2.2, Table 2.3).

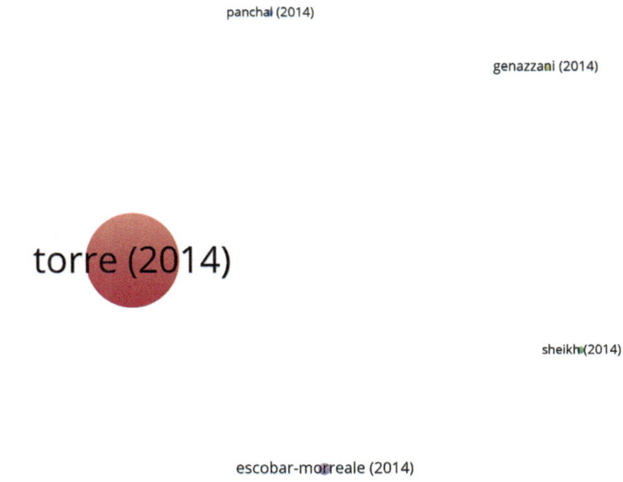

Fig. 2.2 Citation analysis for "PCOS" or "polycystic ovary syndrome"

Table 2.3 Citation analysis associated with "PCOS" or "polycystic ovary syndrome"

Sr. no.	Document	Citations	Links
1	Della Torre (2014) [17]	100	0
2	Escobar-Morreale (2014) [18]	13	0
3	Genazzani et al. (2014) [19]	3	0
4	Nagori (2014) [20]	2	0
5	Sheikh (2014) [21]	1	0

This "total link strength" represents co-authorship links with other countries. A total link strength value of zero indicates that there are no links for coauthorship. Within the dataset, Italy leads with three publications and a high citation count of 103. This demonstrates its significant impact on the research. The United States has two articles and only one citation, which is comparatively lower than that in Italy. Spain has only one scientific paper, but 13 citations, highlighting the importance of this paper. Other countries, such as India, Germany, Poland, and Romania, have published one research paper each and have a different number of citations. This reflects the major variation within the countries in PCOS-related research output and its impact (Table 2.4).

2.3.3 Analysis for the Keywords "Nutrition*" and "PCOS" or "Polycystic Ovary Syndrome"

There were 4 minimum occurrences, and 15 keywords were found within the literature (Fig. 2.3).

There were 4 minimum occurrences, and 15 keywords were found in the literature (Table 2.5).

Table 2.4 Country-wise publication analysis associated with "PCOS" or "polycystic ovary syndrome"

Sr. no.	Country	Documents	Citations	Total link strength
1	Italy	3	103	0
2	United States	2	1	0
3	Germany	1	0	0
4	India	1	2	0
5	Poland	1	0	0
6	Romania	1	0	0
7	Spain	1	13	0

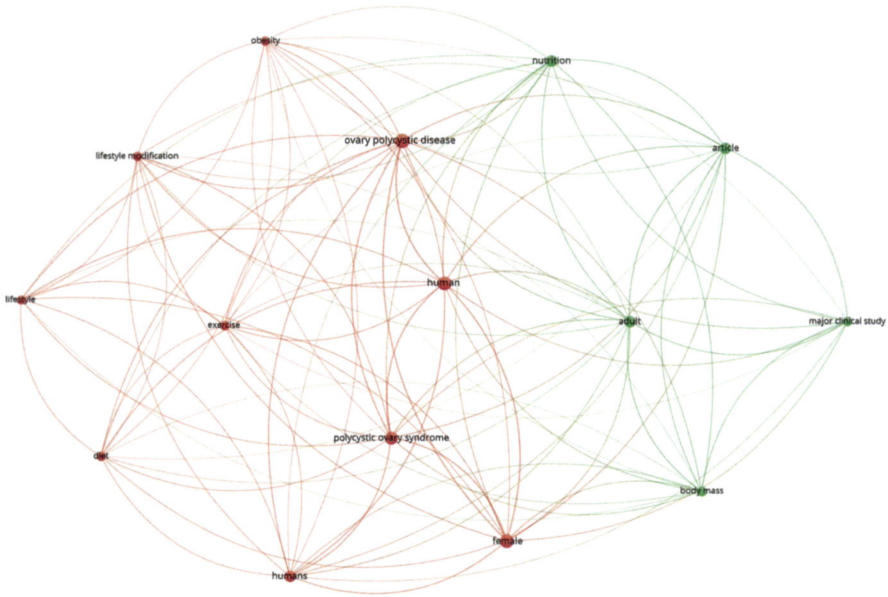

Fig. 2.3 Literature nodes and associations for "nutrition*" and "PCOS" or "Polycystic Ovary Syndrome"

Apart from humans, obesity, adults, and female were the most frequent keywords, focusing on PCOS in adult women for its association with obesity. Lifestyle modification, diet, exercise, and nutrition are also presented, reflecting significant factors in the context of PCOS management (Table 2.6).

Citation analysis reflects the number of times relevant articles have been cited. From the analysis, it can be observed that Silvestris (2019) is the most cited document with 92 citations and can be considered a foundation within the field. This is followed by Javed (2019) with 56 citations, Garruti (2019) with 22, and Kalem (2019) with 1 citation. However, the non-association between the articles is research that can be addressed through collaborative efforts.

Table 2.5 Link strength of the keywords associated with "nutrition*" and "PCOS" or "polycystic ovary syndrome"

Sr. no.	Keyword	Occurrences	Total link strength
1	Human/humans	16	132
2	Ovary polycystic disease	10	80
3	Female	9	75
4	Polycystic ovary syndrome	8	66
5	Adult	6	54
6	Article	6	49
7	Nutrition	6	48
8	Body mass	5	45
9	Diet	4	32
10	Exercise	4	35
11	Lifestyle	4	31
12	Lifestyle modification	4	34
13	Major clinical study	4	34
14	Obesity	4	31

Table 2.6 Link strength of the keywords associated with "nutrition*" and "PCOS" or "polycystic ovary syndrome"-related citations

Sr. no.	Document	Citations	Links
1	Silvestris (2019)	92	0
2	Javed (2019)	56	0
3	Garruti (2019)	22	0
4	De Lima Nunes (2019)	15	0
5	Kuliczkowska-Płaksej (2019)	11	0
6	Boyd (2019)	5	0
7	Silvestrim (2019)	5	0
8	Speelman (2019)	4	0
9	Yavarikia (2019)	3	0
10	Kalem (2019)	1	0

2.3.4 Analysis for the Keyword "Traditional Diet*"

The map includes terms like "article," "diet," "male," "cross-sectional study," "dietary pattern," "human," "female," "physical activity," and "Mediterranean diet." The keywords are connected by curved lines that represent the relationships between them. The keyword "diet" is centrally located and associated with the other keywords, indicating the key focus of the article (Fig. 2.4).

Figure 2.5 depicts the larger nodes reflecting the essential concepts such as "diet," "human," and "Mediterranean diet." The other nodes involve the terms such as "cardiovascular," "mortality," and "questionnaire." Overall, it can be observed that a few clusters are some clusters that are densely connected than others.

There were 2 minimum occurrences, and 32 keywords were found in the literature (Table 2.7).

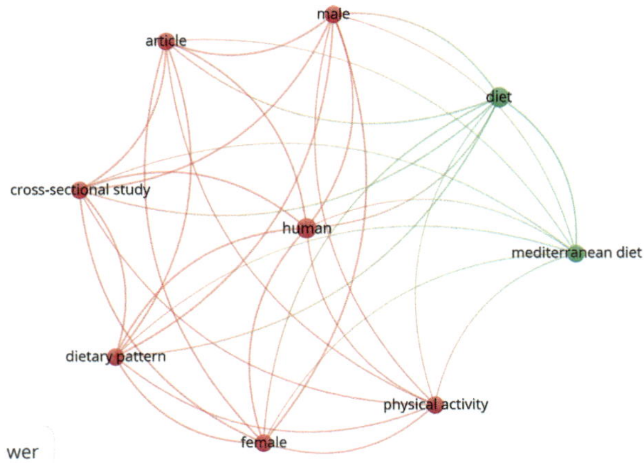

Fig. 2.4 Literature nodes and associations for "traditional diet*"

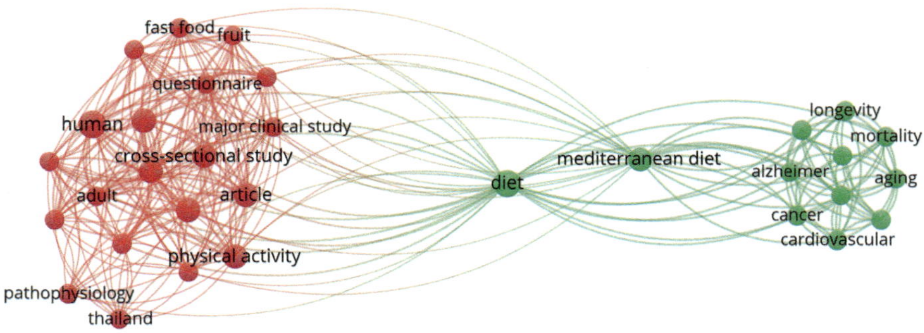

Fig. 2.5 Literature nodes and associations for "traditional diet"

2.3.5 Traditional Dietary Pattern in the Last Decade (2014–2024)

Of the 334 keywords, 22 met the threshold for the 3 minimum number of occurrences of the keyword (Fig. 2.6).

From Table 2.8, it can be concluded that physical activity, the Mediterranean diet, and dietary patterns seem to be key areas of interest in the literature.

Table 2.7 Link strength of the keywords associated with "traditional diet*"

Sr. no.	Keyword	Occurrences	Total link strength
1	Adult	2	30
2	Aging	2	22
3	Alzheimer	2	22
4	Article	3	44
5	Cancer	2	22
6	Cardiovascular	2	22
7	Chronic	2	22
8	Cross-sectional studies	2	30
9	Cross-sectional study	3	44
10	Dementia	2	22
11	Diet	4	52
12	Dietary pattern	3	44
13	Fast food	2	30
14	Feeding behavior	2	28
15	Female	3	44
16	Food frequency questionnaire	2	30
17	Fruit	2	30
18	Human	4	45
19	Humans	2	30
20	Lifestyle	2	22
21	Longevity	2	22
22	Major clinical study	2	30
23	Male	3	44
24	Mediterranean diet	3	36
25	Morbidity	2	22
26	Mortality	2	22
27	Obesity	2	30
28	Pathophysiology	2	15
29	Physical activity	3	28
30	Questionnaire	2	30
31	Thailand	2	14
32	Vegetable	2	30

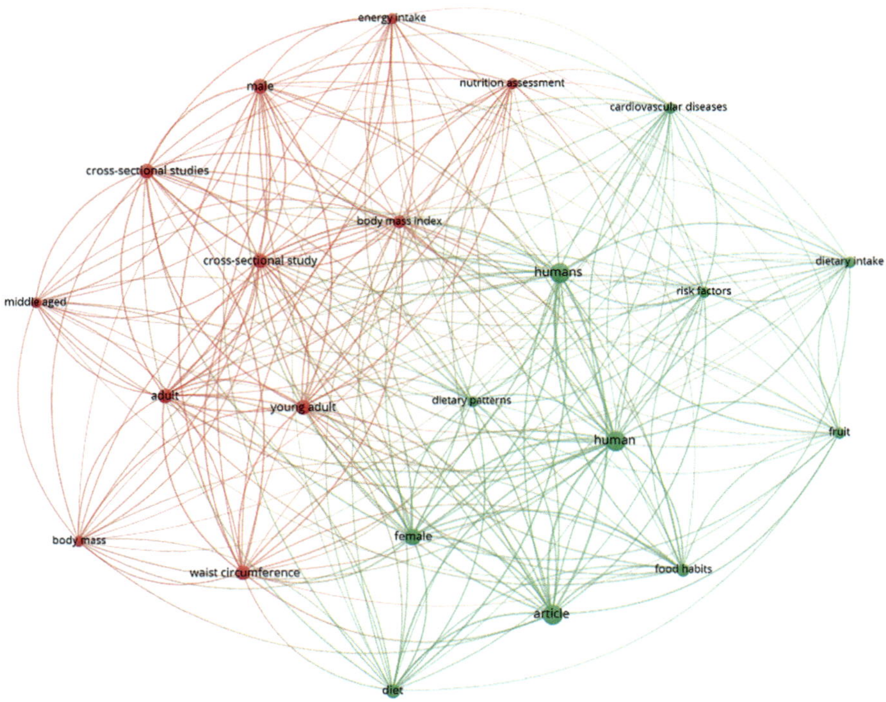

Fig. 2.6 Literature nodes and associations for "traditional dietary pattern in the last decade (2014–2024)"

2.3.6 Recent Trends in Traditional Dietary 2019–2024

A total of 245 articles were found to match the criteria. Of the 209 keywords, for the 3 minimum number of occurrences of the keyword, 9 meet the threshold (Fig. 2.7, Table 2.9).

Physical activity and the Mediterranean diet are the most discussed in the literature.

Table 2.8 Link strength of the keywords associated with "traditional dietary pattern in the last decade (2014–2024)"

Sr. no.	Keyword	Occurrences	Total link strength
1	Young adult	5	75
2	Waist circumference	5	75
3	Risk factors	3	43
4	Nutrition assessment	3	48
5	Middle aged	3	45
6	Male	5	75
7	Humans	9	94
8	Human	9	94
9	Fruit	3	29
10	Food habits	4	53
11	Female	6	84
12	Energy intake	3	45
13	Dietary patterns	3	40
14	Dietary intake	3	30
15	Diet	5	56
16	Cross-sectional study	5	75
17	Cross-sectional studies	5	75
18	Cardiovascular diseases	3	38
19	Body mass index	4	61
20	Body mass	3	44
21	Article	9	94
22	Adult	5	75

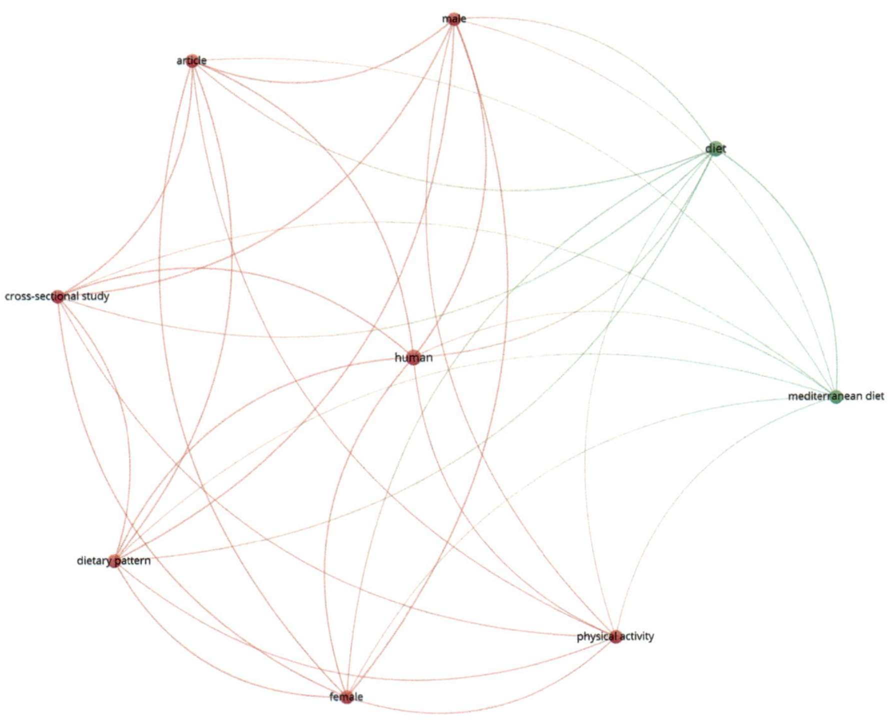

Fig. 2.7 Literature nodes and associations for "traditional dietary 2019–2024"

Table 2.9 Link strength of the keywords associated with "traditional dietary" (2019–2024)

Sr. no.	Keyword	Occurrences	Total link strength
1	Physical activity	3	14
2	Mediterranean diet	3	9
3	Male	3	20
4	Human	4	20
5	Female	3	20
6	Dietary pattern	3	20
7	Diet	4	15
8	Cross-sectional study	3	20
9	Article	3	20

2.4 Discussion

2.4.1 Prevalence of PCOS

The prevalence of PCOS varies in regional, ethnic, and diagnostic contexts. The World Health Organization (WHO) has estimated the prevalence of PCOS 8–13% [3]. As to an epidemiological study conducted in 2019, the prevalence of PCOS in India ranged from 3.7% to 22.5% [6]. In a study done in 2018, the prevalence of PCOS was reported to be 13.54% [22]. A review found the condition prevalence as per the Rotterdam's criteria ranging from 4.2% to 22.5%. However, this prevalence is similar to that in studies conducted in the southern part of India, and limited studies have been conducted in the northern part of India [23]. Compared to the Rotterdam criteria, the PCOS community prevalence calculated using NIH criteria was 3.7% [24]. In another study, the prevalence was found to be 22.5% as per the Rotterdam study compared to the 10.7% as observed as per "Androgen Excess Society criteria" [25]. Variations in prevalence exist between urban and rural populations. The PCOS prevalence rate was 6%, and urban women were at a higher risk of the condition than the rural population [26].

2.4.2 Clinical Features of PCOS

Symptoms of PCOS are observed prior to puberty, can vary among women, and can be periodic. The affected population presents concerns about having "irregular menstrual cycles, anovulation, and acne" [2]. The key symptoms include heavy, prolonged, or unpredictable periods, acne or oily skin, excessive body hair (hirsutism), baldness as observed in men, and weight gain, especially around the belly region [1].

It creates hormonal imbalances, excessive androgen levels, and cysts in the ovaries. Irregular periods of anovulation can cause infertility [3]. Individuals with "androgen excess and oligomenorrhea/amenorrhea" are the risk factors for the condition [2]. Women with PCOS have elevated levels of testosterone, estrogen, luteinizing hormone, insulin, and anti-Müllerian hormone [3].

2.4.3 Associated Factors of PCOS

Although the manifestations of PCOS develop early, it is unfortunately diagnosed during adulthood. The disease is multifactorial and is associated with hereditary conditions along with the lifestyle of individuals. High-calorie intake and lack of exercise have been established to trigger contributors to the condition. Higher socio-economic status and heredity of diabetes mellitus were also associated with a higher prevalence of PCOS. Seven factors are associated with PCOS, as discussed in the literature.

Emotional disturbances such as mood and anxiety are common disorders associated with PCOS. Hence, the researchers recommended that it is good practice to incorporate interview questions, such as patients' real-life situations and tools for assessing depression, mainly in diagnostic procedures to understand and study the psychological characteristics of women, and if psychological or psychiatric counseling or assessment can be accomplished [27].

Hirsutism is the most common sign of hyperandrogenism in PCOS patients. The modified Ferriman–Gallwey (mFG) is widely used to assess hirsutism in PCOS women and which also considered to be an important tool in measuring the androgen level for diagnostic purposes [28].

Infertility is the result of immunological and metabolic abnormalities triggered by endocrine disorders. In women with PCOS, the attributing factors for infertility are impaired ovulation, implantation, and low-grade inflammation [29].

Menstrual symptoms: Research shows that the inclination of fasting glucose level as well as hormonal alteration is found to be significant in women with PCOS. Clinical procedures like anthropometric and biochemical profile analysis are recommended to detect these menstrual symptoms at an early stage [30].

Predicting PCOS in women during the menstrual cycle using advanced diagnostic tools, such as serum AMH, body mass index, and serum androstenone, provides extra ease in detecting and diagnosing PCOS at a very early stage and provides an added advantage for long-term management of PCOS. In addition, strongly recommend to priorities the policy at the country level to focus on the nutrition-based treatment solution for the countries having escalation in the PCOS cases [31], thus, enhancing the quality of life in women suffering from PCOS [32]. Acne is the most common dermatological finding used to clinically correlate women with PCOS [33].

2.4.4 Quality of Life in PCOS

Quality of life has been found to have adverse effects in PCOS patients. This hampers an individual's physical, psychological, and social domains [34]. During disease management, the assessment of health-related quality of life among the population affected by this chronic condition is crucial. Evidence of quality of life can be pivotal in the prevention and enhancement of managerial practices. Moreover, psychological counseling should be conducted alongside medical treatment [35].

Likewise, PCOS symptoms can be attributed to stressful lives, psychological issues, and reproductivity. Furthermore, decreased quality of life was observed in PCOS patients with depressive symptoms which gives rise to psychological morbidity in PCOS patients [36]. In addition, infertility is a significant factor in decreasing overall health-related quality of life in patients with PCOS [34]. Furthermore, several studies have discussed associated factors accountable for women with PCOS, especially youth, found to have compromised their quality of life.

Modification of lifestyle and choosing appropriate nutrients, including herbs and physical activity, can enhance the QOL of PCOS patients and subsequently reduce depression and loss of motivation and decrease the symptoms of PCOS [37]. Social pressure is directly correlated with the quality of life in patients with PCOS; constant criticism will harm PCOS patients which gives rise to poor QOL [36, 38].

Parental criticism is another interpretation of PCOS in women, mainly youth. Continuous criticism leads to a lack of compassion and support from parents and their relatives. These gestures direct the PCOS patients into an introverted character as well as self-isolation finally ending up with poor quality of life [36].

An inverse correlation was found between high-level education and high-level humiliation among women with PCOs [35, 36]; in contrast, reports have found that lower literacy has a poor QOL [39].

Body mass index is inversely proportional to the quality of life of patients with PCOS [39]. Likewise, employment was also found negatively correlated with quality of life in women with PCOS in contrast with the homemaker or the nonworking women [40]. Socioeconomic status is mainly low- to middle-income class category with poor quality of life in comparison with high-income class women with PCOS. A positive family history is associated with poor QoL in PCOS due to distress that has been experienced and witnessed among family members [34, 40].

2.5 Impact of Nutritional Approach in PCOS

Nutritional management is the cornerstone of polycystic ovary syndrome treatment. A well-structured diet can help mitigate disease symptoms, regulate the menstrual cycle, and improve insulin sensitivity. The contributions of proteins, fats, and carbohydrates were not found to have any significant impact on the condition. However, with a reduction in calorie intake, the diets with low GI were found to be effective compared to the high GI diets. However, whole foods, lean proteins, and healthy fats can be recommended, as they provide vital bodily nutrients [41]. Lean proteins provide a high amount of protein with less fat. Consumption of lean proteins found in diets such as fish, tofu, and legumes can strengthen the muscles and enhance the energy levels [42]. In addition, healthy fats such as those found in avocado and nuts enhance the hormonal balance and reduce inflammation [43].

The incorporation of omega-3 fatty acids and reduction of saturated fatty acids are beneficial for positive health outcomes among patients. Other sources of α-linolenic acid can also be effective dietary components for the management of PCOA. An additional form of reduced GI intake diet is the ketogenic diet, which reduces carbohydrate consumption and helps to improve the menstrual cycle and moderation of the blood sugar level and body weight [37]. The initial line of treatment for women with PCOS is lifestyle modification; however, it does not replace pharmaceutical treatment. Clinical guidelines for a number of illnesses include regular physical exercise, maintaining healthy body weight, adhering to good eating habits, and abstaining from tobacco use as key components in the prevention and treatment of metabolic disorders [44].

Women with PCOS should consume more folic acid, calcium, cobalamin, vitamins D and C, and dietary fiber as part of their dietary therapy. Reduced consumption of total lipids, saturated fatty acids, and cholesterol is recommended, because these substances influence ovarian dysfunction by contributing to the development of diabetes and cardiovascular disorders. Some individuals should additionally take potassium, magnesium, and zinc supplements in their diet. Treatment for women with PCOS who have been diagnosed based on the Rotterdam criteria should primarily focus on introducing a well-balanced diet [45]. Study also revealed that zinc deficiency may be linked to the long-term metabolic consequences of polycystic ovarian syndrome and may have a role in its etiology [46]. Micronutrients such as zinc, carotenoids, selenium, chromium, and vitamin E may improve the metabolic state of PCOS patients, while deficiencies in these nutrients may exacerbate metabolic disturbances in PCOS patients with metabolic syndromes [47].

A ketogenic diet (KD) treats fatty liver in obese women with PCOS and liver dysfunction, improves the menstrual cycle, lowers blood sugar and body weight, and strengthens liver function [48]. This study was conducted to assess the impact of nutritional therapy in the management of patients with PCOS undergoing IVF. They recommended lifestyle changes and weight loss as effective tactics. Among these strategies, the Mediterranean diet (MD) or very-low-calorie ketogenic diet (VLCKD) is a viable choice. Their study showed that an extremely low-calorie ketogenic diet was successful [49]. The use of various dietary modifications of flax seeds was found to be effective in the literature, and a study on rats showed that dietary flax seed oil improved PCOS in rats by acting on the microbiota—inflammatory axis—sex steroid hormones. This finding could aid in understanding the pathophysiology and could possibly be used as a low-cost PCOS intervention [50]. Twice-daily flaxseed oil omega-3 fatty acid (1000 mg capsule) supplementation significantly improved insulin levels, hirsutism, triglycerides, VLDL-cholesterol, and CRP levels in a 12-week study on women with PCOS, indicating positive effects on insulin metabolism and specific metabolic markers [51].

The most important treatment for PCOS is a balanced diet that supports insulin management; as a result, drinking infusions of some herbs, such as *Aloe vera*, cinnamon (*Cinnamomum verum*), green tea (*Camellia sinensis*), chamomile (*Matricaria chamomilla*), and white mulberry (Morus alba), would be a suitable complement therapy [52]. Marjoram tea has been shown to have positive effects on the hormonal profiles of women with PCOS by lowering adrenal androgen levels and improving insulin sensitivity [53]. Another class of herbs, green mint (*Mentha spicata* L.), has an antiandrogenic effect and promotes follicular formation in ovarian tissue, making it particularly recommended for women with PCOS who have biochemical evidence of elevated androgen levels [54].

Curcumin, an active phytochemical found in turmeric (*Curcuma longa*), is biologically active. It appears that curcumin effectively lessens the difficulties associated with oxidative stress in patients with PCOS [55]. Cinnamon contains a high concentration of phytochemicals, which may have anti-inflammatory, antibacterial, antioxidant, and cardioprotective properties [56]. Studies have suggested that consumption of approximately 1.5 g of cinnamon powder can be beneficial for women with PCOS [57].

A Mediterranean diet can assist women in managing PCOS symptoms and reaching a healthy weight by adding leafy greens (spinach, kale, escarole, endive, lettuce, etc.), tomatoes, mushrooms, peppers, broccoli, cauliflower, snow peas, celery, and fennel. Whole grains, including barley, sorghum, brown rice, and whole grain-based bread and pasta, can help PCOS sufferers avoid blood sugar increases. Individuals consuming an excessive number of foods high in inflammation can worsen the symptoms of PCOS and increase the chance of developing heart disease, among many other conditions to which people with PCOS are susceptible. Women should avoid eating fried food, fatty food, red meat, processed foods, sugary beverages, refined foods, white rice, etc. [58].

Given that there is no optimal carbohydrate intake for women with PCOS, dietary carbohydrates can be adopted in any range (approximately 40–55%) based on the individual's nutritional evaluation, metabolic objectives, dietary habits, and preferences. For women with PCOS, diets that are high in fat and moderately low in carbohydrates can improve metabolic parameters, lower fasting insulin levels, and increase insulin sensitivity. Research indicates that following a low-carbohydrate, high-protein diet could help PCOS patients lose weight and enhance their metabolic and reproductive health. Sustaining long-term adherence to a low-GI diet is difficult despite the fact that it is recommended for cardiovascular health and satiety [47].

2.6 Traditional Dietary Approaches for Managing PCOS

A well-balanced food plan for PCOS can help control its condition and reduce its symptoms. Some vitamins and minerals, such as calcium, zinc, selenium, and chromium picolinate, as well as vitamins D, E, and K, inositol, folate, and B-12, may help manage PCOS. Furthermore, substances that resemble vitamins, such as α-lipoic acid and bioflavonoids, may be beneficial. The addition of nutritional supplements to PCOS has potential benefits with melatonin, probiotics, ω-3 fatty acids, and cinnamon, among other formulations. Adding these nutrients to the diet can support overall health and hormonal balance [59].

2.6.1 Herbs That Promote Fertility Cycles

Hormonal imbalances and variations in prolactin levels have a major effect on the estrous cycle. Ovulatory cycles and PCOS treatment benefit from lowering prolactin levels and restoring hormonal balance. These two actions may lessen the development of cysts, dissolve existing cysts, and enhance the ovulatory cycles. Two herbs that have been shown to help PCOS patients are vitex and turmeric, which lengthen the ovulatory periods [60].

2.6.1.1 *Vitex agnus-castus*

It has been utilized in herbal therapy for the past two millennia. Menstrual cycle irregularities and premenstrual syndrome, including cyclical mastalgia, postmenopausal hot flashes, and insufficiency of the corpus luteum, are indicative of an imbalance in estrogen levels [61–63]. Vitex fruits are mostly composed of labdane-type diterpenoids, such as viteagnusin, vitexilactone, rotundifuran, and vitex lactam A, and monoterpenoids, such as bornyl acetate, limonene, 1,8-cineol, α-pinene, and β-pinene [64, 65]. Furthermore, the specific activity of the flavonoid apigenin on estrogen receptor β (ERβ) stimulates the ovulatory cycle [66]. All the aforementioned methods may help treat PCOS by further facilitating the reduction of ovarian cyst production.

2.6.1.2 *Curcuma longa*

Used as a spice throughout Asia. It is also known as Indian saffron, yellow root, yellow ginger, *Amomum curcuma* Jacq, *Curcuma domestica* Loir, and *Curcuma domestica* Valerie. A thorough explanation of the chemical components of turmeric can be found elsewhere [67]. Many primary and secondary metabolites have been identified in turmeric, and over 250 phytoconstituents have been identified. These include terpenes (1.5–5%), proteins (5–10%), polysaccharides (60–70%), and resins. The main secondary metabolites of turmeric, known as curcuminoids (2.5–8%), are its resins, which also give the plant its color and the majority of its biological characteristics. The three most significant components that were extracted were curcuminoids, which included curcumin (diferuloylmethane) (71.50–94%), desmethoxycurcumin (6–19.4%), and bisdemethoxycurcumin (0.30–9.10%). It is mainly composed of phenolic compounds, including eugenol, ferulic acid, ascorbic acid, vanillic acid, caffeic acid, syringic acid, protocatechuic acid, and p-coumaric acid, and terpenoids, including carotene, γ-turmerone, camphene, β-sesquiphellandrene, γ-terpinene, and turmerone (Fig. 2.5) [68]. Curcuminoids have a major impact on PCOS treatment. They reduce the follicular sheath and enhance ovulation and corpus luteum development. Turmeric enhances histological characteristics of polycystic ovaries. In addition, curcuminoids cause women with PCOS to have higher serum estrogen levels and lower progesterone levels [69]. Additionally, its hypoglycemic, antioxidant, antihyperlipidemic, and estrogenic properties help manage PCOS and prevent ovarian cell malfunction, which in turn improves ovulation and conception.

2.6.2 Herbs That Have Antiandrogen Effects

One of the main causes of PCOS is elevated blood androgen levels. Consequently, antiandrogen medications have been used to treat PCOS. Owing to their antiandrogenic properties, herbs such as *Glycyrrhiza glabra*, *Linum usitatissimum*, *Mentha spicata*, *Cocos nucifera*, and *Punica granatum* may be helpful in the treatment of PCOS.

2.6.2.1 *Glycyrrhiza glabra*

It supports the body's biosynthesis and estrogen release while acting as a strong antiandrogen. The flavonoids found in *Glycyrrhiza* have an antiandrogenic effect because they interact with estrogenic receptors and exhibit estrogenic action. Furthermore, flavonoids can aid in the release of insulin, which lowers blood sugar and helps treat PCOS [70]. Licorice has additional therapeutic uses in addition to treating PCOS, including treating cough suppression *Glycyrrhiza glabra* and having antibacterial and antiviral properties.

2.6.2.2 *Linum usitatissimum*

Saturated and unsaturated fatty acids, lignans, 3–6% mucilage, 25% proteins, and 30–40% fixed oils. Secoisolariciresinol and secoisolariciresinol diglycoside-SDG are the two major lignans, whereas L-galactose, D-xylose, D-galacturonic acid, and L-rhamnose are abundant in the fiber mucilage. The body's production of estrogen is regulated by the secondary metabolites of lignin, which also support menstruation and fertility [71]. Similarly, they significantly lower blood levels of testosterone and androgen, both of which are beneficial in treating PCOS [72].

2.6.2.3 *Mentha spicata*

Mentha spicata has long been used for culinary applications. These substances decrease the amount of hirsutism and the levels of free by decreasing atretic follicles and increasing graafian follicles, and spearmint helps PCOS patients with ovarian cysts. It possesses anticancer, antidiabetic, and anti-inflammatory properties [73, 74]. Mentha controls the ratio of FSH to LH in the blood. This may be helpful in treating PCOS based on the blood control of LH/FSH. Spearmint possesses antiandrogen properties, as demonstrated by preclinical investigations [75].

2.6.2.4 *Cocos nucifera*

Oil is rich in phenolic components, including flavonoids and saponins, in the roots [76]. The flavonoid found in cocos lowers blood glucose levels and has hypoglycemic properties. In addition, sex hormone levels in the blood, including FSH and LH, are regulated by *C. nucifera* [77]. Similarly, it also increases the weight of the uterus while suppressing the weight of the ovary. This might help to avoid ovarian cyst formation based on hormone control. Menstrual cycle abnormalities in India are treated with oral infusions of coconut inflorescences [78].

2.6.2.5 *Punica granatum*

Is a member of the *Punicaceae* family and is rich in sugars, organic acids, pantothenic acid, vitamins B2, C, and B1, and folic acid. Seeds often contain saturated and unsaturated fatty acids. PCOS can be effectively reduced by the phytosterols and phenolic components (flavonoids and catechins) present in the seed extract, and blood levels of free testosterone, serum estrogen, and androstenedione hormone were normalized in women who regularly ate *Punica granatum* [79].

2.6.3 Herbs That Improve Enzyme Activity, Estrus Cyclicity, and Glucose Sensitivity

Decreased insulin sensitivity and high blood glucose levels are among the main symptoms observed in women with PCOS. Consequently, medications that improve insulin sensitivity are a part of the PCOS regimen. Herbs that control the estrous cycle and lower blood sugar, such as *Cinnamomum cassia* and *Aloe vera*, may be beneficial. They work via the same mechanism [60].

2.6.3.1 *Cinnamomum cassia*

Cinnamomum cassia contains a wide range of polyphenolic compounds, including linalool, eugenol, eugenol, eugenol acetate, methyl eugenol, and benzaldehyde [80]. Found in cinnamon are 80.59% carbs, 59.55–53.1% dietary fiber, 9.5–10.5% moisture, 3.89–4.65% protein, 3.55% ash, and vitamins [61]. In addition to encouraging glucose absorption and liver glycogen production, phenolic chemicals control blood insulin levels [81]. In PCOS-afflicted women, cinnamon extract enhances insulin selectivity. Cinnamon's procyanidins and polyphenols stimulate the insulin signaling pathway, which is what causes the hypoglycemic impact. As an adjuvant, cinnamon is used in PCOS treatment with oral supplementation in the luteal phase, which may help control progesterone levels. Similarly, regular use of cinnamon can successfully decrease polycystic ovarian syndrome and aid in restoring the menstrual cycle [82]. These components possess strong antioxidant and anti-inflammatory properties. They decrease malondialdehyde (MDA) and increase the chance of becoming pregnant, but they also increase the blood levels of glutathione peroxidase (GPX), catalase (CAT), and superoxide dismutase (SOD) [22]. Additionally, it reduces the concentrations of insulin, triglycerides (TG), total cholesterol (TC), low-density lipoprotein (LDL), and fasting blood glucose [83].

2.6.3.2 *Aloe vera*

Aloe vera is a plant belonging to the Liliaceae family and contains minerals, flavonoids, phytosterols, anthraquinone derivatives, and polyphenols, among its secondary metabolites. The main components of *A. vera* are aloe-emodin and barbaloin. Women treated with *Aloe vera* gel showed enhanced steroidogenic activity and partial reversion of estrous cyclicity. Furthermore, it promotes the flow of the steroidogenesis pathway, which in turn increases the synthesis of estrogens. In addition to inhibiting the production of cholesterol in the liver, it can reinstate glucose sensitivity, estrus cycle, and lipoprotein plasma levels [84]. *Aloe vera* helps treat PCOS caused by metabolic abnormalities because it also regulates blood cholesterol and glucose levels [85, 86].

2.6.4 Plants That Increase FSH and Reduce LH Secretions

High LH and low FSH levels are common complications of PCOS. Therefore, medications that can increase FSH levels and decrease LH concentrations are helpful in the management of PCOS. Owing to their beneficial effects, herbs such as *Cimicifuga racemosa*, *Panax ginseng*, and *Foeniculum vulgare* can be used to treat PCOS [60].

2.6.4.1 *Cimicifuga racemosa*

These are responsible for the suppression of ovarian cysts. These substances selectively bind to pituitary and hypothalamic estrogen receptors (ERα). LH production decreases when substances bind to α-estrogen receptors in the pituitary gland. In addition to increasing the likelihood of conception in patients who had ever used clomiphene during the menstrual cycle, flavonoids significantly reduced the blood levels of LH [87].

2.6.4.2 *Pimpinella anisum* L.

Pimpinella anisum L. is use in the relief of oligomenorrhea and enhances the quality of life of women receiving PCOS treatment. The phytoestrogenic qualities of the phenolic components may be more significant in the control and enhancement of menstrual cycles and LH/FSH secretion in PCOS-affected women, as well as in the relief of PCOS-related symptoms [30].

2.6.4.3 *Trigonella foenum-graecum*

Fenugreek fruit contains 8–10% moisture, 45% carbon, 15–28% protein, 6–12% fat, 4–8% ash, 8–16% fiber, and 0.2–0.3% essential oil [88]. β-Pinene, β-caryophyllene, camphor, and neryl acetate are the main ingredients in fenugreek seed oil, which inhibits cysts, and fenugreek seeds have a high concentration of sesquiterpenes, n-alkanes, and certain oxygenated components when it comes to volatile oil [89]. They also contain alkaloids (choline, trigonelline, and carpaine), saponins (fenugrin, foenugracin, trigonoesides, glycoside, yamogenin, smagenin, yuccagenin, sarsasapogenin, hederagin, tigonenin, and diosgenin), phytosterols, terpenoids, and flavonoids (naringenin, saponaretin, lilyn, kaempferol, isovitexin, orientin, vitexin, isoorientin, luteolin, and quercetin) [90].

2.6.5 Effective Inducers of Ovulation

Infertility or frequent pregnancy termination because of the patient's low carrying capacity is the most frequent side effect of PCOS. Therefore, ovulation-stimulating medications are a part of the PCOS therapy regimen. Herbs that stimulate ovulation and have a similar effect, such as *Tribulus terrestris* and *Zingiber officinalis*, may help treat PCOS [60].

2.6.5.1 *Zingiber officinale*

Strong antioxidants include shogaol, gingerol, zingerone, and small quantities of oily resin ginger. These substances have been shown to have antiprostaglandin action by reducing the synthesis of arachidonic acid and blocking the synthesis of prostaglandins [91]. The fertility index, serum testosterone level, testicular weight, and seminal vesicle weight increased when ginger was consumed. In males, it also enhances sperm motility and count. The unique pharmacological and physiological properties of ginger flavonoids and phenolic chemicals may help maintain the proper ratio of progesterone to estrogen. They might also control blood levels of sex hormones [92]. Ginger may be utilized to treat PCOS because its phytoestrogen component balances the ratio of estrogen to progesterone [93].

2.7 Conclusion, Limitations, Recommendations, and Future Directions

The World Health Organization (WHO) has estimated the prevalence of PCOS 8–13%. In India, the prevalence ranges from 3.7% to 22.5%. Although the manifestations of PCOS develop early, it is unfortunately diagnosed during adulthood. The disease is multifactorial and is associated with hereditary conditions along with the lifestyle of individuals. Among the population with PCOS, quality of life has been found to have adverse effects. This hampers an individual's physical, psychological, and social domains. Dietary interventions as a first-line treatment for patients with PCOS(PCOS) have been evaluated, but the optimal diet has not been determined. Proper diet and the maintenance of adequate nutritional status are of great importance in the prevention of this disorder, and therapeutics and dietary habits play an important role in the recovery of patients with PCOS.

2.7.1 Limitations of the Study

Overall, the quality of evidence is still low to moderate for PCOS research. Much more research is now required on this often overlooked yet prevalent. Variations in regional health systems were taken into account and acknowledged, and a procedure for adapting translation resources and guidelines was also given [94].

2.7.2 Implications: Managerial/Policy/Societal

Women with PCOS benefit from diets with lower rates of obesity and insulin resistance (IR); nevertheless, to create a customized and long-lasting nutritional intervention, the condition of obesity and IR should be assessed early. Further research is needed to determine the long-term safety, effectiveness, and health benefits of food management in patients with PCOS [95]. Giving doctors and patients precise guidance on best practices that are based on the most reliable research, opinions of knowledgeable interdisciplinary experts, and patient preferences. A thorough multimodal distribution and translation program has been developed, and an integrated assessment program has been created to complement the research recommendations made by the Guideline [94]. Studies have revealed that junk food exacerbates PCOS symptoms, and maintaining a balanced diet is essential for controlling the illness. A well-balanced diet is a useful strategy to encourage people to choose better foods. It can undoubtedly help in PCOS control if it contains certain food components, including fruits, vegetables, whole grains, low-fat dairy, and healthy fatty acids [59]. Complete treatment of polycystic ovarian syndrome necessitates the knowledge and skills of several different types of providers owing to its complexity. Most healthcare professionals concurred that multidisciplinary clinics will eventually improve the prognosis of patients with PCOS. Although physicians seem excited about the chance to adopt a multidisciplinary strategy, it is necessary to identify the perceived obstacles that prevent clinics from becoming multidisciplinary. Lobbying for insurance reimbursement and educating the medical community, including physicians and dietitians, about the value of specialized nutrition counseling are two areas that require further attention. The best method to guarantee that PCOS patients have access to lifestyle interventions—which are thought to be the first-line treatment for PCOS—is probably to have access to dietitians who are knowledgeable about PCOS [96].

2.7.3 Recommendations

Women with PCOS can benefit from adopting a healthy lifestyle, getting adequate exercise, and eating the correct food. Because an ideal diet has not yet been found, there is no one for women with PCOS. It has been demonstrated that a low-GI diet works better than an equivalent diet in terms of fiber and nutrients. PCOS can also be mitigated by eating a diet rich in omega-3 fatty acids and MI. Weight loss improves insulin sensitivity, sex hormone-binding globulin (SHBG) levels, and androgen synthesis, all of which improve menstrual cycles and increase fertility in PCOS-affected women. Tasks must be completed [97]. Although there is no set diet for PCOS, experts advise adhering to a lower-calorie meal plan that has either low-carbohydrate or low-glycemic-index carbohydrates. The greatest foods for those with PCOS include vegetables, fruits high in fiber, whole grains, lean proteins, and monounsaturated fats. If PCOS is present, stay away from processed foods, fatty foods, baked goods, sweets, and excessive amounts of salt or sugar [98]. Finally, from the time of diagnosis, women with PCOS should follow the same dietary guidelines under the supervision of registered dietitians, gynecologists, fertility specialists, and endocrinologists. This will help patients understand how diet and lifestyle factors contribute to the disorder and how non-pharmacological means can modify them for a better prognosis [95]. In addition, the following advice can assist you in adhering to a PCOS diet: Make slight dietary modifications. Read food labels carefully and make better choices. To maintain control over the components, meals were prepared at home. When dining out, choose items that are baked or grilled. If necessary, obtain advice from a qualified nutritionist or physician. A well-structured PCOS diet plan, nutritional supplementation, strength training, weight management, lifestyle adjustments, stress management, and abstinence from junk food are all part of a comprehensive approach to the treatment of PCOS. Women with PCOS can enhance general well-being, reduce symptoms, and improve hormonal balance in women with PCOS. To ensure that the treatment plan is customized to each patient's needs, it is imperative to communicate with medical professionals before making any significant lifestyle adjustments.

2.7.4 Future Directions

Future research should concentrate on areas where PCOS remains poorly understood, especially in the areas of traditional dietary approaches for PCOS. Currently, there are no viable treatments for this condition. Therefore, the provision of symptomatic relief to patients is recommended. Further research is required to evaluate and confirm the effects of long-term dietary management of PCOS.

References

1. NHS. Polycystic ovary syndrome. 11 Oct 2022. https://www.nhs.uk/conditions/polycystic-ovary-syndrome-pcos/.
2. Witchel SF, Oberfield SE, Peña AS. Polycystic ovary syndrome: pathophysiology, presentation, and treatment with emphasis on adolescent girls. J Endocr Soc. 2019;3(8):1545–73. https://doi.org/10.1210/js.2019-00078.
3. WHO. Polycystic ovary syndrome. 2023. https://www.who.int/news-room/fact-sheets/detail/polycystic-ovary-syndrome.
4. Deswal R, Narwal V, Dang A, Pundir CS. The prevalence of polycystic ovary syndrome: a brief systematic review. J Hum Reprod Sci. 2020;13(4):261–71. https://doi.org/10.4103/jhrs.JHRS_95_18.
5. Nidhi R, Padmalatha V, Nagarathna R, Amritanshu R. Prevalence of polycystic ovarian syndrome in indian adolescents. J Pediatr Adolesc Gynecol. 2011;24(4):223–7. https://doi.org/10.1016/j.jpag.2011.03.002.
6. Ganie MA, Vasudevan V, Wani IA, Baba MS, Arif T, Rashid A. Epidemiology, pathogenesis, genetics & management of polycystic ovary syndrome in India. Indian J Med Res. 2019;150(4):333–44. https://doi.org/10.4103/ijmr.IJMR_1937_17.
7. Polycystic ovary syndrome (PCOS). Johns Hopkins Medicine. https://www.hopkinsmedicine.org/health/conditions-and-diseases/polycystic-ovary-syndrome-pcos. Accessed 22 Apr 2024.
8. Glycemic index: what it is and how to use it. https://www.healthline.com/nutrition/glycemic-index. Accessed 22 Apr 2024.
9. In vitro fertilization (IVF)—Mayo Clinic. https://www.mayoclinic.org/tests-procedures/in-vitro-fertilization/about/pac-20384716. Accessed 22 Apr 2024.
10. Guarnotta V, Emanuele F, Amodei R, Giordano C. Very low-calorie ketogenic diet: a potential application in the treatment of hypercortisolism comorbidities. Nutrients. 2022;14(12):2388. https://doi.org/10.3390/nu14122388.

11. Harvard T.H. Chan School of Public Health. Diet review: Mediterranean diet. The Nutrition Source. 16 Jan 2018. https://www.hsph.harvard.edu/nutritionsource/healthy-weight/diet-reviews/mediterranean-diet/.
12. Follicle-stimulating hormone (FSH): what it is and function. Cleveland Clinic. https://my.clevelandclinic.org/health/articles/24638-follicle-stimulating-hormone-fsh. Accessed 22 Apr 2024.
13. Definition of luteinizing hormone—NCI Dictionary of Cancer Terms—NCI. 2 Feb 2011. https://www.cancer.gov/publications/dictionaries/cancer-terms/def/luteinizing-hormone.
14. Khan SA, Magd H, Khatri B, Arora S, Sharma N. Critical success factors of Internet of Things and digital marketing. In: Naim A, Devi V, editors. Global applications of the Internet of Things in digital marketing. IGI Global; 2023. p. 233–53. https://doi.org/10.4018/978-1-6684-8166-0.ch012.
15. Magd H, Khan SA, Khatri B, Sharma N, Arora S. Understanding the relationship between IoT and digital marketing: a bibliometric analysis. In: Naim A, Devi V, editors. Global applications of the Internet of Things in digital marketing. IGI Global; 2023. p. 123–40. https://doi.org/10.4018/978-1-6684-8166-0.ch007.
16. Sharma N, Khatri B, Khan SA. Exploring the past and identifying the future research agenda for social media and tourist behavior: a bibliometric analysis. In: Ramos C, Costa T, Severino F, Calisto M, editors. Social media strategies for tourism interactivity. IGI Global; 2024. p. 261–84. https://doi.org/10.4018/979-8-3693-0960-5.ch011.
17. Della Torre S, Benedusi V, Fontana R, Maggi A. Energy metabolism and fertility: a balance preserved for female health. Nat Rev Endocrinol. 2014;10(1):13–23. https://doi.org/10.1038/nrendo.2013.203.
18. Escobar-Morreale HF. Reproductive endocrinology: menstrual dysfunction—a proxy for insulin resistance in PCOS? Nat Rev Endocrinol. 2014;10(1):10–1. https://doi.org/10.1038/nrendo.2013.232.
19. Genazzani AD, Prati A, Despini G, Marini G, Ricchieri F. PCOS from lifestyle to the use of inositol and insulin sensitizers. In: Genazzani AR, Brincat M, editors. Frontiers in gynecological endocrinology, From symptoms to therapies, vol. 1. Springer International Publishing; 2014. p. 59–67. https://doi.org/10.1007/978-3-319-03494-2_7.
20. Nagori C. Correlation of ovarian and stromal volumes to fasting and postprandial insulin levels in polycystic ovarian syndrome patients. Int J Infertil Fetal Med. 2014;5(1):12–4. https://doi.org/10.5005/jp-journals-10016-1073.
21. Sheikh M. Role of ultrasound in the assessment of female infertility. Donald School J Ultrasound Obstet Gynecol. 2014;8(2):184–200. https://doi.org/10.5005/jp-journals-10009-1354.
22. Desai N, Tiwari RT, Patel SS. Prevalence of polycystic ovary syndrome and its associated risk factors among adolescent and young girls in ahmedabad region. Indian J Pharm Pract. 2018;11(3):119–25. https://doi.org/10.5530/ijopp.11.3.27.
23. Bharali MD, Rajendran R, Goswami J, Singal K, Rajendran V. Prevalence of polycystic ovarian syndrome in India: a systematic review and meta-analysis. Cureus. 2022;14(12):e32351. https://doi.org/10.7759/cureus.32351.
24. Gill H, Tiwari P, Dabadghao P. Prevalence of polycystic ovary syndrome in young women from North India: a community-based study. Indian J Endocrinol Metab. 2012;16(Suppl 2):S389–92. https://doi.org/10.4103/2230-8210.104104.
25. Joshi B, Mukherjee S, Patil A, Purandare A, Chauhan S, Vaidya R. A cross-sectional study of polycystic ovarian syndrome among adolescent and young girls in Mumbai, India. Indian J Endocrinol Metab. 2014;18(3):317–24. https://doi.org/10.4103/2230-8210.131162.
26. Vidya Bharathi R, Swetha S, Neerajaa J, Varsha Madhavica J, Janani DM, Rekha SN, et al. An epidemiological survey: effect of predisposing factors for PCOS in Indian urban and rural population. Middle East Fertil Soc J. 2017;22(4):313–6. https://doi.org/10.1016/j.mefs.2017.05.007.
27. Veltman-Verhulst SM, Boivin J, Eijkemans MJC, Fauser BJCM. Emotional distress is a common risk in women with polycystic ovary syndrome: a systematic review and meta-analysis of 28 studies. Hum Reprod Update. 2012;18(6):638–51. https://doi.org/10.1093/humupd/dms029.

28. Spritzer PM, Marchesan LB, Santos BR, Fighera TM. Hirsutism, normal androgens and diagnosis of PCOS. Diagnostics. 2022;12(8):1922. https://doi.org/10.3390/diagnostics12081922.
29. Kicińska AM, Maksym RB, Zabielska-Kaczorowska MA, Stachowska A, Babińska A. Immunological and metabolic causes of infertility in polycystic ovary syndrome. Biomedicines. 2023;11(6):1567. https://doi.org/10.3390/biomedicines11061567.
30. Christodoulopoulou V, Trakakis E, Pergialiotis V, Peppa M, Chrelias C, Kassanos D, Papantoniou N. Clinical and biochemical characteristics in PCOS women with menstrual abnormalities. J Family Reprod Health. 2016;10(4):184–90.
31. Xu H, Feng G, Alpadi K, Han Y, Yang R, Chen L, Li R, Qiao J. A model for predicting polycystic ovary syndrome using serum AMH, menstrual cycle length, body mass index and serum androstenedione in Chinese reproductive aged population: a retrospective cohort study. Front Endocrinol. 2022;13:821368. https://doi.org/10.3389/fendo.2022.821368.
32. Shahmoradi L, Azadbakht L, Farzi J, Kalhori SRN, Yazdipour AB, Solat F. Nutritional management recommendation systems in polycystic ovary syndrome: a systematic review. BMC Womens Health. 2024;24(1):234. https://doi.org/10.1186/s12905-024-03074-3.
33. Fauser BCJM, Tarlatzis BC, Rebar RW, Legro RS, Balen AH, Lobo R, Carmina E, Chang J, Yildiz BO, Laven JSE, Boivin J, Petraglia F, Wijeyeratne CN, Norman RJ, Dunaif A, Franks S, Wild RA, Dumesic D, Barnhart K. Consensus on women's health aspects of polycystic ovary syndrome (PCOS): the Amsterdam ESHRE/ASRM-Sponsored 3rd PCOS Consensus Workshop Group. Fertil Steril. 2012;97(1):28–38.e25. https://doi.org/10.1016/j.fertnstert.2011.09.024.
34. Tabassum F, Sinha HH, Dhar K, Jyoti C, Akhtar MS, Chopra VS. Assessment of psycho-emotional distress due to age, body mass index, and marital status in polycystic ovary syndrome in North Indian population. Int J Womens Health Reprod Sci. 2020;8(4):368–75. https://doi.org/10.15296/ijwhr.2020.59.
35. Sánchez-Ferrer ML, Adoamnei E, Prieto-Sánchez MT, Mendiola J, Corbalán-Biyang S, Moñino-García M, Palomar-Rodríguez JA, Torres-Cantero AM. Health-related quality of life in women with polycystic ovary syndrome attending to a tertiary hospital in Southeastern Spain: a case-control study. Health Qual Life Outcomes. 2020;18(1):232. https://doi.org/10.1186/s12955-020-01484-z.
36. Peerwani G, Rozi S, Lakhdir MPA, Zuberi N, Asad N. Association of depressive symptoms and quality of life in Pakistani youth (15–24 years) with polycystic ovarian syndrome: a web-based analytical cross-sectional study. Front Glob Womens Health. 2023;4:967883. https://doi.org/10.3389/fgwh.2023.967883.
37. Szczuko M, Kikut J, Szczuko U, Szydłowska I, Nawrocka-Rutkowska J, Ziętek M, Verbanac D, Saso L. Nutrition strategy and life style in polycystic ovary syndrome—narrative review. Nutrients. 2021;13(7):2452. https://doi.org/10.3390/nu13072452.
38. Taghavi SA, Bazarganipour F, Hugh-Jones S, Hosseini N. Health-related quality of life in Iranian women with polycystic ovary syndrome: a qualitative study. BMC Womens Health. 2015;15(1):111. https://doi.org/10.1186/s12905-015-0272-4.
39. Ching HL, Burke V, Stuckey BGA. Quality of life and psychological morbidity in women with polycystic ovary syndrome: body mass index, age and the provision of patient information are significant modifiers. Clin Endocrinol. 2007;66(3):373–9. https://doi.org/10.1111/j.1365-2265.2007.02742.x.
40. Rzońca E, Bień A, Wdowiak A, Szymański R, Iwanowicz-Palus G. Determinants of quality of life and satisfaction with life in women with polycystic ovary syndrome. Int J Environ Res Public Health. 2018;15(2):376. https://doi.org/10.3390/ijerph15020376.
41. Chudzicka-Strugała I, Gołębiewska I, Banaszewska B, Brudecki G, Zwoździak B. The role of individually selected diets in obese women with PCOS—a review. Nutrients. 2022;14(21):4555. https://doi.org/10.3390/nu14214555.
42. Barrea L, Frias-Toral E, Verde L, Ceriani F, Cucalón G, Garcia-Velasquez E, Moretti D, Savastano S, Colao A, Muscogiuri G. PCOS and nutritional approaches: differences between lean and obese phenotype. Metab Open. 2021;12:100123. https://doi.org/10.1016/j.metop.2021.100123.

43. Xenou M, Gourounti K. Dietary patterns and polycystic ovary syndrome: a systematic review. Maedica. 2021;16(3):516–21. https://doi.org/10.26574/maedica.2020.16.3.516.
44. Del Pup L, Cagnacci A. IMPROVE lifestyle in polycystic ovary syndrome: a systematic strategy. Gynecol Endocrinol. 2021;37(10):875–8. https://doi.org/10.1080/09513590.2021.1871892.
45. Szczuko M, Skowronek M, Zapalowska-Chwyc M, Starczewski A. Quantitative assessment of nutrition in patients with polycystic ovary syndrome (PCOS). Rocz Panstw Zakl Hig. 2016;67(4):419. http://agro.icm.edu.pl/agro/element/bwmeta1.element.agro-aa12b997-29ff-428c-9ca7-1a51d1018361.
46. Guler I, Himmetoglu O, Turp A, Erdem A, Erdem M, Onan MA, Taskiran C, Taslipinar MY, Guner H. Zinc and homocysteine levels in polycystic ovarian syndrome patients with insulin resistance. Biol Trace Elem Res. 2014;158(3):297–304. https://doi.org/10.1007/s12011-014-9941-7.
47. Pandey M, Niroula K, Pandey M, Niroula K. Optimizing nutrition for PCOS management: a comprehensive guide. IntechOpen; 2024. https://doi.org/10.5772/intechopen.114149.
48. Shishehgar F, Mirmiran P, Rahmati M, Tohidi M, Ramezani Tehrani F. Does a restricted energy low glycemic index diet have a different effect on overweight women with or without polycystic ovary syndrome? BMC Endocr Disord. 2019;19(1):93. https://doi.org/10.1186/s12902-019-0420-1.
49. Meneghini C, Bianco C, Galanti F, Tamburelli V, Dal Lago A, Licata E, Gallo M, Fabiani C, Corno R, Miriello D, Rago R. The impact of nutritional therapy in the management of overweight/obese PCOS patient candidates for IVF. Nutrients. 2023;15(20):20. https://doi.org/10.3390/nu15204444.
50. Wang T, Sha L, Li Y, Zhu L, Wang Z, Li K, Lu H, Bao T, Guo L, Zhang X, Wang H. Dietary α-linolenic acid-rich flaxseed oil exerts beneficial effects on polycystic ovary syndrome through sex steroid hormones—microbiota—inflammation axis in rats. Front Endocrinol. 2020;11 https://doi.org/10.3389/fendo.2020.00284.
51. Mirmasoumi G, Fazilati M, Foroozanfard F, Vahedpoor Z, Mahmoodi S, Taghizadeh M, Esfeh NK, Mohseni M, Karbassizadeh H, Asemi Z. The effects of flaxseed oil omega-3 fatty acids supplementation on metabolic status of patients with polycystic ovary syndrome: a randomized, double-blind, placebo-controlled trial. Exp Clin Endocrinol Diab. 2018;126(4):222–8. https://doi.org/10.1055/s-0043-119751.
52. Popova A, Mihaylova D. A review of the medicinal plants in Bulgaria—collection, storage, and extraction techniques. Asian J Pharm Clin Res. 2018;11:28–35. https://doi.org/10.22159/ajpcr.2018.v11i3.22994.
53. Haj-Husein I, Tukan S, Alkazaleh F. The effect of marjoram (Origanum majorana) tea on the hormonal profile of women with polycystic ovary syndrome: a randomised controlled pilot study. J Hum Nutr Diet. 2016;29(1):105–11. https://doi.org/10.1111/jhn.12290.
54. Grant P. Spearmint herbal tea has significant anti-androgen effects in polycystic ovarian syndrome. A randomized controlled trial. Phytother Res. 2010;24(2):186–8. https://doi.org/10.1002/ptr.2900.
55. Heshmati J, Moini A, Sepidarkish M, Morvaridzadeh M, Salehi M, Palmowski A, Mojtahedi MF, Shidfar F. Effects of curcumin supplementation on blood glucose, insulin resistance and androgens in patients with polycystic ovary syndrome: a randomized double-blind placebo-controlled clinical trial. Phytomedicine. 2021;80:153395. https://doi.org/10.1016/j.phymed.2020.153395.
56. Gruenwald J, Freder J, Armbruester N. Cinnamon and health. Crit Rev Food Sci Nutr. 2010;50(9):822–34. https://doi.org/10.1080/10408390902773052.
57. Hajimonfarednejad M, Nimrouzi M, Heydari M, Zarshenas MM, Raee MJ, Jahromi BN. Insulin resistance improvement by cinnamon powder in polycystic ovary syndrome: a randomized double-blind placebo controlled clinical trial. Phytother Res. 2018;32(2):276–83. https://doi.org/10.1002/ptr.5970.
58. PCOS diet. 1 Feb 2023. https://www.hopkinsmedicine.org/health/wellness-and-prevention/pcos-diet.

59. A holistic approach to natural management of PCOS: how to cure PCOS naturally. https://www.asterdmhealthcare.com/health-library/a-holistic-approach-to-natural-management-of-pcos-how-to-cure-pcos-naturally.
60. Lakshmi JN, Babu AN, Kiran SSM, Nori LP, Hassan N, Ashames A, Bhandare RR, Shaik AB. Herbs as a source for the treatment of polycystic ovarian syndrome: a systematic review. BioTech. 2023;12(1):4. https://doi.org/10.3390/biotech12010004.
61. Liu J, Burdette JE, Xu H, Gu C, Van Breemen RB, Bhat KPL, Booth N, Constantinou AI, Pezzuto JM, Fong HHS, Farnsworth NR, Bolton JL. Evaluation of estrogenic activity of plant extracts for the potential treatment of menopausal symptoms. J Agric Food Chem. 2001;49(5):2472–9. https://doi.org/10.1021/jf0014157.
62. Merz P-G, Gorkow C, Schrödter A, Rietbrock S, Sieder C, Loew D, Dericks-Tan JSE, Taubert HD. The effects of a special Agnus castus extract (BP1095E1) on prolactin secretion in healthy male subjects. Exp Clin Endocrinol Diabetes. 2009;104(06):447–53. https://doi.org/10.1055/s-0029-1211483.
63. Webster DE, Lu J, Chen S-N, Farnsworth NR, Wang ZJ. Activation of the μ-opiate receptor by Vitex agnus-castus methanol extracts: implication for its use in PMS. J Ethnopharmacol. 2006;106(2):216–21. https://doi.org/10.1016/j.jep.2005.12.025.
64. Sorensen JM, Katsiotis ST. Variation in essential oil yield and composition of Cretan *Vitex agnus castus* L. fruits. J Essent Oil Res. 1999;11(5):599–605. https://doi.org/10.1080/10412905.1999.9701221.
65. Zhelev I, Petkova Z, Kostova I, Damyanova S, Stoyanova A, Dimitrova-Dyulgerova I, Antova G, Ercisli S, Assouguem A, Kara M, Almeer R, Sayed AA. Chemical composition and antimicrobial activity of essential oil of fruits from Vitex agnus-castus L., growing in two regions in Bulgaria. Plants. 2022;11(7):896. https://doi.org/10.3390/plants11070896.
66. Shishodia S, Singh T, Chaturvedi MM. Modulation of transcription factors by curcumin. In: Aggarwal BB, Surh Y-J, Shishodia S, editors. The molecular targets and therapeutic uses of curcumin in health and disease, vol. 595. Springer; 2007. p. 127–48. https://doi.org/10.1007/978-0-387-46401-5_4.
67. Wojcik M, Krawczyk M, Wojcik P, Cypryk K, Wozniak LA. Molecular mechanisms underlying curcumin-mediated therapeutic effects in type 2 diabetes and cancer. Oxidative Med Cell Longev. 2018;2018:1–14. https://doi.org/10.1155/2018/9698258.
68. Tanvir EM, Hossen MS, Hossain MF, Afroz R, Gan SH, Khalil MI, Karim N. Antioxidant properties of popular turmeric (*Curcuma longa*) varieties from Bangladesh. J Food Qual. 2017;2017:1–8. https://doi.org/10.1155/2017/8471785.
69. Jiménez-Osorio AS, Monroy A, Alavez S. Curcumin and insulin resistance—molecular targets and clinical evidences. Biofactors. 2016;42(6):561–80. https://doi.org/10.1002/biof.1302.
70. Bency Baby T, Smitha Rani, Remya K, Rasheed SP, Azeem AK. Polycystic ovarian syndrome: therapeutic potential of herbal remedies—a review. https://www.florajournal.com/archives/2016/vol4issue5/PartB/5-1-2-689.pdf.
71. Jelodar G, Masoomi S, Rahmanifar F. Hydroalcoholic extract of flaxseed improves polycystic ovary syndrome in a rat model. Iran J Basic Med Sci. 2018;21(6) https://doi.org/10.22038/ijbms.2018.25778.6349.
72. Eftekhari A, Khusro A, Ahmadian E, Dizaj SM, Hasanzadeh A, Cucchiarini M. Phytochemical and nutra-pharmaceutical attributes of Mentha spp.: a comprehensive review. Arab J Chem. 2021;14(5):103106. https://doi.org/10.1016/j.arabjc.2021.103106.
73. Rooney S, Pendry B. Phytotherapy for polycystic ovarian syndrome: a review of the literature and evaluation of practitioners' experiences. J Herb Med. 2014;4(3):159–71. https://doi.org/10.1016/j.hermed.2014.05.001.
74. Wang J, Ji J, Song Z, Zhang W, He X, Li F, Zhang C, Guo C, Wang C, Yuan C. Hypocholesterolemic effect of emodin by simultaneous determination of in vitro and in vivo bile salts binding. Fitoterapia. 2016;110:116–22. https://doi.org/10.1016/j.fitote.2016.03.007.
75. Chen X, Tao C, Wang J, He B, Xu J. Meta-analysis of therapeutic efficacy and effects of integrated traditional Chinese and Western medicine on coagulation and fibrinolysis system in patients with threatened abortion and polycystic ovary syndrome. Am J Transl Res. 2022;14(5):2768–78.

76. Costa CTC, Bevilaqua CML, Morais SM, Camurça-Vasconcelos ALF, Maciel MV, Braga RR, Oliveira LMB. Anthelmintic activity of Cocos nucifera L. on intestinal nematodes of mice. Res Vet Sci. 2010;88(1):101–3. https://doi.org/10.1016/j.rvsc.2009.05.008.
77. Lima EBC, Sousa CNS, Meneses LN, Ximenes NC, Santos Júnior MA, Vasconcelos GS, Lima NBC, Patrocínio MCA, Macedo D, Vasconcelos SMM. Cocos nucifera (L.) (Arecaceae): a phytochemical and pharmacological review. Braz J Med Biol Res. 2015;48(11):953–64. https://doi.org/10.1590/1414-431x20154773.
78. Bhandary MJ, Chandrashekar KR, Kaveriappa KM. Medical ethnobotany of the Siddis of Uttara Kannada district, Karnataka, India. J Ethnopharmacol. 1995;47(3):149–58. https://doi.org/10.1016/0378-8741(95)01274-H.
79. Hossein K, Leila K, Ebrahim T, Nazanin S, Farzad P, Elham R, Mohammad P, Zahra H. The effect of pomegranate juice extract on hormonal changes of female Wistar rats caused by polycystic ovarian syndrome. Biomed Pharmacol J. 2015;8(2):971–7. https://doi.org/10.13005/bpj/849.
80. Jayaprakasha GK, Rao LJ, Sakariah KK. Chemical composition of volatile oil from Cinnamomum zeylanicum buds. Z Nat C. 2002;57(11–12):990–3. https://doi.org/10.1515/znc-2002-11-1206.
81. Evans P, Halliwell B. Micronutrients: oxidant/antioxidant status. Br J Nutr. 2001;85(Suppl 2):S67–74.
82. Muchuweti M, Kativu E, Mupure CH, Chidewe C, Ndhlala AR, Benhura MAN. Phenolic composition and antioxidant properties of some spices. Am J Food Technol. 2007;2(5):414–20. https://doi.org/10.3923/ajft.2007.414.420.
83. Ainehchi N, Khaki A, Ouladsahebmadarek E, Hammadeh M, Farzadi L, Farshbaf-Khalili A, Asnaashari S, Khamnei H, Khaki AA, Shokoohi M. The effect of clomiphene citrate, herbal mixture, and herbal mixture along with clomiphene citrate on clinical and para-clinical parameters in infertile women with polycystic ovary syndrome: a randomized controlled clinical trial. Arch Med Sci. 2020;16(6):1304–18. https://doi.org/10.5114/aoms.2020.93271.
84. Desai BN, Maharjan RH, Nampoothiri LP. Aloe barbadensis Mill. formulation restores lipid profile to normal in a letrozole-induced polycystic ovarian syndrome rat model. Pharmacognosy Res. 2012;4(2):109–15. https://doi.org/10.4103/0974-8490.94736.
85. Badgujar SB, Patel VV, Bandivdekar AH. *Foeniculum vulgare* Mill: a review of its botany, phytochemistry, pharmacology, contemporary application, and toxicology. Biomed Res Int. 2014;2014:1–32. https://doi.org/10.1155/2014/842674.
86. Farideh ZZ, Bagher M, Ashraf A, Akram A, Kazem M. Effects of chamomile extract on biochemical and clinical parameters in a rat model of polycystic ovary syndrome. J Reprod Infertil. 2010;11(3):169–74.
87. Herrmann K, Nagel CW. Occurrence and content of hydroxycinnamic and hydroxybenzoic acid compounds in foods. Crit Rev Food Sci Nutr. 1989;28(4):315–47. https://doi.org/10.1080/10408398909527504.
88. Girardon P, Bessiere J, Baccou J, Sauvaire Y. Volatile constituents of fenugreek seeds. Planta Med. 1985;51(6):533–4. https://doi.org/10.1055/s-2007-969591.
89. Ahmad A, Alghamdi SS, Mahmood K, Afzal M. Fenugreek a multipurpose crop: potentialities and improvements. Saudi J Biol Sci. 2016;23(2):300–10. https://doi.org/10.1016/j.sjbs.2015.09.015.
90. Khanna A, John F, Das S, Thomas J, Rao J, Maliakel B, Im K. Efficacy of a novel extract of fenugreek seeds in alleviating vasomotor symptoms and depression in perimenopausal women: a randomized, double-blinded, placebo-controlled study. J Food Biochem. 2020;44(12):e13507. https://doi.org/10.1111/jfbc.13507.
91. Atashpour S, Kargar Jahromi H, Kargar Jahromi Z, Maleknasab M. Comparison of the effects of Ginger extract with clomiphene citrate on sex hormones in rats with polycystic ovarian syndrome. Int J Reprod Biomed. 2017;15(9):561–8.
92. Ali BH, Blunden G, Tanira MO, Nemmar A. Some phytochemical, pharmacological and toxicological properties of ginger (Zingiber officinale Roscoe): a review of recent research. Food Chem Toxicol. 2008;46(2):409–20. https://doi.org/10.1016/j.fct.2007.09.085.

93. Poojari P, Paramanya A, Singh D, Ali A. Polycystic ovarian syndrome: causes and therapies by herbal medicine. In: Herbal medicines. Elsevier; 2022. p. 435–51. https://doi.org/10.1016/B978-0-323-90572-5.00028-7.
94. Teede HJ, Tay CT, Laven JJE, Dokras A, Moran LJ, Piltonen TT, Costello MF, Boivin J, Redman LM, Boyle JA, Norman RJ, Mousa A, Joham AE. Recommendations from the 2023 international evidence-based guideline for the assessment and management of polycystic ovary syndrome. J Clin Endocrinol Metabol. 2023;108(10):2447–69. https://doi.org/10.1210/clinem/dgad463.
95. Che X, Chen Z, Liu M, Mo Z. Dietary interventions: a promising treatment for polycystic ovary syndrome. Ann Nutr Metab. 2021;77(6):313–23. https://doi.org/10.1159/000519302.
96. Wolf W, Wattick R, Murray P, Clemmer M, Olfert M. Future implications of using registered dietitians in multidisciplinary polycystic ovary syndrome treatment. Healthcare. 2018;6(4):144. https://doi.org/10.3390/healthcare6040144.
97. Zehravi M, Maqbool M, Ara I. Healthy lifestyle and dietary approaches to treating polycystic ovary syndrome: a review. Open Health. 2022;3(1):60–5. https://doi.org/10.1515/openhe-2022-0008.
98. Grassi A. PCOS diet: what to eat to manage symptoms. https://www.verywellhealth.com/what-is-the-best-diet-for-pcos-2616314. Accessed 19 Apr 2024.

The Role of Nutrients in PCOS: An Exploration of Key Nutrients and Their Impact on PCOS Symptoms

3

Palvi Sharma, Rakesh Kumar, Meenu Gupta, and Jyotsna Rani

3.1 Introduction

Polycystic ovary syndrome, also known as PCOS, is a hormonal condition that primarily affects women who are fertile. It's characterized by a combination of symptoms related to reproductive, metabolic, and endocrine functions. Eight to thirteen percent of women in the world who are of reproductive age are thought to suffer from PCOS, the most prevalent endocrine disorder. PCOS is a multifaceted disorder that involves irregularities in metabolism, endocrine system, and reproduction. These abnormalities include reduced fertility, ovulatory disturbance, hyperandrogenism, and an increased risk of obesity, insulin resistance, hepatic steatosis, and dyslipidemia [1]. This condition affects 5–20% of women, depending on the diagnostic criteria, and is associated with irregular menstrual periods, polycystic ovaries, hyperandrogenism, insulin resistance, and obesity [2]. Its symptoms include anomalies related to hormones and reproduction, such as irregular or nonexistent periods, weight gain, acne, male pattern baldness, and problems with conception. Additionally, PCOS increases the chance of getting diseases like cardiovascular disorders, abnormal cholesterol levels, high blood pressure, type 2 diabetes, and several malignancies, including endometrial and breast cancer [3]. Although the precise etiology of PCOS is still unknown, a combination of genetic, environmental,

P. Sharma (✉)
Department of Computer Science and Engineering, Model Institute of Engineering and Technology, Jammu, Jammu & Kashmir, India

R. Kumar · M. Gupta
Department of Computer Science and Engineering, Chandigarh University, Chandigarh, Punjab, India

J. Rani
Obstetrics and Gynaecology, Dr. B. R. Ambedkar State Institute of Medical Sciences, Mohali, Punjab, India

R. Kumar et al. (eds.), *AI-Based Nutritional Intervention in Polycystic Ovary Syndrome (PCOS)*, https://doi.org/10.1007/978-981-96-2120-0_3

prenatal androgen exposure, and epigenetic factors are probably responsible. The development and management of PCOS are greatly influenced by a number of environmental factors, including stress, smoking, physical activity, and food choices, as shown in Fig. 3.1.

All women with PCOS, regardless of weight, have insulin resistance [4]. Previous studies indicates that insulin is a major factor in the overproduction of androgens, specifically influencing the ovarian theca cells, which results in higher levels of these hormones in PCOS-affected women than in non-PCOS women. There is a suggestion that insulin stimulates the CYP-17 gene, which is implicated in the generation of androgens. Furthermore, insulin stops follicle maturation by making ovarian granulosa cells more sensitive to luteinizing hormone (LH) too quickly. Hormonal imbalances are exacerbated by the combined effects of insulin and LH, which further promote the synthesis of androstenedione [5]. Additionally, through insulin-like growth factor (IGF-1), insulin indirectly affects steroidogenesis. In addition to insulin, elevated levels of IGF-1 in follicular fluid also encourage early ovarian follicle atresia and enhanced androgen production. The interactions between insulin and insulin-like growth factor (IGF-1) intensify the symptoms indicated earlier. Additionally, studies show that the liver reduced synthesis of sex hormone-binding globulin (SHBG), a result of insulin's inhibitory impact, contributing to the higher testosterone levels in the blood of women with PCOS. Therefore, the main strategy for controlling the condition is to modify lifestyle factors including familial upbringing, economic standing, cultural background (including religion and custom), education level, ethnicity, and age, which have an impact on women's eating habits [6–8]. Further, adding different nutrients to their diet can help women with PCOS control their symptoms and maintain overall health. These include high-fiber foods that can help control blood sugar levels and enhance insulin sensitivity, such as fruits, vegetables, whole grains, legumes, and nuts. Walnuts, flaxseeds, and fatty fish are good sources of omega-3 fatty acids, which have anti-inflammatory

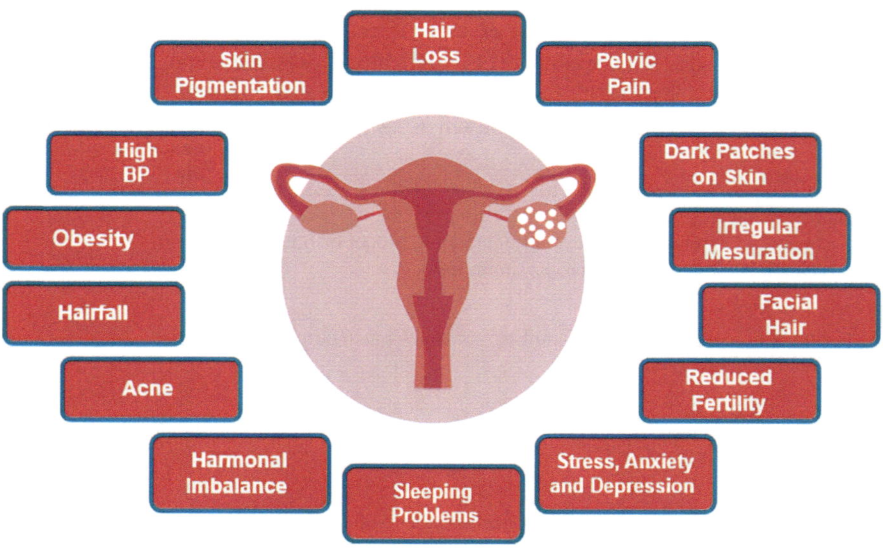

Fig. 3.1 Symptoms of PCOS

qualities that may help lessen PCOS-related inflammation. Additionally, monounsaturated fats from foods like avocados, almonds, seeds, and olive oil can help regulate weight and enhance insulin sensitivity. Lean protein sources including fish, poultry, tofu, and lentils can help to stabilize blood sugar levels and increase satiety when they are included in meals and snacks [9–11]. Antioxidant-rich foods, such as bell peppers, spinach, kale, and berries, can help fight inflammation and oxidative stress. For the metabolism of glucose and general health, an adequate diet of vitamins and minerals is essential, especially vitamin D, magnesium, zinc, and chromium. Foods high in isothiol, such as nuts, citrus fruits, beans, and lentils, can help balance hormones and increase insulin sensitivity [12]. Additionally, foods high in folate, such leafy greens, citrus fruits, and beans, can help maintain reproductive health, whereas foods high in calcium, such as dairy, tofu, almonds, and leafy greens, are crucial for maintaining healthy bones, particularly for women with PCOS who are more likely to develop osteoporosis. Effective PCOS management requires a well-balanced diet based on personal needs, preferences, and health objectives, with advice from medical professionals or trained dietitians [13–15].

In order to better understand the nutritional requirements of women with PCOS and create individualized dietary programs that will enhance their health outcomes, AI and DL approaches can be very helpful tools. In order to find patterns and relationships between dietary components and PCOS symptoms, AI and DL approaches can analyze enormous datasets of clinical and nutritional data. These methods can be used to detect frequent nutritional imbalances or deficiencies linked to PCOS, such as high consumption of refined carbohydrates and saturated fats or insufficient intake of certain nutrients like magnesium, vitamin D, and omega-3 fatty acids. However, it's critical to incorporate these technology developments into all-encompassing healthcare strategies that place an emphasis on patient education, holistic treatment, and multidisciplinary cooperation between researchers, dietitians, and healthcare professionals.

Organization of Chapter

The rest of the chapter is organized as: Section 3.2 presents the review process used to extract the relevant articles as per the PRISMA guidelines. Section 3.3 discusses the background study on the identification of PCOS. Section 3.4 highlights the investigations that are extracted from the literature survey. Section 3.5 introduced the methodology used for the identification of PCOS from the ultrasound images. Results and Discussion are discussed in Sect. 3.6. And, finally, Sect. 3.7 concludes the chapter.

3.2 Review Process

In this section, PRISMA guidelines are used for the extraction of relevant articles with respect to the problem statement. Three databases, i.e., IEEE Xplore, Scopus, and Web of Science, are used for the collection of articles. The different steps of the systematic review are shown in Fig. 3.2. A total 678 articles are selected from the year 2016 to 2024 using the keywords "PCOS," "Women," "Nutrients," "Diet,"

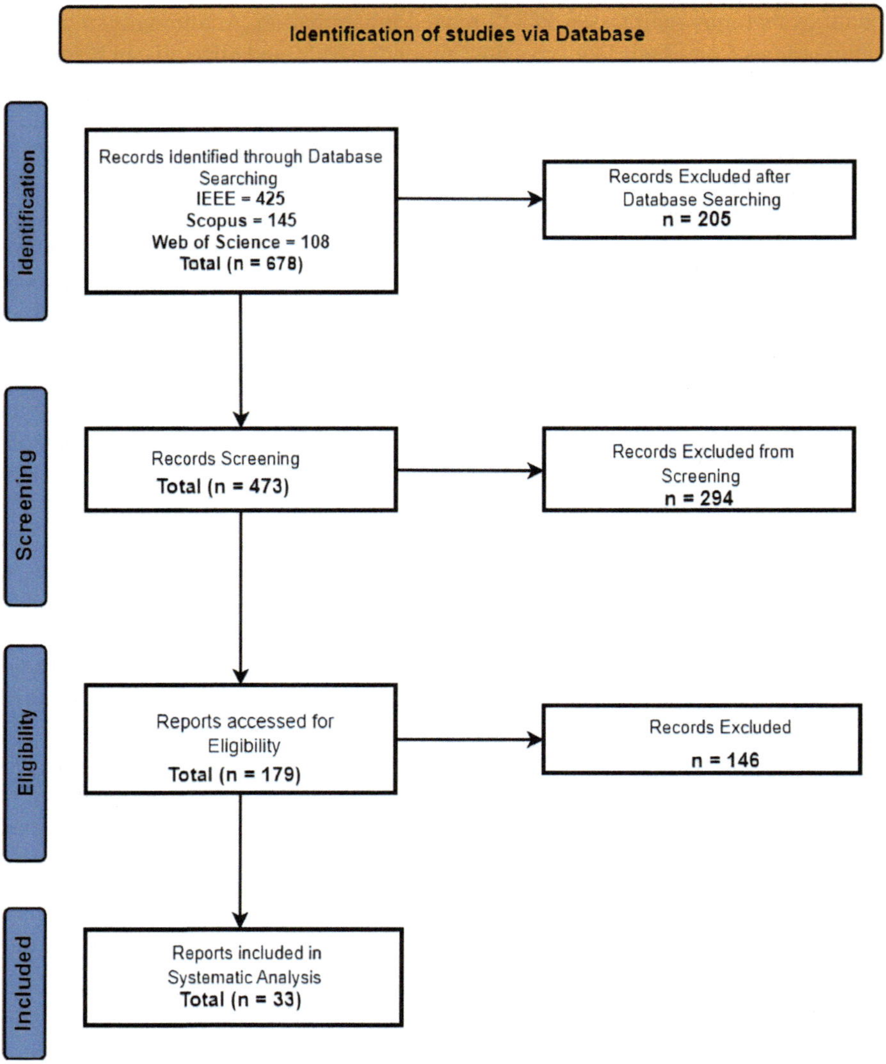

Fig. 3.2 The systematic review process

"Lifestyle Changes," "AI," and "DL." From the selected articles (678 – 205 = 473), 205 articles are discarded because it contains only review papers and duplicate data and some articles are not relevant to the problem statement. After this, 473 articles are selected for the screening process, and 249 articles are eliminated (473 – 249 = 179) because they are not suitable according to the problem statement. Further in the eligibility phase, 146 articles are excluded from the 179 articles (179 – 146 = 33) due to their lack of primary data or lack of relevance to the scope. Finally, 33 articles are selected for the identification of PCOS.

3.3 Background Study

This section discusses the research analysis done by different researchers to identify the PCOS in women with AI and DL technologies.

Zaeemzadeh et al. [4] compared women with and without metabolic syndrome (MetS) to examine dietary consumption of antioxidant micronutrients in PCOS patients. Forty-two participants were selected, 14 of whom were in the case group (PCOS with MetS) and 28 of whom were in the control group (PCOS without MetS). A food frequency questionnaire was used to gauge micronutrient consumption. The findings revealed that PCOS women with MetS had considerably lower intakes of selenium, zinc, chromium, carotenoids, and vitamin E than PCOS women without MetS. According to the results, PCOS patients who consume higher amounts of these nutrients may be more resistant to MetS. Cowan et al. [6] highlighted the importance of adopting a holistic approach to lifestyle management in PCOS, considering not only traditional factors like diet and exercise but also emerging areas of research such as psychological, sleep, and TCIM interventions. Further, authors discussed that women can have more treatment options and more control over their healthcare decisions if these varied techniques are incorporated into future PCOS management classifications. Elmannai et al. [16] discussed the applications of ensemble learning and machine learning (ML) for effective diagnosis with the goal of improving model confidence and transparency through local and global explanations. This work focused on the early treatment of PCOS that can help to prevent long-term consequences like type 2 diabetes. To maximize performance, feature selection techniques are combined with a variety of machine learning models, such as logistic regression, random forest, decision tree, naive Bayes, support vector machine, K-nearest neighbor, XGBoost, and AdaBoost. For increased accuracy, stacking ML models using a meta-learner is advised. To improve machine learning models, Bayesian optimization is utilized, along with SMOTE and ENN approaches, to rectify class imbalance. Results from experiments on a benchmark PCOS dataset show that the best results were obtained by stacking ML with REF feature selection.

Suha and Islam [17] used expanded ML classification technique for the identification of PCOS. The convolutional neural network (CNN) applying cutting-edge methods and transfer learning extracted features from 594 ovarian ultrasound pictures. Then, PCOS and non-PCOS ovaries were classified using stacking ensemble ML, which uses traditional models as base learners and bagging or boosting as a meta-learner. When compared to current ML techniques, this method decreases training time and increases accuracy. For feature extraction, the pre-trained "VGGNet16" model with CNN architecture achieved an accuracy of 99.89% for classification. Lv et al. [18] suggested an automated DL method that focused on scleral alterations as possible markers of PCOS in order to assist in its identification. Authors used a dataset of full-eye images from 721 Chinese women, including 388 PCOS patients. Further, authors used an upgraded U-Net to partition scleral images and a ResNet model to extract deep features. The categorization process then makes use of a multi-instance model. After, the testing and validation the proposed model achieved an average AUC of 0.979 and a classification accuracy of 0.929.

Alamoudi et al. [19] addressed PCOS, a leading cause of female infertility, emphasizing the importance of early diagnosis to manage symptoms and associated health risks. Further, authors proposed inception model for the diagnosis of PCOS. The study presented a dataset with clinical information and ultrasound images for PCOS categorization. After the training of the model, the authors achieved 84.81% accuracy, 69.57% precision, 72.73% F1 score, 76.19% sensitivity, and 87.93% specificity. Next, this model also identified whether or not polycystic kidneys are present in the ultrasound images. Barrera et al. [20] proposed common AI techniques including SVM, K-nearest neighbor, and regression models. Authors also discussed the application of AI and ML in the diagnosis or classification of PCOS, a common but frequently underdiagnosed endocrine condition in women. Different types of datasets were used in the investigations, including genomic and proteomic data, electronic health records, and clinical data. Further, authors compared AI model with the clinical diagnosis and achieved area under the receiver operating curve (ROC) ranging from 73% to 100%, diagnostic accuracy from 89% to 100%, sensitivity from 41% to 100%, specificity from 75% to 100%, positive predictive value (PPV) from 68% to 95%, and negative predictive value (NPV) from 94% to 99%.

Khanna et al. [21] discussed Harris Hawks and Salp Swarm Optimization model for the prediction of PCOS in patients who were fertile. Authors used 541 patients from Kerala, India, as a dataset for heterogeneous ML and DL classifiers. Further, the authors also used explainable AI (XAI) approaches as SHAP, LIME, ELI5, QLattice, and feature significance with random forest to make the model predictions comprehensible and interpretable. After the training, the proposed model achieved 98% accuracy.

Sumathi et al. [22] introduced CNN-based algorithms to identify ovarian cysts and use ultrasound images to differentiate between basic cysts, PCOS, and malignant cysts. The study intends to automate the classification procedure in light of the difficulties associated with manual assessment. For training and testing, the authors used a separate dataset of illnesses linked to PCOS. In the end, the suggested approach classified cysts with an accuracy rate of 85%, showing encouraging outcomes for automating this diagnostic procedure.

Nsugbe [23] proposed decision tree (DT), linear decision analysis (LDA), logistic regression (LR), K-nearest neighbor, and SVM for the diagnosis of the PCOS. The study suggested a prediction approach that first balances synthetic sample production with the Kaggle PCOS dataset. Authors created a probability-based inference technique to gauge and classify patients' PCOS severity. Further, the proposed model achieved 81%, 82%, 81%, 84%, and 82% accuracy for DT, LDA, LR, KNN, and SVM, respectively. Ahmed et al. [24] provided thorough review of PCOS diagnosis approaches, with a particular emphasis on ML techniques. Authors discussed the current algorithms and features, efficiency, methods of analysis, results, and datasets used. Further, authors discussed about the limited size of the dataset, imbalance, and detection rate problems. Authors also introduced the current ML-based

PCOS diagnosis algorithms. Bedi et al. [25] proposed integrated adaptive bilateral filter based framework and attention residual UNet (AResUNet) for the detection of PCOS. Authors also presented a hybrid approach for the early detection of gynecological cancer in women by identifying PCOS. Authors used MMOTU dataset that consisted of 1639 ultrasound images from 294 patients.

Lim et al. [26] introduced seven ML models including K-nearest neighbors (KNN), support vector machine (SVM), decision trees, random forest, logistic regression, voting, and long short term memory (LSTM) networks. This study also provided information for the diagnosis of pulse in traditional Chinese medicine (TCM). Authors used ML techniques to identify and forecast PCOS based on radial pulse wave parameters. Authors used the data of 459 patients which is grouped into 2 categories, i.e., with PCOS and without PCOS. Further, the voting and LSTM models demonstrated the highest performance, achieving a testing accuracy of 72.174% and an F1 score of 0.818, with respective AUC values of 0.715 and 0.722.

Thakre et al. [27] used different ML models like random forest, SVM, logistic regression, Gaussian Naïve Bayes, and K-nearest neighbors for the detection of PCOS using a minimal set of optimal parameters. Further, the authors used the chi-square technique, for the selection of top 30 features out of 41, and these features were incorporated into the feature vector. The Prasoon Kottarathil owned dataset used for testing and training is accessible on Kaggle. After training and testing, the model achieved mean accuracy of 90.91, 88.11, 89.98, 86.95, and 87.64 for random forest, SVM, logistic regression, Gaussian Naïve Bayes, and K-nearest neighbors, respectively. Kaur et al. [28] proposed a novel approach using ultrasound images of ovaries and transfer learning-based DL models to classify PCOS. The proposed model was trained on the large dataset of the ultrasound images and pretrained on the medical images with Inception V3 model. The results suggested that transfer learning enhanced the PCOS detection accuracy and achieved 99.48% accuracy. Tiwari and Maheshwari [29] identified PCOS by the use of DL models called Wavelet ConvNets with ultrasound imaging. For image analysis, Wavelet CNN (Wavelet ConvNets) integrated wavelet transformation with ConvNets. The ultrasound images were subjected to the 2D discrete wavelet transform (2D-DWT) with the Haar wavelet, which produced four sub-bands that each represented a different frequency component. After concatenating these sub-bands, a four-channel feature map was produced and put into the ConvNet for classification. The PCOS-WaveConvNet classifier achieved an accuracy of 99.7%.

Adla et al. [30] used various ML algorithms like LR, SVM, NB, LSVM (linear support vector machine), PSVM (polynomial SVM), RBFSVM (radial basis function SVM), KNN, AdaBoost (AD), linear discriminant classifier (LDC), quadratic discriminant classifier (QDC), and RF for the diagnosis of PCOS. Authors used polycystic ovary syndrome dataset consisting of 541 patient samples. Out of the 541 samples, 177 were diagnosed with the PCOS and 364 were healthy. Further, a hybrid feature selection method was used to minimize the number of features utilizing filters and wrappers after the data had been preprocessed. After training and assessing a number of classification algorithms, the model that performed the best was the support vector machine with a linear kernel and achieved an accuracy of 91.6%, recall of 80.6%, and precision of 93.665%.

Hosain et al. [31] proposed PCONet, a convolutional neural network (CNN) for the identification of polycystic ovaries from ultrasound images. Furthermore, transfer learning was used to refine InceptionV3, a pretrained CNN, for the identical task. Further, authors used 1924 images for the training and 1932 images for the testing. Finally, PCONet achieved 98.12% accuracy, and InceptionV3 achieved 96.56% accuracy on test images.

3.4 Proposed Investigation

In this section, some investigations are extracted based on the literature review that will be helpful for future insights, and the proposed solutions are discussed in Sect. 3.6. Some of the investigations are as follows:

Investigation 1: How can AI-based nutritional interventions be utilized to address PCOS symptoms effectively?

Investigation 2: How do chromium, magnesium, and zinc contribute to insulin sensitivity and blood sugar regulation in women with PCOS?

Investigation 3: How does oxidative stress impact women with PCOS, and what strategies can be employed to mitigate its effects on their health?

Investigation 4: How does the intake of specific nutrients such as vitamin D, vitamin B, fiber, and protein contribute to managing and improving the symptoms of PCOS in women?

3.5 Methodology

There are several important phases involved in training a DL model with a PCOS dataset as shown in Fig. 3.3. First, to ensure quality and consistency, relevant patient information is gathered and preprocessed, including test results, medical history, and demographics. Next, methods for feature extraction or selection are used to determine which factors are most useful for PCOS prediction. After choosing a suitable DL architecture, the model is trained on a split dataset using optimization techniques. To improve model performance, hyperparameter tuning is carried out, and then the model is evaluated using metrics such as accuracy and F1 score. Eventually, the model can be interpreted to understand its decision-making process. Finally, after thorough evaluation and compliance with healthcare regulations, the model can be deployed to aid healthcare professionals in diagnosing PCOS and providing personalized treatments. After completing the training of a DL model for PCOS prediction, it's crucial to consider the role of nutrients in managing and reducing PCOS symptoms. Women with PCOS may benefit from specific nutrients, which have been shown to support insulin sensitivity, hormone balance, and general reproductive health. For example, omega-3 fatty acids, which are frequently included in fish oil, have anti-inflammatory qualities and may assist women with PCOS manage their menstrual cycles and insulin resistance.

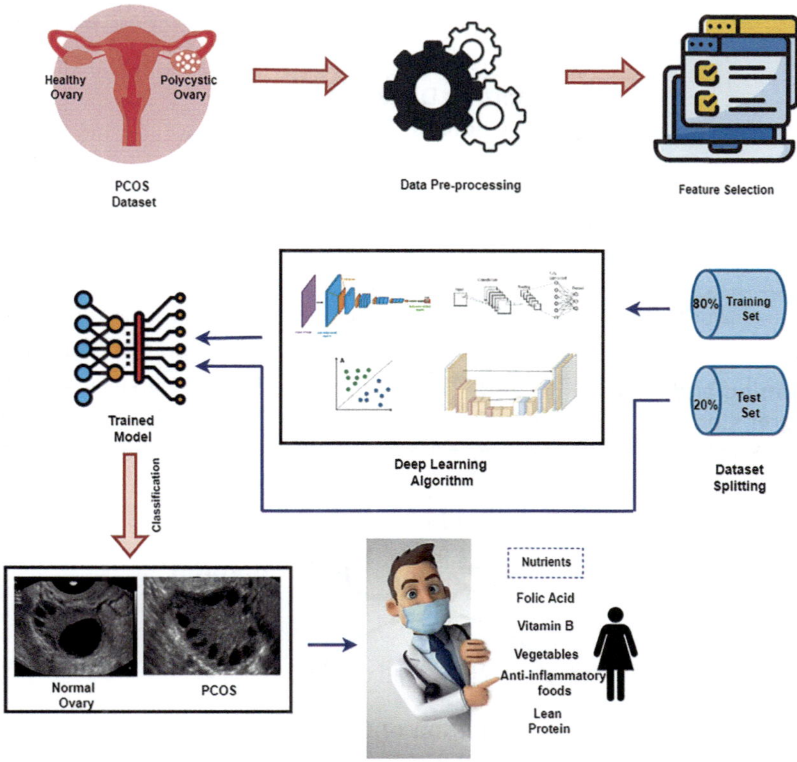

Fig. 3.3 Analysis of the proposed study's architectural framework for predicting PCOS syndrome

3.6 Discussion

This section provides a comprehensive overview of the various investigations undertaken in the study.

Investigation 1: How can AI-based nutritional interventions be utilized to address PCOS symptoms effectively?

P.S. There are multiple methods in which AI-based nutritional treatments might be utilized to effectively manage symptoms of PCOS. In order to find patterns and connections that could either cause PCOS to develop or worsen its symptoms, AI systems can firstly examine enormous volumes of data, including patient demographics, medical histories, dietary preferences, and biomarkers. By tailoring dietary suggestions to each person's unique needs and features, this analysis can assist maximize treatment results. Second, meal plans and dietary recommendations that are customized to meet the unique needs and tastes of every patient can be obtained using AI-powered platforms. Nutrient-dense meals that support hormone balance, control insulin sensitivity, and regulate weight which are all important aspects of controlling PCOS may be the emphasis of

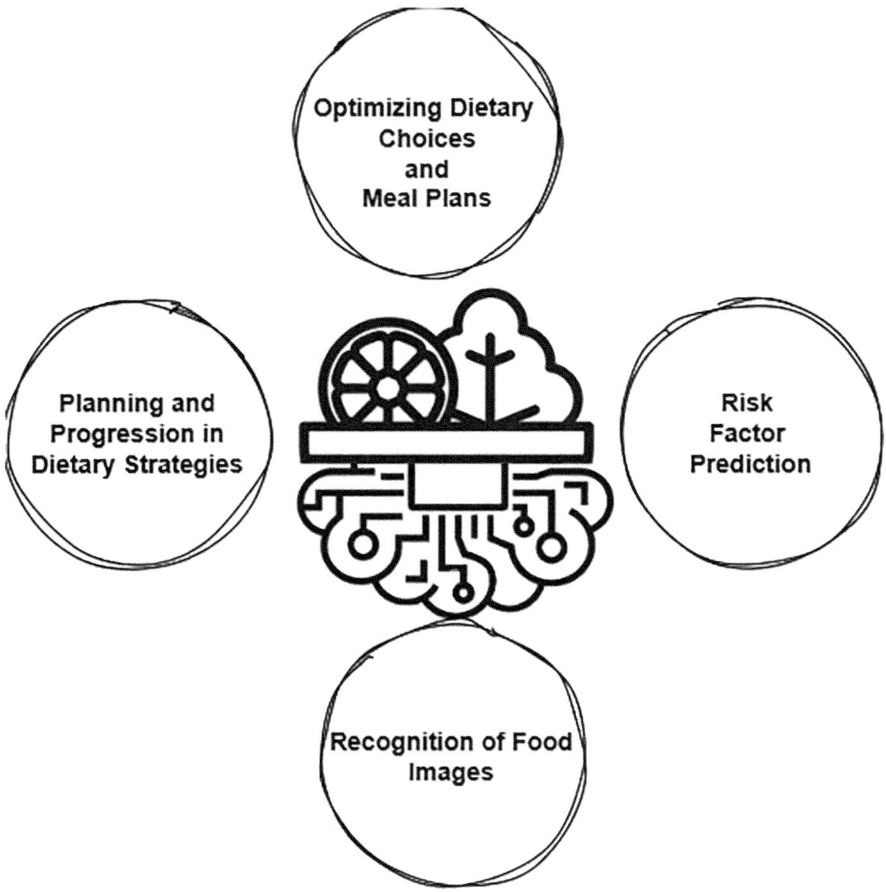

Fig. 3.4 AI-based nutritional interventions

these recommendations. Furthermore, AI is able to adapt to changing needs and provide continuous support by continuously monitoring patient progress and modifying nutritional therapies in real time depending on feedback and changes in health condition. Overall, AI-based nutritional interventions offer a promising approach to managing PCOS by providing personalized, data-driven guidance (as shown in Fig. 3.4) and support to improve symptom management and overall health outcomes.

Investigation 2: How do chromium, magnesium, and zinc contribute to insulin sensitivity and blood sugar regulation in women with PCOS?

P.S. Micronutrients like zinc, magnesium, and chromium are crucial for blood sugar control and insulin sensitivity as shown in Fig. 3.5. This is especially true for women who have PCOS, a disorder that is frequently linked to insulin resistance [32].

Fig. 3.5 Regulation of insulin levels and management of blood sugar levels

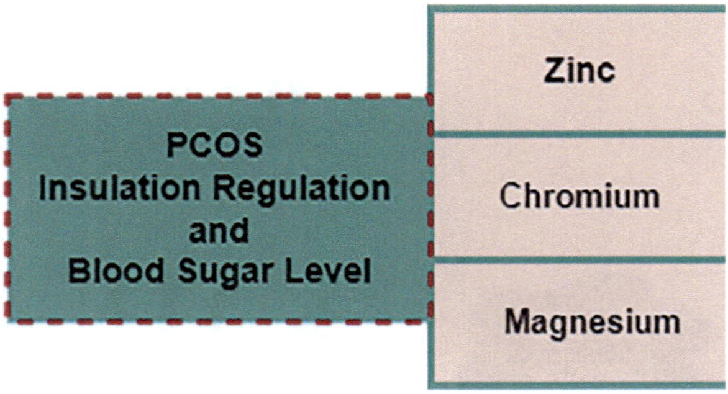

Chromium: Insulin signaling and glucose metabolism are two processes that chromium is related to. It increases insulin's ability to bind to cells, which makes it easier for the body to absorb and metabolize glucose. It has been demonstrated that chromium supplements increase insulin sensitivity in people with insulin resistance, especially PCOS-affected women. Chromium can help control blood sugar levels and lower the risk of issues related to insulin resistance, like type 2 diabetes, by improving insulin sensitivity.

Magnesium: The body uses magnesium for more than 300 metabolic processes, including insulin signaling and glucose metabolism. Since magnesium shortage has been connected to insulin resistance, it is essential to the function of insulin. Magnesium supplementation has been demonstrated to enhance insulin sensitivity and glucose tolerance in PCOS-affected women, possibly lowering their chance of type 2 diabetes and other metabolic issues related to PCOS.

Zinc: Insulin synthesis, storage, and secretion are all impacted by zinc. Furthermore, it influences glucose metabolism and insulin sensitivity. Insulin resistance and decreased glucose tolerance have been linked to zinc deficiency. Zinc supplementation has been demonstrated to increase insulin sensitivity and lower inflammatory indicators in women with PCOS, as these markers are frequently raised in PCOS. Zinc may help women with PCOS regulate their blood sugar levels better by promoting insulin action and lowering inflammation. Zinc, magnesium, and chromium are crucial minerals that support blood sugar control and insulin sensitivity in PCOS-affected women. By taking these micronutrient supplements, one may be able to decrease the risk of PCOS-related metabolic problems and enhance insulin sensitivity and glucose metabolism.

Investigation 3: How does oxidative stress impact women with PCOS, and what strategies can be employed to mitigate its effects on their health?

P.S. The PCOS is significantly influenced by oxidative stress, which is defined as an imbalance between the body's antioxidant defenses and the creation of reactive oxygen species (ROS). Oxidative stress markers are frequently elevated in women with PCOS, and this can lead to a number of conditions related to the illness, such as insulin resistance, inflammation, an increased risk of cardiovascular disease, and infertility [33]. Several strategies (as shown in Fig. 3.6) can be used to reduce the negative impact of oxidative stress on the health of women with PCOS:

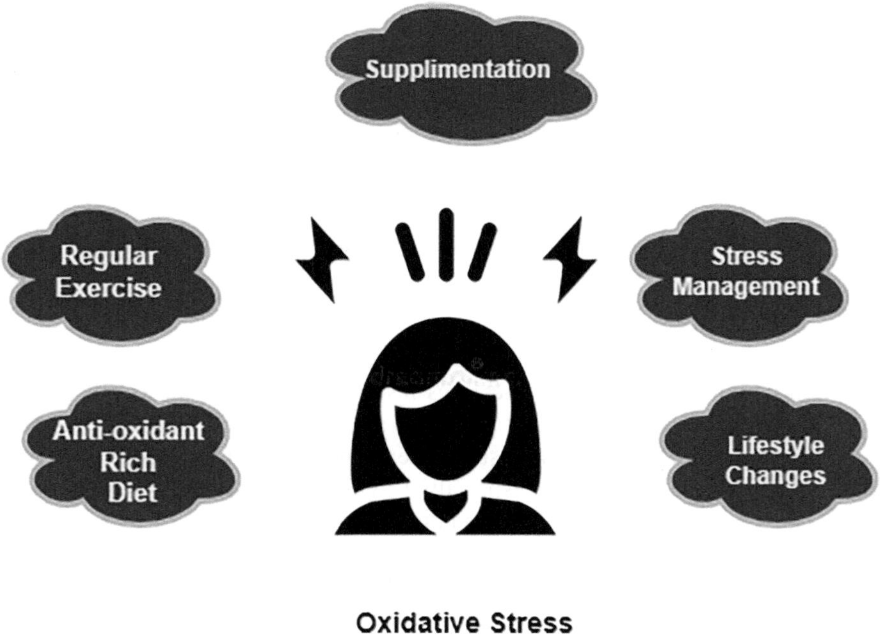

Fig. 3.6 Oxidative stress impact on women

Antioxidant-rich diet: Adopting a diet high in antioxidants can be very beneficial for women with PCOS in controlling the condition's intricate metabolic and reproductive elements. Women with PCOS may be able to reduce inflammation, manage weight, support reproductive health, lower their risk of cardiovascular and metabolic diseases, improve insulin sensitivity, and mitigate oxidative stress by focusing on foods high in antioxidants, such as colorful fruits and vegetables, nuts, seeds, whole grains, legumes, herbs, and spices. This dietary strategy promotes general well-being and addresses important aspects of PCOS, offering a variety of advantages. It is imperative to maintain a balanced diet and seek advice from medical professionals in order to customize nutritional approaches to meet specific requirements and maximize their efficacy in PCOS management.

Supplementation: Women with PCOS may benefit further from antioxidant supplements that target oxidative stress and its related issues. These supplements include vitamin C, vitamin E, selenium, and coenzyme Q10. Coenzyme Q10, sometimes referred to as ubiquinone, is an antioxidant that lowers oxidative damage to cellular components and is essential for the synthesis of mitochondrial energy. Research has indicated that administering these antioxidant supplements to women with PCOS can help improve oxidative stress markers, lower inflammation, and improve insulin sensitivity.

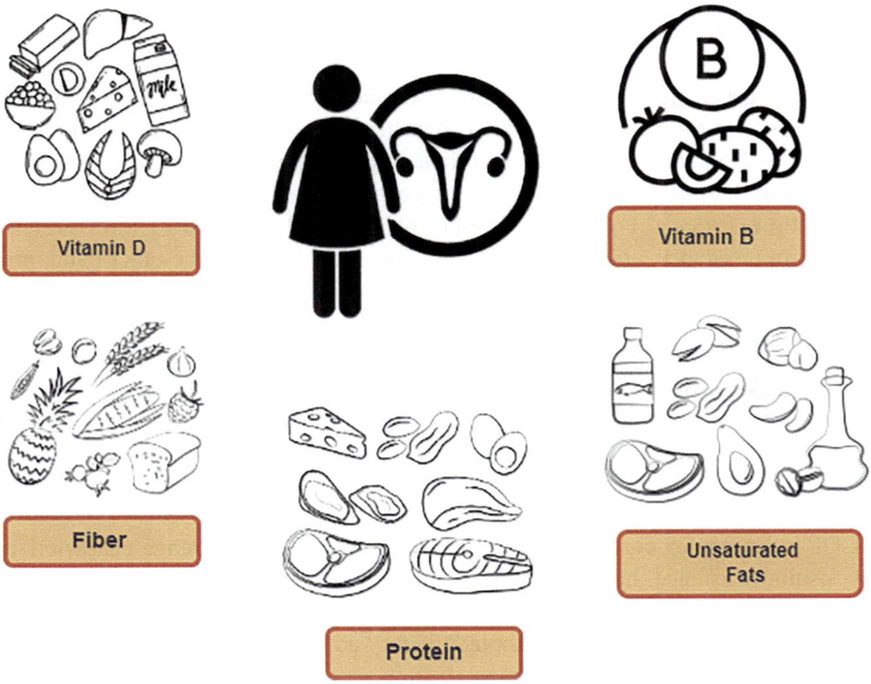

Fig. 3.7 Vitamins needed for women with PCOS

Regular exercise: Regular physical activity has been demonstrated to lower oxidative stress and boost antioxidant enzyme activity in PCOS-affected women. It can be advantageous to include yoga, strength training, or aerobic activity in the regimen.

Stress management: Prolonged stress can raise the amount of oxidative stress. Stress management and oxidative damage reduction are possible with methods including progressive muscle relaxation, deep breathing exercises, and mindfulness meditation.

Lifestyle changes: Reducing alcohol intake, quitting smoking, and exposing women with PCOS to less pollutants in the environment can all help lower their levels of oxidative stress.

By employing these techniques, women diagnosed with PCOS may be able to lower their levels of oxidative stress, enhance their general well-being, and lessen the likelihood of PCOS-related issues. Before implementing any major dietary or lifestyle changes, though, it is imperative to speak with a healthcare professional, particularly someone who is thinking about taking medicine or supplements.

Investigation 4: How does the intake of specific nutrients such as vitamin D, vitamin B, fiber, and protein contribute to managing and improving the symptoms of PCOS in women?

P.S. Key nutrients play essential roles in managing the array of symptoms associated with PCOS. Certain nutrients, such as fiber, protein, vitamin B, and vitamin D, are crucial for controlling and reducing the symptoms of PCOS in females as shown in Fig. 3.7. In order to address frequent problems in PCOS, vitamin D supports insulin sensitivity, controls menstrual cycles, and lowers inflammation [9]. The B vitamins B6, B12, and folate, in particular, help with energy metabolism and hormone balance, which is essential for reducing irregular cycles and insulin resistance. Foods high in fiber help control blood sugar levels, reduce insulin resistance, and aid in weight management [11]. On the other hand, protein aids in blood sugar regulation, muscle building, and hormone synthesis. B vitamin sources like leafy greens and lean meats, vitamin D-rich foods like fatty fish and fortified dairy, fiber rich fruits, vegetables, and whole grains and protein sources like chicken and lentils can all be included in a diet [13].

3.7 Conclusion

PCOS is a complex condition that presents a multifaceted challenge characterized by insulin resistance, hyperandrogenism, and a spectrum of metabolic, endocrine, reproductive, and psychological implications. Even though PCOS is common, its precise cause is yet unknown. Although dietary adjustments, physical activity, and nutritional supplementation are typical therapy approaches, more research is needed to determine the exact effectiveness of these changes and how best to apply them. The results of this study provide insight into the possible therapeutic benefits of certain nutrients, including isoflavonoids, resveratrol, vitamin D, and inositol, in treating the hormonal and metabolic abnormalities linked to PCOS. For individualized treatment plans, however, an in-depth understanding and validation of the formulations, doses, and long-term effectiveness of these interventions are necessary. The results of this study illuminate the possible therapeutic benefits of particular nutrients, opening the door to AI-assisted personalized therapy regimens that necessitate careful formulation, dosage, and long-term effectiveness validation for a comprehensive approach to PCOS management.

References

1. Rodriguez Paris V, Solon-Biet SM, Senior AM, Edwards MC, Desai R, Tedla N, Walters KA. Defining the impact of dietary macronutrient balance on PCOS traits. Nat Commun. 2020;11(1):5262.
2. Faghfoori Z, Fazelian S, Shadnoush M, Goodarzi R. Nutritional management in women with polycystic ovary syndrome: a review study. Diabetes Metab Syndr Clin Res Rev. 2017;11:S429–32.
3. Che X, Chen Z, Liu M, Mo Z. Dietary interventions: a promising treatment for polycystic ovary syndrome. Ann Nutr Metab. 2021;77(6):313–23.
4. Zaeemzadeh N, Jahanian Sadatmahalleh S, Ziaei S, Kazemnejad A, Movahedinejad M, Mottaghi A, Mohamadzadeh N. Comparison of dietary micronutrient intake in PCOS patients with and without metabolic syndrome. J Ovarian Res. 2021;14:1–9.

5. Szczuko M, Skowronek M, Zapalowska-Chwyc M, Starczewski A. Quantitative assessment of nutrition in patients with polycystic ovary syndrome (PCOS). Rocz Panstw Zakl Hig. 2016;67(4):419.
6. Cowan S, Lim S, Alycia C, Pirotta S, Thomson R, Gibson-Helm M, et al. Lifestyle management in polycystic ovary syndrome–beyond diet and physical activity. BMC Endocr Disord. 2023;23(1):14.
7. Calcaterra V, Verduci E, Cena H, Magenes VC, Todisco CF, Tenuta E, Zuccotti G. Polycystic ovary syndrome in insulin-resistant adolescents with obesity: the role of nutrition therapy and food supplements as a strategy to protect fertility. Nutrients. 2021;13(6):1848.
8. Selen H, Yeşilkaya B. The role of dietary supplements and lifestyle changes in reducing polycystic ovary syndrome complications. Hacettepe Univ Faculty Health Sci J. 2021;8(3):453–65.
9. Rawat A. Polycystic ovarian syndrome: role of nutrition, vitamins, and minerals—myoinositol and vitamin D3. J S Asian Fed Obstet Gynaecol. 2020;12(2):63–4.
10. Farshchi H, Rane A, Love A, Kennedy RL. Diet and nutrition in polycystic ovary syndrome (PCOS): pointers for nutritional management. J Obstet Gynaecol. 2007;27(8):762–73.
11. Dubey P, Reddy S, Boyd S, Bracamontes C, Sanchez S, Chattopadhyay M, Dwivedi A. Effect of nutritional supplementation on oxidative stress and hormonal and lipid profiles in PCOS-affected females. Nutrients. 2021;13(9):2938.
12. Szczuko M, Sankowska P, Zapalowska-Chwyc M, Wysokinski P. Studies on the quality nutrition in women with polycystic ovary syndrome (PCOS). Rocz Panstw Zakl Hig. 2017;68(1):61.
13. Papavasiliou K, Papakonstantinou E. Nutritional support and dietary interventions for women with polycystic ovary syndrome. Nutr Diet Suppl. 2017;9:63–85.
14. Barrea L, Verde L, Camajani E, Cernea S, Frias-Toral E, Lamabadusuriya D, Muscogiuri G. Ketogenic diet as medical prescription in women with polycystic ovary syndrome (PCOS). Curr Nutr Rep. 2023;12(1):56–64.
15. Barrea L, Marzullo P, Muscogiuri G, Di Somma C, Scacchi M, Orio F, Savastano S. Source and amount of carbohydrate in the diet and inflammation in women with polycystic ovary syndrome. Nutr Res Rev. 2018;31(2):291–301.
16. Elmannai H, El-Rashidy N, Mashal I, Alohali MA, Farag S, El-Sappagh S, Saleh H. Polycystic ovary syndrome detection machine learning model based on optimized feature selection and explainable artificial intelligence. Diagnostics. 2023;13(8):1506.
17. Suha SA, Islam MN. An extended machine learning technique for polycystic ovary syndrome detection using ovary ultrasound image. Sci Rep. 2022;12(1):17123.
18. Lv W, Song Y, Fu R, Lin X, Su Y, Jin X, Huang G. Deep learning algorithm for automated detection of polycystic ovary syndrome using scleral images. Front Endocrinol. 2022;12:789878.
19. Alamoudi A, Khan IU, Aslam N, Alqahtani N, Alsaif HS, Al Dandan O, Al Bahrani R. A deep learning fusion approach to diagnosis the polycystic ovary syndrome (PCOS). Appl Comput Intell Soft Comput. 2023;2023 https://doi.org/10.1155/2023/9686697.
20. Barrera FJ, Brown ED, Rojo A, Obeso J, Plata H, Lincango EP, Shekhar S. Application of machine learning and artificial intelligence in the diagnosis and classification of polycystic ovarian syndrome: a systematic review. Front Endocrinol. 2023;14:1106625.
21. Khanna VV, Chadaga K, Sampathila N, Prabhu S, Bhandage V, Hegde GK. A distinctive explainable machine learning framework for detection of polycystic ovary syndrome. Appl Syst Innov. 2023;6(2):32.
22. Sumathi M, Chitra P, Prabha RS, Srilatha K. Study and detection of PCOS related diseases using CNN. In: IOP conference series: materials science and engineering, Feb 2021, vol. 1070(1). IOP Publishing; 2021. p. 012062.
23. Nsugbe E. An artificial intelligence-based decision support system for early diagnosis of polycystic ovaries syndrome. Healthc Anal. 2023;3:100164.
24. Ahmed S, Rahman MS, Jahan I, Kaiser MS, Hosen AS, Ghirime D, Kim SH. A review on the detection techniques of polycystic ovary syndrome using machine learning. IEEE Access. 2023;11:86522.

25. Bedi P, Goyal SB, Rajawat AS, Kumar M. An integrated adaptive bilateral filter-based framework and attention residual U-net for detecting polycystic ovary syndrome. Decision Anal J. 2024;10:100366.
26. Lim J, Li J, Feng X, Feng L, Xia Y, Xiao X, Xu Z. Machine learning classification of polycystic ovary syndrome based on radial pulse wave analysis. BMC Complement Med Ther. 2023;23(1):409.
27. Thakre V, Vedpathak S, Thakre K, Sonawani S. PCOcare: PCOS detection and prediction using machine learning algorithms. Biosci Biotechnol Res Commun. 2020;13(14):240–4.
28. Kaur N, Gupta G, Kaur P. Transfer-based deep learning technique for PCOS detection using ultrasound images. In: 2023 International conference on network, multimedia and information technology (NMITCON), Sept 2023. IEEE; 2023. p. 1–6.
29. Tiwari S, Maheshwari P. PCOS-WaveConvNet: a wavelet convolutional neural network for polycystic ovary syndrome detection using ultrasound images. In: 2023 9th International conference on information technology trends (ITT), May 2023. IEEE; 2023. p. 117–22.
30. Adla YAA, Raydan DG, Charaf MZJ, Saad RA, Nasreddine J, Diab MO. Automated detection of polycystic ovary syndrome using machine learning techniques. In: 2021 Sixth international conference on advances in biomedical engineering (ICABME), Oct 2021. IEEE; 2021. p. 208–12.
31. Hosain AS, Mehedi MHK, Kabir IE. Pconet: a convolutional neural network architecture to detect polycystic ovary syndrome (PCOS) from ovarian ultrasound images. In: 2022 International conference on engineering and emerging technologies (ICEET), Oct 2022. IEEE; 2022. p. 1–6.
32. Günalan E, Yaba A, Yılmaz B. The effect of nutrient supplementation in the management of polycystic ovary syndrome-associated metabolic dysfunctions: a critical review. J Turk German Gynecol Assoc. 2018;19(4):220.
33. Rudnicka E, Duszewska AM, Kucharski M, Tyczyński P, Smolarczyk R. Oxidative stress and reproductive function: oxidative stress in polycystic ovary syndrome. Reproduction. 2022;164(6):F145–54.

4 AI-Powered Personalized Nutrition: How AI Can Customize Nutrition Plans Based on Individual PCOS Profiles

Ushaa Eswaran, Vivek Eswaran, Keerthna Murali, and Vishal Eswaran

4.1 Introduction

Polycystic ovary syndrome (PCOS) is a common yet complex endocrine disorder affecting women of reproductive age. It is characterized by a constellation of symptoms including ovarian dysfunction, hyperandrogenism, and polycystic ovarian morphology, often accompanied by metabolic complications such as obesity, insulin resistance, and inflammation. PCOS not only imposes a significant clinical burden but also carries substantial economic and psychological impacts, with annual costs per patient exceeding $12,000 in certain settings [1].

The heterogeneity that marks the presentation of PCOS, ranging from mild irregular cycles to full-fledged metabolic syndrome, poses a significant challenge in its management. Additionally, the intricate gene-environment interactions driving the pathogenesis of PCOS contribute to its complexity. Despite its high prevalence and disruptive lifelong symptomatology, most existing management approaches fail to address the nuanced, personalized needs of distinct PCOS phenotypes [2].

U. Eswaran (✉)
Department of ECE, Mahalakshmi Tech Campus, Chennai, Tamil Nadu, India

V. Eswaran
Medallia, Austin, TX, USA

K. Murali
Dell EMC, CKAD, AWS CSAA, Austin, TX, USA

V. Eswaran
CVS Health Centre, Dallas, TX, USA

R. Kumar et al. (eds.), *AI-Based Nutritional Intervention in Polycystic Ovary Syndrome (PCOS)*, https://doi.org/10.1007/978-981-96-2120-0_4

Mainstay strategies for PCOS management comprise lifestyle modifications encompassing diet, physical activity, weight management, and psychological support [3]. However, a glaring gap persists in translating broad guidelines into precise, phenotype-targeted prescriptions that align recommended dietary changes with the distinctive metabolic terrain underlying each PCOS variant. This likely contributes to suboptimal adherence and efficacy of conventional therapy [4].

The emerging field of precision nutrition, fueled by advances in artificial intelligence (AI) and machine learning (ML), holds immense potential to bridge this void. By harnessing the power of these technologies, personalized dietary recommendations can be tailored based on an individual's unique PCOS phenotype, capturing the intrinsic heterogeneity in pathophysiology. This chapter proposes a blueprint leveraging explainable AI (XAI) techniques to provide personalized nutrition therapy for PCOS, encompassing data gathering, phenotype dissection, mapping nutrition to outcomes, continual optimization, and addressing adoption barriers.

Figure 4.1 [5] shows an AI-powered precision nutrition pipeline for PCOS management which is a comprehensive flow diagram illustrating the proposed AI-driven pipeline for providing personalized nutrition recommendations to women with PCOS. It could depict the various stages, including data collection, phenotype dissection using explainable AI, mapping nutrition to phenotypes, continual optimization, and addressing adoption challenges.

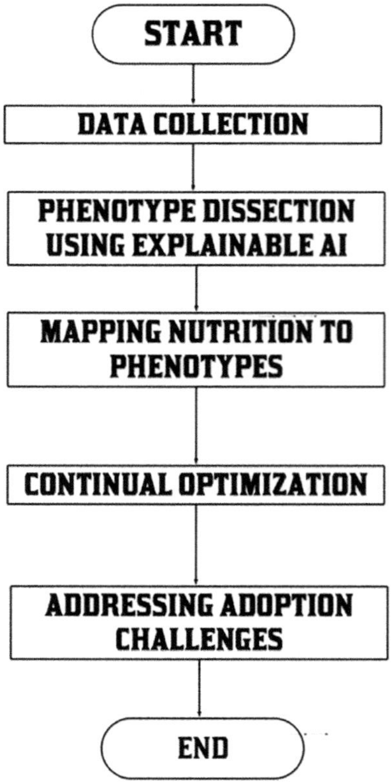

Fig. 4.1 AI-powered precision nutrition pipeline for PCOS management

Advancing Precision Nutrition for PCOS via AI

The growing field of precision nutrition [6] endeavors to bridge this void by harnessing advances in artificial intelligence (AI) and machine learning [7] to enable customized dietary recommendations based on an individual's phenotypic profile. Early successes demonstrating improved engagement and outcomes have been reported in areas like prediabetes and cardiovascular health. A similar model tailored to capture the intrinsic heterogeneity in PCOS pathophysiology holds immense yet untapped potential to enhance the lives of millions of women [8].

The chapter delves into the compiling of an exhaustive PCOS database by assimilating multidimensional inputs across pertinent domains, including symptom tracking, clinical evaluation, biochemical assays, dietary assessment, gut microbiome mapping, and multi-omics profiling. Subsequently, it explores the application of XAI algorithms to dissect distinctive phenotypes and connect them to optimal nutrition via machine learning models. The chapter also addresses the continual optimization of recommendations through phenotype-targeted randomized controlled trials (RCTs) and the integration of patient-reported outcomes. Finally, it delineates opportunities and challenges surrounding the adoption of AI-enabled personalized nutrition prescriptions, such as clinician engagement, user experience, and access barriers.

This chapter proposes a blueprint leveraging explainable AI (XAI) techniques to provide personalized nutrition therapy for PCOS by systematically

1. Compiling an exhaustive PCOS database via multi-domain data gathering
2. Dissecting distinctive phenotypes through XAI algorithms
3. Connecting phenotype to optimal nutrition via ML
4. Continual optimization of recommendations via RCTs
5. Overcoming adoption barriers

Objectives of the Chapter

The objectives of the chapter are:

- To propose an AI-based precision nutrition model for providing customized dietary recommendations for PCOS by systematically assimilating multi-domain data.
- To explore the use of explainable AI techniques for deciphering pathology and dissecting distinctive PCOS phenotypes.
- To outline a methodology for mapping dietary components to outcomes via machine learning algorithms and continually updating recommendations.
- And, to delineate opportunities and challenges around advancing the adoption of AI-enabled personalized nutrition prescriptions for PCOS management.

Organization of the Chapter

The rest of the chapter is organized as: Section 4.2 discusses the compilation of an exhaustive PCOS database through multi-domain data gathering, including symptom tracking, clinical evaluation, biochemical assays, dietary assessment, gut microbiome mapping, and multi-omics profiling. Section 4.3 explores the use of explainable AI techniques, such as SHAP analysis and local interpretable model-agnostic explanations (LIME), to dissect distinctive PCOS phenotypes. Section 4.4 outlines the process of mapping nutrition recommendations to PCOS phenotypes using machine learning models and advanced personalized nutrition strategies. Section 4.5 discusses the continual optimization of therapeutic recommendations through phenotype-targeted randomized controlled trials (RCTs) and the integration of patient-reported outcomes. Section 4.6 delineates opportunities and challenges in advancing the adoption of AI-enabled personalized nutrition prescriptions, including clinician engagement, user experience, and access barriers. And, finally, Sect. 4.7 concludes the chapter with future scope.

4.2 Understanding Polycystic Ovary Syndrome (PCOS)

4.2.1 Compiling an Exhaustive PCOS Database

The first milestone lies in portraying a holistic snapshot of one's unique PCOS phenotype. This requires assimilating multidimensional inputs across pertinent domains encompassing the following:

4.2.1.1 Symptom Tracking

Symptoms tracking is a process that begins with the systematic monitoring of the lived experiences of women with PCOS, self-reported via mobile applications, wearables, and journals. Key areas include:

To compile an exhaustive PCOS database, it is crucial to systematically monitor and track the various symptoms experienced by women with PCOS. This can be done through self-reporting using mobile applications, wearables, and journals [9]. The following key areas to be considered are as follows:

Menstrual disturbances: Menstrual irregularities are a hallmark of PCOS. Women may experience oligomenorrhea (infrequent periods), amenorrhea (absence of periods), or abnormal uterine bleeding. Tracking the frequency and duration of menstrual cycles, along with any associated symptoms, can provide valuable insights into the hormonal imbalances present in each individual.

Signs of androgen excess: Hyperandrogenism is a common characteristic of PCOS. Symptoms such as hirsutism (excessive hair growth), acne, and alopecia (hair loss) should be monitored and quantified. Assessing the severity and distribution of these symptoms can help determine the degree of androgen excess and guide personalized treatment approaches.

Fertility health: PCOS is often associated with difficulties in conceiving and maintaining pregnancy. Tracking conception rates, pregnancy outcomes, and any relevant reproductive health parameters can provide valuable information about the impact of PCOS on fertility. This data can help tailor interventions to improve reproductive outcomes for women with PCOS.

Anthropometric changes: Weight and body composition changes are frequently observed in women with PCOS. Monitoring changes in body weight, body mass index (BMI), waist circumference, and body fat percentage can provide insights into the metabolic disturbances associated with PCOS. This information can guide personalized weight management strategies and help optimize overall health outcomes.

Dermatological manifestations: Certain dermatological manifestations, such as acanthosis nigricans (darkening and thickening of the skin) and skin tags, may be more prevalent in individuals with PCOS. Quantifying the presence and severity of these manifestations can contribute to a more comprehensive understanding of PCOS phenotypes and associated metabolic abnormalities.

Psychological well-being: PCOS can have a significant impact on psychological well-being, leading to increased rates of anxiety, depression, and reduced quality of life. Assessing psychological symptoms using validated scales or questionnaires can help identify individuals who may require additional support and interventions targeting mental health.

By systematically tracking and quantifying these various dimensions of PCOS, a comprehensive database can be created. This database will provide a detailed and individualized snapshot of each person's unique PCOS phenotype, allowing for more personalized and targeted interventions. Additionally, it can serve as a valuable resource for research and further understanding of the condition.

4.2.1.2 Clinical Evaluation

In addition to symptom tracking, a detailed clinical evaluation by the healthcare team is imperative for compiling an exhaustive PCOS database. The 2018 international guidelines on PCOS provide a framework for stratifying PCOS into four phenotypes, each with distinct clinical characteristics:

Frank PCOS: This phenotype represents the classic presentation of PCOS and is characterized by the presence of all three key features: oligo-/anovulation, hyperandrogenism, and polycystic ovarian morphology (PCOM). Oligo-/anovulation refers to infrequent or absent menstrual periods, while hyperandrogenism manifests as clinical signs such as hirsutism, acne, and alopecia. PCOM is identified through ultrasound imaging, which reveals the presence of multiple small follicles in the ovaries. Women with Frank PCOS typically exhibit all three features, providing a clear diagnosis.

Ovulatory PCOS: In this phenotype, women exhibit hyperandrogenism and PCOM but have regular ovulation. They do not experience oligo-/anovulation. This subgroup highlights the heterogeneity of PCOS and suggests that other factors beyond ovulation disturbances contribute to the development of PCOS-related features. Women with ovulatory PCOS may have normal menstrual cycles but still present with hyperandrogenism and polycystic ovaries, indicating the importance of considering other clinical and biochemical features alongside imaging findings.

Non-PCOM PCOS: This phenotype is characterized by the presence of oligo-/anovulation and hyperandrogenism, but without PCOM on ultrasound. These individuals exhibit the hormonal and menstrual irregularities associated with PCOS but may not demonstrate the characteristic ovarian morphology. This highlights the importance of considering clinical and biochemical features alongside imaging findings in diagnosing PCOS. Non-PCOM PCOS may indicate a subset of individuals who have hormonal and metabolic disturbances without the characteristic polycystic ovarian morphology.

Suspected PCOS: This phenotype is characterized by the presence of oligo-/anovulation and PCOM, but without significant hyperandrogenism. These individuals exhibit some features of PCOS but do not meet the criteria for hyperandrogenism. It is essential to consider alternative causes of oligo-/anovulation in these cases, such as thyroid disorders or hyperprolactinemia. Suspected PCOS may require further evaluation and monitoring before a definitive diagnosis can be made.

Table 4.1 summarizes the key clinical features, hormonal profiles, and metabolic parameters associated with various PCOS subtypes, such as frank PCOS, ovulatory PCOS, non-PCOM PCOS, and suspected PCOS. The table provides a clear overview of the heterogeneity within PCOS and aid in understanding the distinct phenotypes discussed in the chapter.

In addition to phenotypic characterization, the clinical evaluation should also encompass an assessment of associated metabolic comorbidities. PCOS is often associated with metabolic disturbances, including obesity, insulin resistance, glucose intolerance, dyslipidemia, and increased cardiovascular risk. Evaluating these metabolic parameters provides a comprehensive understanding of the individual's metabolic health and guides personalized treatment strategies. Assessing factors such as body weight, body mass index (BMI), waist circumference, fasting glucose levels, lipid profile, and cardiovascular risk factors helps identify individuals at higher risk for metabolic complications and informs targeted interventions.

By incorporating a detailed clinical evaluation into the PCOS database, healthcare professionals can gain a deeper understanding of each individual's phenotype and associated metabolic risks. This information enables personalized interventions and tailored management strategies that address the specific needs of each PCOS subtype. It also facilitates the identification of potential comorbidities and enables early intervention and appropriate monitoring to mitigate long-term health risks associated with PCOS.

4.2.1.3 Biochemical Assays: Comprehensive Health Assessment for Personalized Care

Androgen Profile Analysis

The androgen profile encompasses a suite of crucial hormones influencing various physiological functions. Testosterone, androstenedione, and DHEA sulphate, prominent androgens, regulate muscle mass, bone density, libido, and overall

Table 4.1 Phenotypic characteristics of different PCOS subtypes

Subtype	Clinical features	Hormonal profiles	Metabolic parameters
Frank PCOS	– Irregular menstrual cycles	– Elevated levels of androgens (testosterone, DHEAS) [10]	– Insulin resistance [10]
	– Clinical or biochemical hyperandrogenism	– LH:FSH ratio >2:1 [10]	– Increased risk of type 2 diabetes [10]
	– Polycystic ovaries on ultrasound (PCOM)	– Increased LH levels [10]	– Dyslipidemia (elevated LDL, decreased HDL) [10]
	– Exclusion of other androgen excess disorders	– Normal or elevated FSH levels [10]	
Ovulatory PCOS	– Irregular menstrual cycles	– Elevated LH:FSH ratio [11]	– Mild insulin resistance [11]
	– Clinical or biochemical hyperandrogenism	– Normal androgen levels [11]	– Increased risk of cardiovascular diseases [11]
	– Normal ovarian morphology on ultrasound	– Normal LH levels [11]	– Abdominal obesity [11]
	– Exclusion of other causes of hyperandrogenism	– Normal FSH levels [11]	
Non-PCOM PCOS	– Irregular menstrual cycles	– Normal LH:FSH ratio [12]	– Variable insulin sensitivity [12]
	– Clinical or biochemical hyperandrogenism	– Normal androgen levels [12]	– Normal lipid profile [12]
	– Normal ovarian morphology on ultrasound	– Normal LH and FSH levels [12]	– Risk factors vary based on metabolic profile [12]
Suspected PCOS	– Irregular menstrual cycles	– Variable hormonal profiles	– Variable metabolic parameters
	– Clinical signs of hyperandrogenism	– Inconclusive hormonal tests	– Requires further investigation

vitality. Variations in these hormones may signal issues like hypogonadism, affecting reproductive health, bone density, and energy levels. An in-depth analysis aids in identifying hormonal imbalances, guiding therapeutic interventions and lifestyle modifications for optimal well-being.

Case Study 1: Hormonal Imbalance and Reproductive Health

Sarah, a 30-year-old woman, presented with irregular menstrual cycles and fertility concerns. Hormonal assays revealed elevated LH levels and decreased FSH, indicating potential PCOS. This information guided Sarah's treatment, including lifestyle modifications and medication, leading to regular cycles and improved fertility outcomes.

Gonadotropins: FSH and LH Concentrations

FSH and LH play pivotal roles in reproductive health, regulating ovulation, menstrual cycles, and sperm production. Fluctuations in these hormones may indicate infertility, polycystic ovary syndrome (PCOS), or pituitary gland disorders. Accurate measurements enable early detection and management of reproductive issues, supporting family planning and fertility treatments.

Case Study 2: Metabolic Health and Cardiovascular Risk

John, a 45-year-old man, had a family history of heart disease. His lipid panel and glycemic indices showed elevated LDL cholesterol and borderline high blood sugar. Based on these results, John adopted a balanced diet, exercise regimen, and lipid-lowering medication. Regular monitoring indicated significant improvements in his cholesterol levels and blood sugar control, reducing his cardiovascular risk.

Insulin and Glycemic Indices, Lipid Panel

These tests offer a comprehensive view of metabolic health. Insulin and glycemic indices assess blood sugar regulation, identifying prediabetes or diabetes risks. Lipid panels indicate cardiovascular health by evaluating cholesterol and triglyceride levels. Monitoring these parameters helps prevent metabolic disorders, guiding dietary adjustments, and medication, reducing the risk of heart disease and diabetes-related complications.

Case Study 3: Inflammatory Markers and Chronic Disease

David, a 55-year-old patient, experienced persistent joint pain and fatigue. Biochemical assays revealed elevated CRP and IL-6 levels. Further investigations confirmed rheumatoid arthritis. Treatment, including anti-inflammatory medication and lifestyle modifications, managed David's symptoms and halted disease progression.

Inflammatory Markers: CRP, IL-6

CRP and IL-6 levels serve as indicators of inflammation, associated with various chronic diseases like heart disease, arthritis, and autoimmune disorders. Elevated levels may signal infection, tissue damage, or inflammatory conditions, necessitating further investigation and targeted treatments to mitigate associated health risks.

Case Study 4: Nutritional Deficiencies Impacting Health

Emma, a 40-year-old woman, complained of chronic fatigue and bone pain. Assessments showed severely low vitamin D levels and borderline folate levels. Supplementation and dietary changes addressed these deficiencies, alleviating her fatigue and improving bone health.

Vitamin D, B12, and Folate Status

Assessing these vitamins helps detect deficiencies that impact bone health, neurological function, and immune response. Vitamin D deficiency can lead to bone diseases, while B12 and folate deficiencies are linked to anemia, neuropathy, and cardiovascular issues. Monitoring and correcting these deficiencies through supplementation and dietary modifications are crucial for overall health and disease prevention.

Case Study 5: Biomarkers Guiding Treatment Response

Susan, a 35-year-old woman with PCOS, displayed elevated testosterone levels alongside insulin resistance markers per initial hormonal assays. She was prescribed an insulin-sensitizing medication alongside lifestyle changes. Follow-up assays after 6 months revealed significant improvements in her insulin levels and lipid profile. However, testosterone continued to remain high. This biomarker data guided modification of her treatment plan, now emphasizing antiandrogen therapy to better target hormonal imbalance.

Case Study 6: Informing Dietary Modifications

Emily, a 27-year-old newly diagnosed with PCOS, underwent a comprehensive hormonal workup. While her androgen levels were normal, assessments showed vitamin D deficiency, elevated triglycerides, and elevated inflammatory marker CRP. Emily also complained of fatigue. Based on her biomarker data, the nutritionist advised vitamin D and omega-3 fatty acid supplementation alongside anti-inflammatory dietary changes emphasizing plant-based foods. Within 3 months, Emily displayed remarkable improvements in her vitamin D, lipid profile, and energy levels.

Each assay provides a comprehensive snapshot of an individual's health, aiding in early detection, personalized treatment plans, and preventive strategies, fostering optimal health and well-being.

4.2.1.4 Dietary Assessment: Precision Nutrition Tracking and Its Impact

Self-Reported Dietary Histories

Self-reported dietary histories, often gathered through food recalls and records, offer valuable insights into an individual's nutritional status. These methodologies provide a retrospective view of one's dietary habits, aiding in understanding patterns, nutritional deficiencies, and areas for improvement. Incorporating technology-enabled methods enhances precision in tracking calories, macronutrients, micronutrients, and food groups.

Case Study 1: Technology-Enabled Nutritional Tracking

Sarah, a 28-year-old woman diagnosed with PCOS, used a dietary tracking app that monitored macronutrients and micronutrients. The app highlighted her high intake of refined carbohydrates and low consumption of fiber. With personalized guidance based on the app's analysis, Sarah made dietary modifications, increasing fiber-rich foods and reducing refined carbs. This significantly improved her glycemic control and energy levels.

Real-Time Example: Health Tracking Wearables
Wearable devices with nutritional tracking capabilities, such as smartwatches, analyze an individual's dietary choices, providing real-time feedback. These devices offer instant insights into calorie consumption, nutrient intake, and adherence to dietary guidelines. Users can adjust their dietary habits based on these insights, promoting healthier eating behaviors.

Dietary Trends in PCOS
Common dietary tendencies in PCOS often include high consumption of refined carbohydrates, low intake of fiber, saturated fats, and inadequate amounts of fruits and vegetables. These patterns can exacerbate hormonal imbalances and metabolic issues characteristic of PCOS.

Case Study 2: Impact of Dietary Modifications
Mark, a 32-year-old diagnosed with PCOS, had a diet high in refined sugars and low in fiber. Guided by a nutritionist, Mark shifted to a balanced diet comprising whole grains, lean proteins, and increased vegetable intake. Over time, this dietary shift aided in stabilizing his blood sugar levels and regulating his hormonal profile, mitigating PCOS symptoms.

Technology-Enabled Precision Nutrition
Utilizing technology for dietary assessment enables accurate and detailed tracking of nutritional intake. Apps and devices allow individuals to precisely monitor calorie intake, macro- and micronutrient composition, and adherence to recommended food groups.

Real-Time Example: AI-Powered Nutrition Apps
AI-driven nutrition apps analyze dietary patterns, recommending personalized meal plans and suggesting healthier food alternatives. These apps use machine learning algorithms to assess an individual's dietary choices, offering tailored nutritional advice and meal options.

Role in Holistic Health Management
Accurate dietary assessments are integral in managing various health conditions, including PCOS. They form the cornerstone for personalized nutrition interventions, aiding in optimizing hormonal balance, managing weight, and improving overall well-being. Incorporating technology-enhanced methodologies augments the accuracy and accessibility of dietary tracking, empowering individuals in their health journey.

Each individual's dietary assessment, combined with precision nutrition tracking, forms a critical component in managing health conditions and promoting overall well-being. Leveraging technology for enhanced dietary monitoring offers promising avenues for personalized health management and improved lifestyle choices.

4.2.1.5 Gut Microbiome Mapping

The gut microbiome's role in health, particularly its impact on metabolic conditions like polycystic ovary syndrome (PCOS), has gained significant attention. PCOS, a hormonal disorder affecting reproductive-age women, often comes with metabolic disturbances such as insulin resistance, obesity, and inflammation [13].

Recent research, as outlined in, suggests that the gut microbiome plays a pivotal role in influencing metabolic health outcomes in PCOS. Techniques like 16S rRNA profiling enable scientists to delve into the composition and functionality of the gut microbial community. This sequencing method allows for the identification of microbial richness (the number of different species present), diversity (the variety of species), and the specific genera that potentially affect insulin sensitivity and inflammation.

For instance, a case study published in the journal *Gut* conducted microbial profiling in women with and without PCOS. The results showcased significant differences in the gut microbiota composition between the two groups. Women with PCOS exhibited lower microbial diversity and altered abundance of certain bacterial genera, notably lower levels of beneficial bacteria like *Bifidobacterium* and higher levels of potentially harmful bacteria like *Lactobacillus*.

Moreover, a longitudinal study followed the dietary and lifestyle changes of women diagnosed with PCOS. Over time, shifts in their gut microbiome were observed alongside improvements in metabolic health markers. Those who adopted a diet rich in fiber, prebiotics, and probiotics demonstrated an increase in microbial diversity and an enhancement in insulin sensitivity.

Real-time examples highlight the potential for personalized interventions targeting the gut microbiome to manage PCOS-related metabolic complications. For instance, a patient with PCOS struggling with insulin resistance might undergo microbiome analysis. Based on the findings, a targeted intervention could involve personalized dietary recommendations, incorporating specific probiotics or prebiotics and lifestyle modifications. Over time, follow-up assessments could reveal changes in the gut microbiota alongside improvements in metabolic health parameters.

16S rRNA sequencing represents a powerful culture-independent technique that enables comprehensive profiling of microbial composition within the gut microbiome. It focuses on the 16S rRNA gene present in bacteria and archaea which contains hypervariable regions that provide species-specific signature sequences.

The methodology relies on isolating microbial DNA from an individual's stool sample. Next, the 16S rRNA gene is targeted using polymerase chain reaction (PCR) to amplify this region. This is followed by high-throughput next generation sequencing, generating vast datasets encompassing millions of DNA reads.

Sophisticated computational pipelines and reference databases facilitate taxonomic classification by mapping the sequenced reads to microbial species based on the unique 16S signature sequences. The final taxonomic assignment provides insights into the microbial richness (number of species), diversity (variety of species), and relative abundances of different genera and species inhabiting the individual's gut.

Certain limitations in taxonomic resolution exist for closely related species. Nevertheless, the 16S rRNA survey delivers a comprehensive snapshot of the gut microbiome composition, providing crucial insights into dysbiosis linked to health conditions like PCOS. Identifying key genera with pro- or anti-inflammatory effects helps match individuals to personalized therapeutic modules including pre-/probiotics.

This high-resolution view of the microbial inhabitants within the gut offered by 16S sequencing is invaluable in understanding microbiome-disease associations, guiding phenotype-targeted interventions.

These studies underscore the intricate interplay between the gut microbiome and metabolic health in PCOS. They also offer promising avenues for future interventions that focus on modulating the gut microbiota to ameliorate metabolic complications associated with this syndrome [14].

4.2.1.6 Multi-omics Profiling Unveiling the Complexity of PCOS: A Comprehensive Approach

Polycystic ovary syndrome (PCOS) represents a multifaceted endocrine disorder affecting women of reproductive age. To unravel the intricate web of factors contributing to its manifestations, the integration of various high-throughput methodologies encompassing genomics, epigenomics, transcriptomics, proteomics, and metabolomics has emerged as a groundbreaking approach, as emphasized in [15, 16].

Consider a longitudinal study encompassing a diverse cohort of women diagnosed with PCOS. This study employed a multi-omics strategy to unravel the underlying molecular mechanisms associated with the syndrome. The genomic analysis identified specific genetic variants associated with steroid synthesis and insulin metabolism, elucidating the genetic underpinnings contributing to the clinical presentations observed in these individuals [17].

For instance, variations in genes encoding enzymes critical for androgen biosynthesis were detected in a subset of women displaying hyperandrogenism, a hallmark feature of PCOS. This genomic insight shed light on the molecular pathways contributing to the excess androgen production observed in these patients [18].

Simultaneously, epigenomic investigations revealed distinctive DNA methylation patterns in genes related to insulin signaling pathways. These epigenetic modifications provided crucial insights into the dysregulation of insulin metabolism commonly observed in individuals with PCOS, further deepening our understanding of the syndrome's molecular intricacies [19].

Transcriptomic analysis offered valuable information by uncovering differential gene expression profiles in tissues relevant to PCOS pathology, such as ovarian or adipose tissue. These expression patterns highlighted specific pathways implicated in irregular menstrual cycles and metabolic disturbances characteristic of the syndrome.

Moreover, proteomic profiling facilitated the identification of pivotal proteins involved in hormonal regulation or metabolic pathways, revealing alterations in protein levels associated with insulin signaling or androgen metabolism in women with PCOS [20].

Further complementing these findings, metabolomic analysis unveiled distinctive metabolic signatures associated with PCOS. Aberrations in certain metabolites linked to insulin resistance, lipid metabolism, and inflammation were identified, providing a unique metabolic fingerprint characteristic of the syndrome.

The integration of multi-omics data, in conjunction with detailed clinical parameters, lifestyle factors, and gut microbiome composition, enabled a comprehensive phenotypic characterization of individuals with PCOS. This holistic approach not only elucidated the intricate molecular landscape contributing to the syndrome but also paved the way for personalized therapeutic plans tailored to address the specific molecular and physiological dysfunctions identified in each patient [21, 22].

For instance, a patient presenting with PCOS exhibiting insulin resistance along with specific genetic variants related to insulin metabolism might receive a highly customized treatment plan. This plan could encompass tailored lifestyle modifications, personalized dietary interventions, exercise regimens, and pharmacological therapies meticulously designed to address the individual's unique genetic predispositions and metabolic imbalances [23].

The integration of multi-omics profiling with clinical data holds immense promise in advancing precision medicine for conditions like PCOS. By allowing for precise and individualized therapeutic strategies based on the unique molecular underpinnings of each patient's condition, this approach represents a significant leap toward more effective management and treatment of complex disorders.

4.3 Dissecting PCOS Subtypes via Explainable AI

The multidimensional dataset aggregated in the previous step must be mined to unravel key phenotypic patterns and associated risks. Conventional analytics fall short in deciphering complex interactions within heterogeneous PCOS data. Explainable AI (XAI) offers a sophisticated solution via techniques like the following:

4.3.1 SHAP Analysis Unveiling Individualized PCOS Manifestations: Case-Based Insights

PCOS represents a multifaceted condition with diverse manifestations and varied impacts on different individuals. Utilizing SHAP analysis within predictive models tailored for PCOS allows for the identification of key features driving specific adverse outcomes, providing a personalized understanding of the syndrome's complexities.

SHAP (SHapley Additive exPlanations) is a game-theoretic approach that calculates the contribution of each feature to the model's prediction. It provides an interpretable and consistent attribution method, allowing for the identification of influential features at both the global and local levels. The SHAP value for a feature represents the change in the predicted outcome when that feature is included or excluded from the model.

The equation is as follows:

$$\varphi\_i = \Sigma\_S \subseteq F\{i\}\left(|S|!(|F| - |S| - 1)!/|F|!\right) * \left(f\left(S \cup \{i\}\right) - f\left(S\right)\right)$$

where φ_i is the SHAP value for feature i, F is the set of all features, and $f(S)$ is the model prediction for the subset of features S.

This equation calculates the SHAP value for a specific feature by considering all possible subsets of features and the change in the model's prediction when that feature is added or removed. The SHAP value is a weighted sum of these changes, with the weights determined by the combination of features and their importance.

By analyzing the SHAP values for each feature, researchers can identify the features that have the most significant impact on the model's predictions for specific individuals or subgroups within the PCOS population. This information can be invaluable for understanding the unique manifestations of PCOS and tailoring personalized treatment and management strategies.

Figure 4.2 [24, 25] illustrates the concept of SHAP analysis and its application in PCOS. It showcases how SHAP attributes importance to specific features in predicting adverse outcomes for individual PCOS cases, aiding in personalized understanding and management strategies.

Python code below is used to generate the SHAP summary plot for identifying influential features in PCOS. This code utilizes the SHAP library along with a random forest classifier model to perform the analysis.

```
import sys
!{sys.executable} -m pip install shap

import shap
import matplotlib.pyplot as plt
import numpy as np
```

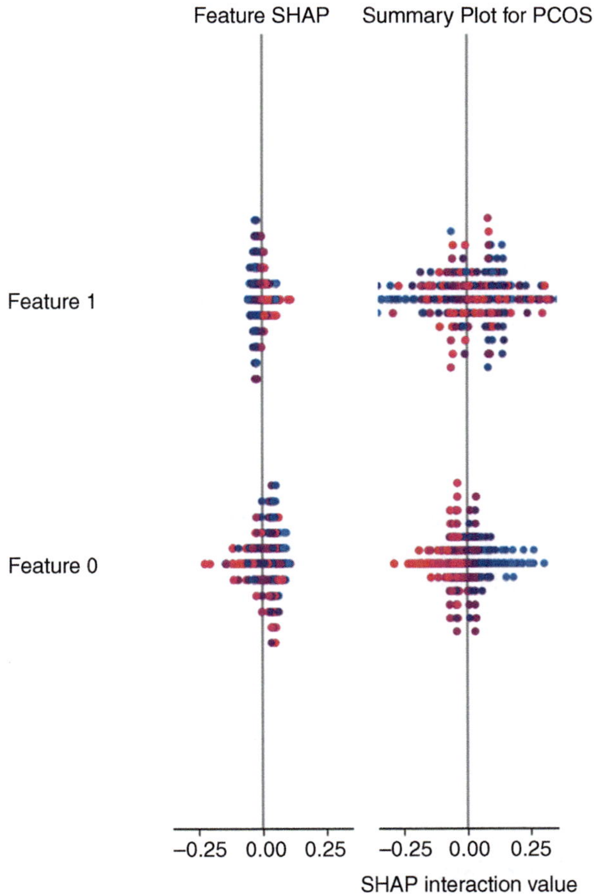

Fig. 4.2 SHAP analysis for identifying influential features in PCOS

```
from sklearn.ensemble import RandomForestClassifier
from sklearn.datasets import make_classification
from sklearn.model_selection import train_test_split

# Generate sample data
X, y = make_classification(n_samples=1000, n_features=10,
n_informative=5, random_state=42)

# Split data into train and test sets
X_train, X_test, y_train, y_test = train_test_split(X, y,
test_size=0.2, random_state=42)

# Train a Random Forest model
model = RandomForestClassifier(random_state=42)
model.fit(X_train, y_train)
```

```
# Calculate SHAP values
explainer = shap.TreeExplainer(model)
shap_values = explainer.shap_values(X_test)

# Check if SHAP values are None
if shap_values is None:
    print("SHAP values are None. Please check your model
and data.")
else:
  # Create a SHAP summary plot
  shap.summary_plot(shap_values, X_test, plot_type="bar",
show=False)
  plt.title("SHAP Summary Plot for PCOS")
  plt.tight_layout()
  plt.show()
```

4.3.1.1 Code to Generate SHAP Analysis for Identifying Influential Features in PCOS

This code generates a SHAP summary plot depicting the importance of different features in predicting outcomes for individual PCOS cases. The plot provides insights into the influential features driving the model's predictions, aiding in the interpretation and understanding of PCOS manifestations.

For example, if elevated levels of anti-Müllerian hormone (AMH) are identified as a crucial feature driving the prediction of subfertility in a particular PCOS case, clinicians can provide targeted fertility counseling and interventions based on this insight.

4.3.1.2 Case Study: SHAP Analysis in Predicting and Understanding PCOS Manifestations

Imagine a cohort of women diagnosed with PCOS, each exhibiting unique clinical presentations. Employing SHAP analysis within predictive models trained on diverse datasets, researchers aimed to uncover key features influencing adverse outcomes in individual PCOS cases [11].

Patient A

Clinical profile: This patient showcases elevated levels of anti-Müllerian hormone (AMH), a common characteristic of PCOS.

SHAP analysis outcome: The SHAP analysis applied to this patient's data reveals the substantial contribution of elevated AMH levels to the model's prediction of subfertility. By attributing higher importance to AMH levels, the model elucidates the strong correlation between elevated AMH and the likelihood of subfertility. This insight empowers clinicians to provide targeted fertility counseling and personalized management strategies, recognizing the association between elevated AMH and increased subfertility risk in this individual.

Patient B

Clinical profile: This patient presents with acanthosis nigricans, a dermatological condition often linked to insulin resistance.

SHAP analysis outcome: In this case, SHAP analysis highlights acanthosis nigricans as a critical feature driving the model's prediction of escalating diabetes risk. The model assigns significant importance to this feature, signaling its strong association with an increased propensity for developing diabetes. This revelation prompts proactive measures such as intensified glucose monitoring, tailored lifestyle modifications, and potentially early intervention strategies to mitigate the risk of diabetes progression.

These case examples vividly illustrate how SHAP analysis discerns specific features driving adverse outcomes in individual PCOS cases. By attributing importance to different features and delineating their impact on predictive models, SHAP analysis equips clinicians with insights to anticipate and intervene in a more personalized manner.

Armed with SHAP analysis insights, healthcare providers can offer tailored counseling, proactive monitoring, and individualized interventions addressing the unique risks and manifestations associated with PCOS in each patient. This tailored approach might involve fertility treatments, intensified metabolic monitoring, lifestyle modifications, or early pharmacological interventions, tailored to the high-impact features identified for each individual.

Ultimately, SHAP analysis stands as a pivotal tool in personalized medicine, facilitating precise risk assessment, prognostication, and bespoke interventions in managing PCOS and its associated complications. This approach empowers clinicians to tailor interventions to individual needs, thereby enhancing patient care and outcomes in the realm of PCOS management.

4.3.2 Local Interpretable Model-Agnostic Explanations (LIME)

LIME is an algorithm that locally approximates complex model predictions to pinpoint influential variables [23]. If obesity and vitamin D deficiency are identified by LIME analysis as key factors driving depression in a woman with PCOS, tailored interventions can be initiated.

In essence, XAI functionality offers granular visibility into paths exacerbating complications within a given patient's unique PCOS footprint. This sets the stage for targeted decision-making. The potential of local interpretable model-agnostic explanations (LIME) in understanding and addressing the complexities of polycystic ovary syndrome (PCOS) in individual cases is increasingly recognized.

4.3.2.1 LIME Unveiling Personalized PCOS Complications: Case-Based Insights

PCOS represents a complex interplay of various factors, making its management challenging. Employing LIME, an algorithm focused on locally approximating complex model predictions, allows for the identification of influential variables in individual cases, paving the way for targeted interventions tailored to a patient's unique PCOS presentation.

4.3.2.2 Case Study: Leveraging LIME Analysis for Tailored Interventions in PCOS

Imagine a scenario involving a group of women diagnosed with PCOS, each exhibiting diverse clinical profiles and manifestations of the syndrome. Researchers utilized LIME to dissect influential factors driving specific complications within each patient's PCOS footprint.

Patient A

Clinical profile: This patient demonstrates obesity and concomitant vitamin D deficiency alongside symptoms of depression.

LIME analysis outcome: LIME analysis reveals that, within this patient's unique PCOS context, obesity and vitamin D deficiency emerge as pivotal factors significantly impacting the model's prediction of depression. The algorithm highlights the influential roles of these factors in exacerbating depressive symptoms in this individual.

Patient B

Clinical profile: This patient presents with irregular menstrual cycles, hyperandrogenism, and insulin resistance.

LIME analysis outcome: For this patient, LIME analysis emphasizes hyperandrogenism and insulin resistance as the primary drivers influencing the model's prediction of metabolic disturbances. By spotlighting these features within the patient's PCOS landscape, LIME highlights their substantial contribution to the observed metabolic imbalances.

These case examples illustrate how LIME enables the identification of influential variables within each patient's unique PCOS context, shedding light on the factors exacerbating specific complications.

The insights gleaned from LIME analysis empower healthcare providers to initiate targeted interventions tailored to individual PCOS footprints. For instance, armed with the understanding that obesity and vitamin D deficiency significantly impact depression in Patient A, clinicians can craft personalized interventions. These interventions might involve tailored lifestyle modifications, such as specialized dietary plans, exercise regimens, and vitamin D supplementation, aimed at mitigating depressive symptoms in this individual.

Similarly, for Patient B, interventions could be focused on managing hyperandrogenism and insulin resistance through tailored pharmaceutical approaches, lifestyle modifications, and hormonal therapies, addressing the specific metabolic disturbances exacerbated by these factors.

In essence, the eXplainable Artificial Intelligence (XAI) functionality offered by LIME provides granular visibility into the pathways exacerbating complications within a patient's unique PCOS presentation. This sets the stage for targeted decision-making and the implementation of tailored interventions, thereby enhancing the precision and effectiveness of PCOS management strategies tailored to each individual's needs.

4.4 Mapping Nutrition Recommendations to PCOS Phenotypes

Advanced Personalized Nutrition in PCOS: Mapping Diet-Disease Variants [26].

4.4.1 Understanding PCOS Subtypes and Phenotypic Diversity

PCOS is a heterogeneous condition, displaying various subtypes with distinct phenotypic presentations. These subtypes may manifest as hyperinsulinemia, be inflammatory, or present with diverse hormonal and metabolic profiles. Recognizing these variations is crucial for tailoring effective nutritional interventions.

4.4.1.1 Machine Learning Models in Identifying Diet-Disease Patterns

Researchers utilize machine learning models to analyze vast datasets encompassing dietary components and clinical outcomes in different PCOS subgroups. These models sift through extensive data to uncover correlations between specific dietary elements and the response within distinct PCOS phenotypes. One of the commonly used machine learning models for this purpose is logistic regression.

Equation is as follows:

$$\log\left(p/(1-p)\right) = \beta\_0 + \beta\_1x\_1 + \beta\_2x\_2 + \cdots + \beta\_nx\_n$$

where p is the probability of a particular outcome (e.g., improved insulin sensitivity), β_0 is the intercept, and β_1, β_2, ..., β_n are the coefficients associated with the predictor variables x_1, x_2, ..., x_n (e.g., dietary components).

This logistic regression equation models the relationship between the predictor variables (dietary components) and the probability of a specific outcome (e.g., improved insulin sensitivity) in a PCOS subgroup. The coefficients (β_1, β_2, ..., β_n) represent the strength and direction of the association between each dietary component and the outcome. A positive coefficient indicates that an increase in the corresponding dietary component is associated with a higher probability of the outcome, while a negative coefficient suggests the opposite.

By training such machine learning models on vast datasets spanning different PCOS phenotypes, researchers can uncover intricate patterns and correlations between dietary elements and clinical responses. These insights facilitate the development of personalized nutritional interventions tailored to the unique metabolic, hormonal, or inflammatory profiles of distinct PCOS subtypes.

4.4.1.2 Case Studies Highlighting Phenotype-Specific Nutritional Interventions

Case Study: Mapping Nutrition to PCOS Inflammatory Phenotype

This case study explores the application of mapping dietary components to specific dysregulated pathways underlying an inflammatory PCOS phenotype, with the goal of tailoring anti-inflammatory nutritional interventions.

Context: A subset of women with PCOS exhibit a predominantly inflammatory profile, characterized by elevated levels of inflammatory markers such as C-reactive protein (CRP), interleukin-6 (IL-6), and tumor necrosis factor-alpha (TNF-α). This chronic low-grade inflammation is associated with metabolic disturbances, including insulin resistance and an increased risk of cardiovascular complications.

Methodology: Researchers employed machine learning techniques to establish connections between various dietary components and their potential influence on inflammatory pathways implicated in PCOS pathogenesis. Specifically, they focused on identifying foods and nutrients with anti-inflammatory properties that could modulate key signaling cascades, such as the nuclear factor-kappa B (NF-κB) pathway, which plays a pivotal role in regulating inflammatory responses.

One dietary component that emerged as a promising candidate was omega-3 fatty acids, particularly those found in fish oil and certain plant sources like flaxseeds and walnuts. Extensive research has demonstrated the anti-inflammatory effects of omega-3 fatty acids, mediated through their ability to inhibit the production of pro-inflammatory cytokines and modulate the activity of transcription factors like NF-κB.

Results: A cohort of women diagnosed with the inflammatory PCOS phenotype was recruited and prescribed a dietary intervention enriched with omega-3 fatty acid sources. Over the course of several months, these individuals underwent regular assessments of inflammatory markers, lipid profiles, and clinical parameters related to PCOS symptomatology.

The findings revealed a significant reduction in circulating levels of CRP, IL-6, and TNF-α among participants adhering to the omega-3-rich dietary regimen. Additionally, improvements were observed in insulin sensitivity, lipid profiles, and subjective reports of PCOS-related symptoms, such as menstrual irregularities and hirsutism.

Implications: This case study demonstrates the potential of leveraging AI-driven approaches to map dietary components to specific pathways dysregulated in distinct PCOS phenotypes. By identifying and incorporating anti-inflammatory foods like omega-3 fatty acids into personalized nutritional plans, healthcare providers can offer targeted interventions for women exhibiting an inflammatory PCOS profile.

Moreover, the observed improvements in metabolic parameters and symptom alleviation highlight the potential benefits of this precision nutrition approach in mitigating the adverse effects of chronic inflammation associated with PCOS. By addressing the underlying inflammatory pathways through tailored dietary modifications, this strategy holds promise for improving overall health outcomes and quality of life for women with this inflammatory PCOS subtype.

Case Study: Targeting Insulin Resistance in Hyperinsulinemia PCOS

In a study focusing on women with hyperinsulinemia PCOS, machine learning models identified a positive correlation between diets rich in myoinositol and improved insulin sensitivity. Consequently, a targeted dietary intervention emphasizing myoinositol-rich foods was prescribed to a subset of these patients [27].

Over time, this cohort showed remarkable improvements in insulin sensitivity markers. These findings underscored the potential of phenotype-specific dietary modifications, guided by machine learning insights, in mitigating insulin resistance within this PCOS subtype.

Case Study: Alleviating Inflammation in Inflammatory PCOS Subtype

Similarly, machine learning analysis among women exhibiting predominantly inflammatory PCOS suggested the efficacy of anti-inflammatory diets. Patients following personalized anti-inflammatory dietary plans rich in omega-3 fatty acids, antioxidants, and anti-inflammatory foods displayed reductions in inflammatory markers and improved symptomatology associated with inflammation.

Real-Time Implementation: Personalized Nutritional Therapy

In a clinical setting, a woman diagnosed with PCOS undergoes thorough phenotypic profiling revealing her subtype characterized by hyperinsulinemia. Utilizing machine learning models that have identified dietary responses linked to this phenotype, a tailored nutritional plan emphasizing myoinositol-rich foods is prescribed.

Follow-up assessments reveal substantial improvements in her insulin sensitivity and metabolic health parameters. This real-time application validates the efficacy of phenotype-specific dietary interventions guided by machine learning-derived insights in addressing the metabolic disturbances inherent in her PCOS subtype.

Impact and Future Implications

These case studies and real-time implementations highlight the potential of machine learning-driven approaches in tailoring nutritional interventions for PCOS subtypes. By delineating phenotype-specific diet-disease patterns, personalized nutritional strategies can be devised to target the unique metabolic, hormonal, or inflammatory features within distinct PCOS subgroups.

This novel approach to personalized nutrition holds promise for improving PCOS management, offering tailored dietary interventions aimed at addressing the specific underlying dysfunctions associated with each subtype. This not only enhances the effectiveness of nutritional therapies but also signifies a significant leap toward precision medicine in PCOS care.

4.4.2 Mapping Diet to Pathways

Mapping diet to pathways dysregulated in polycystic ovary syndrome (PCOS) pathophysiology offers a fascinating avenue to align nutritional interventions with the specific physiological dysfunctions seen in different PCOS phenotypes. This approach, as outlined, involves establishing connections between foods and the pathways implicated in PCOS pathogenesis, such as steroidogenesis, insulin metabolism, and inflammation [28].

4.4.2.1 Precision Nutrition Targeting PCOS Pathways

Understanding Pathophysiological Pathways in PCOS

PCOS manifests through various pathophysiological pathways, including alterations in steroidogenesis, insulin metabolism, and inflammation. Recognizing these pathways is crucial for tailoring precise nutritional interventions [29].

Establishing Relationships Between Foods and Pathways

Researchers explore the relationships between dietary components and the dysregulated pathways in PCOS. For instance, investigations might reveal that spearmint tea exhibits the potential to modulate steroidogenesis, specifically by reducing free testosterone levels in hyperandrogenic phenotypes.

Table 4.2 enlists various dietary components (e.g., spearmint tea, myoinositol, omega-3 fatty acids) and their potential effects on specific pathways dysregulated in PCOS, such as steroidogenesis, insulin metabolism, and inflammation. It would support the discussion on mapping nutrition to pathways and serve as a reference for tailoring dietary interventions based on individual PCOS phenotypes.

Table 4.2 Dietary components and their influence on PCOS-related pathways

Dietary component	Influence on PCOS-related pathways	References
Spearmint tea	Potential to reduce androgen levels by inhibiting steroidogenesis	[30]
Myoinositol	Improves insulin sensitivity and ovarian function	[31]
Omega-3 fatty acids	Reduces inflammation and improves lipid profiles	[32]

4.4.2.2 Case Studies Illustrating Pathway-Specific Nutritional Interventions

Case Study 1: Modulating Androgen Levels in Hyperandrogenic PCOS
In a study focusing on women with hyperandrogenic PCOS, researchers identified a potential link between dietary consumption of spearmint tea and reductions in free testosterone levels. A cohort of patients with hyperandrogenism incorporated spearmint tea into their diets.

Subsequent assessments showcased a noticeable decline in free testosterone levels among these individuals. This highlights the potential of targeted nutritional interventions to modulate specific pathways, such as androgen metabolism, within this PCOS subtype.

Case Study 2: Modulating Insulin Sensitivity
Similarly, in another study focusing on insulin-resistant PCOS subtypes, researchers identified foods or dietary patterns that positively influence insulin metabolism. A cohort of individuals with insulin resistance incorporated specific foods or dietary interventions known to enhance insulin sensitivity.

Follow-up assessments revealed improvements in insulin sensitivity markers, validating the role of targeted nutrition in modulating the insulin metabolism pathway within this PCOS subgroup.

Real-Time Application: Personalized Nutritional Therapy
A woman diagnosed with PCOS undergoes thorough phenotypic characterization, revealing specific dysregulations in steroidogenesis and insulin metabolism. Machine learning models connect these pathological traits within her PCOS profile with the highest probability nutritional therapies for desired clinical improvement.

Based on this analysis, a personalized nutritional plan is tailored for her, incorporating spearmint tea to address hyperandrogenism and specific dietary modifications to improve insulin sensitivity.

Over time, follow-up assessments demonstrate improvements in androgen levels and insulin sensitivity markers, validating the efficacy of precision nutritional therapy tailored to address the dysregulated pathways identified within her PCOS profile.

Impact and Future Implications
By linking foods to dysregulated pathways in PCOS, precision nutrition approaches pave the way for tailored interventions targeting specific pathophysiological features within different PCOS subtypes. This personalized approach not only enhances the effectiveness of nutritional therapies but also signifies a significant advancement toward precision medicine in PCOS care. It establishes a foundation for machine learning-driven pipelines connecting pathological traits in a woman's PCOS profile with targeted nutritional therapies for optimal clinical improvements.

4.5 Continual Optimization of Recommendations

The continual optimization of therapeutic recommendations in nutrition science is an evolving process, particularly through the integration of empirical evidence derived from phenotype-targeted randomized controlled trials (RCTs). These trials provide valuable insights into the responsiveness of specific disease subtypes to different dietary interventions, allowing for the refinement of predictive models guiding nutritional therapies.

4.5.1 Role of Phenotype-Targeted RCTs in Refinement

4.5.1.1 Designing Targeted Trials

Researchers design RCTs tailored to specific disease phenotypes within conditions like PCOS. These trials aim to evaluate the efficacy of diverse dietary interventions on distinct subtypes, elucidating which dietary patterns yield optimal outcomes for each phenotype.

4.5.1.2 Case Study: RCT Findings and Therapeutic Recommendations

Imagine an RCT focused on comparing the effects of different dietary interventions in managing metabolic complications among women with PCOS. The trial evaluates the impact of a high-fiber diet versus a low-carbohydrate diet on insulin sensitivity in two distinct subgroups: hyperinsulinemia PCOS and insulin-resistant PCOS.

The findings reveal that while both dietary approaches demonstrate improvements in insulin sensitivity, the high-fiber diet showcases superior outcomes in individuals with hyperinsulinemia PCOS, whereas the low-carbohydrate diet proves more effective for those with insulin-resistant PCOS.

4.5.1.3 Integration of RCT Data into Predictive Models

The data from this RCT are incorporated into predictive models guiding nutritional interventions for PCOS. The updated model now discerns that, based on the RCT evidence, a high-fiber diet is preferred for managing insulin sensitivity in hyperinsulinemic PCOS, while a low-carbohydrate diet is recommended for individuals with insulin-resistant PCOS.

4.5.1.4 Real-Time Application: Adapting Interventions

In clinical practice, a woman diagnosed with PCOS and hyperinsulinemic features receives a tailored nutritional plan emphasizing a high-fiber diet, aligning with the updated recommendations derived from RCT data. Over time, assessments show improvements in her insulin sensitivity, validating the efficacy of this phenotype-targeted dietary intervention based on empirical evidence.

4.5.1.5 Impact and Future Directions

The continual integration of empirical evidence from phenotype-targeted RCTs into predictive models refines and optimizes nutritional interventions. This adaptive approach ensures that dietary recommendations evolve in line with the latest evidence, enhancing the precision and effectiveness of dietary therapies for specific disease subtypes within conditions like PCOS. It lays the groundwork for ongoing advancements in personalized nutrition and precision medicine.

4.5.2 Incorporating Patient-Reported Outcomes

The integration of patient-reported outcomes (PROs) into nutritional interventions for conditions like polycystic ovary syndrome (PCOS) plays a pivotal role in creating patient-centered, personalized approaches to therapy.

4.5.2.1 Significance of Patient-Reported Outcomes in Nutritional Interventions

Understanding Patient Perspectives

PROs encompass subjective experiences, symptoms, and overall well-being reported by patients undergoing specific dietary interventions. In the context of PCOS management, these outcomes offer invaluable insights into patient-reported symptom improvements, adherence challenges, and overall satisfaction with the prescribed dietary plans.

Case Study: Integrating Patient Feedback

In a clinical trial focusing on personalized dietary interventions for women with PCOS, participants were provided individualized nutritional plans based on predictive models. They were encouraged to actively report their experiences, including changes in symptoms, ease of following the diet plan, and any difficulties encountered during adherence.

Real-Time Application: Patient-Centric Personalization

In clinical practice, a woman diagnosed with PCOS adheres to an individualized dietary plan tailored to her specific phenotype and symptomatology. Throughout the intervention, she engages in a participatory framework that allows her to provide feedback on her diet plan's suitability and its impact on her symptoms.

Her PROs reveal that while the dietary plan effectively improved some symptoms, such as reducing acne and regulating menstrual cycles, she faced challenges in adhering to certain dietary restrictions due to lifestyle constraints. This feedback is integrated into the AI-powered algorithm guiding nutritional recommendations.

Benefits and Future Implications

The integration of PROs into nutritional decision support systems represents a shift toward patient-centered care in PCOS management. This approach ensures that dietary interventions evolve not only based on clinical evidence but also on the practical experiences and needs of individuals living with PCOS.

By incorporating patient perspectives through PROs, nutritional interventions become more responsive to individual experiences and preferences. This continual enrichment ensures that dietary recommendations are more effectively tailored, enhancing adherence and overall success in managing PCOS symptoms.

Furthermore, this patient-driven approach fosters a collaborative healthcare environment, where patients actively participate in their care decisions. It empowers individuals with PCOS to contribute to the optimization of their own treatment plans, ultimately leading to more personalized, effective, and sustainable outcomes in PCOS management.

4.6 Opportunities and Challenges in Advancing Adoption

The proposed vision of AI-enabled, personalized nutrition prescriptions for women with PCOS shows immense potential for transformative impact. By effectively bridging bench-to-bedside gaps, it can enhance clinical outcomes, patient satisfaction, and caregiver productivity around this ambiguous condition. However, pragmatic challenges threaten adoption:

4.6.1 Clinician Engagement

Clinician engagement is crucial for the successful integration of AI-driven algorithms in healthcare settings, particularly when there's concern about potential replacement of expertise. Addressing physician hesitancy proactively through the seamless integration of AI into clinical workflows and continuous learning opportunities can facilitate acceptance and adoption of AI technologies, as indicated in recent studies and healthcare reports.

4.6.1.1 Understanding Clinician Hesitancy

Concerns and Resistance
Physicians might express concerns regarding the reliance on AI algorithms, fearing that it could diminish their clinical judgment or impact patient care negatively. Proactive measures are necessary to address these concerns and ensure a collaborative integration of AI technologies.

Case Study: Integrating AI into Clinical Practice
In a hospital setting, an AI-driven algorithm designed to assist in managing PCOS is introduced. Initially, clinicians exhibit hesitancy in adopting algorithmic recommendations due to concerns about potential expertise replacement.

Real-Time Application: Ergonomic Integration and Continued Learning
The healthcare facility organizes training sessions and workshops to educate clinicians on the algorithm's functioning, its strengths and limitations, and how it complements clinical expertise. They demonstrate the algorithm's role as a supportive tool, enhancing decision-making rather than replacing it.

4.6.1.2 Benefits and Learning Opportunities

Continued Education and Training
Regular educational sessions, case discussions, and practical demonstrations help clinicians understand the AI algorithm's rationale and its contributions to PCOS management. These learning opportunities ensure that clinicians are well-versed in utilizing AI as an adjunct tool in their decision-making process.

Ergonomic Integration
The AI algorithm is seamlessly integrated into the existing clinical workflows. During patient consultations, physicians use the algorithm to access personalized nutritional recommendations based on the patient's PCOS subtype. This information supplements their clinical judgment and contributes to a more comprehensive treatment plan.

Impact and Future Implications
By proactively addressing physician hesitancy and emphasizing the supportive role of AI within clinical practice, healthcare organizations foster an environment where clinicians perceive AI as a tool augmenting their expertise rather than replacing it. This approach enhances trust in AI-driven recommendations, ultimately leading to improved patient care and outcomes in PCOS management.

This collaborative integration ensures that AI technologies complement clinician expertise, leading to more informed decision-making and improved patient care, marking a significant step toward effective and efficient PCOS management.

4.6.2 User Experience

Enhancing user experience through intuitive interfaces and user-friendly tools is pivotal for patient centricity in delivering personalized dietary recommendations, especially in the context of conditions like polycystic ovary syndrome (PCOS). Incorporating comprehensible interfaces with visualizations and employing tools like chatbots and virtual assistants can significantly simplify adoption and engagement, as emphasized in recent research and industry reports.

4.6.2.1 Case Study: User Experience Optimizing Adherence

This case study focuses on the role of user-centric design principles and optimized user experiences in enhancing adherence and engagement with personalized dietary interventions for PCOS management.

Context: Adherence to dietary recommendations is a significant challenge in the management of chronic conditions like PCOS. Factors such as lack of understanding, complexity of dietary guidelines, and poor user experiences can contribute to suboptimal adherence rates, ultimately diminishing the effectiveness of personalized nutritional interventions.

Methodology: A team of researchers and developers collaborated to create a mobile health application specifically designed for women with PCOS. The app incorporated user-centric design principles, including visually intuitive interfaces, interactive guidance through chatbots or virtual assistants, and gamification elements to enhance user engagement.

The app's interface was designed to present personalized dietary recommendations in a visually appealing and easy-to-understand manner, leveraging graphics, icons, and intuitive navigation. Additionally, a conversational chatbot was integrated into the app, allowing users to interact with a virtual assistant and receive real-time guidance, clarifications, and reminders related to their dietary plan.

To further promote adherence, the app incorporated gamification elements, such as earning points or badges for consistently following dietary recommendations, tracking progress, and achieving milestones. These elements aimed to create a sense of accomplishment and motivation, fostering long-term engagement with the personalized nutritional intervention.

Results: A pilot study was conducted involving women with PCOS who were provided access to the user-centric mobile app. Participants were asked to use the app as their primary resource for accessing and adhering to their personalized dietary plans over a period of several months.

The study tracked adherence rates, patient satisfaction, and clinical outcomes related to PCOS symptom alleviation. The results revealed significantly higher adherence rates among participants using the user-centric app compared to those following traditional paper-based dietary guidelines. Additionally, patient satisfaction scores were notably higher, with users reporting a positive and engaging experience while using the app.

Importantly, improved adherence was associated with better clinical outcomes, including improved regulation of menstrual cycles, reduced hirsutism, and improved metabolic parameters like insulin sensitivity and lipid profiles.

Implications: This case study underscores the pivotal role of user experience in driving adherence and engagement with personalized dietary interventions for PCOS management. By incorporating user-centric design principles, intuitive interfaces, interactive guidance, and gamification elements, healthcare providers can create a more engaging and accessible experience for patients, ultimately enhancing adherence and improving clinical outcomes.

Furthermore, the observed improvements in patient satisfaction and symptom alleviation highlight the potential of user-centric approaches to not only promote adherence but also contribute to overall quality of life and well-being for women with PCOS. This case study emphasizes the importance of considering user experiences as a critical factor in the successful implementation and adoption of AI-enabled personalized nutrition strategies.

4.6.2.2 Significance of User Experience in Dietary Personalization

Accessible and Understandable Information

Patients managing PCOS require clear and accessible information regarding their personalized dietary plans. Visual aids and user-friendly interfaces play a vital role in enhancing comprehension and engagement.

Real-Time Application: Intuitive Interfaces and Visualization

In a health app designed for PCOS management, the dietary recommendations for different PCOS subtypes are presented through an interactive and visually appealing interface. Patients can explore their personalized diet plans through graphics-led visualizations that illustrate food categories, portion sizes, and recommended frequencies.

Figures 4.3 and 4.4 depict a mock-up or wireframe of a user-friendly interface for a mobile or web application designed to deliver personalized dietary recommendations for PCOS management. It could showcase features like visually appealing graphics, interactive elements, and virtual assistant integration, highlighting the importance of user experience in enhancing adoption and engagement.

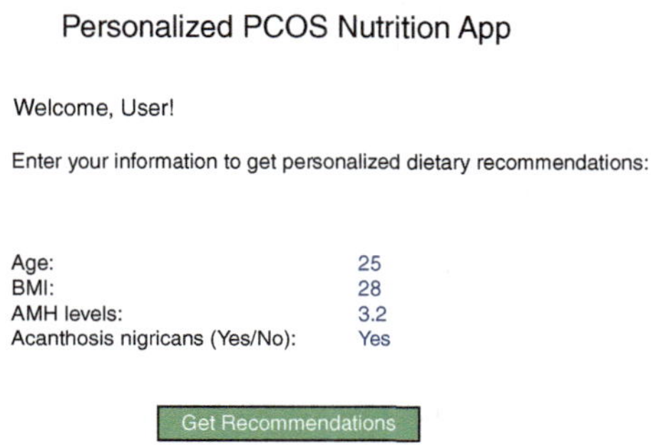

Fig. 4.3 User interface for personalized PCOS nutrition app

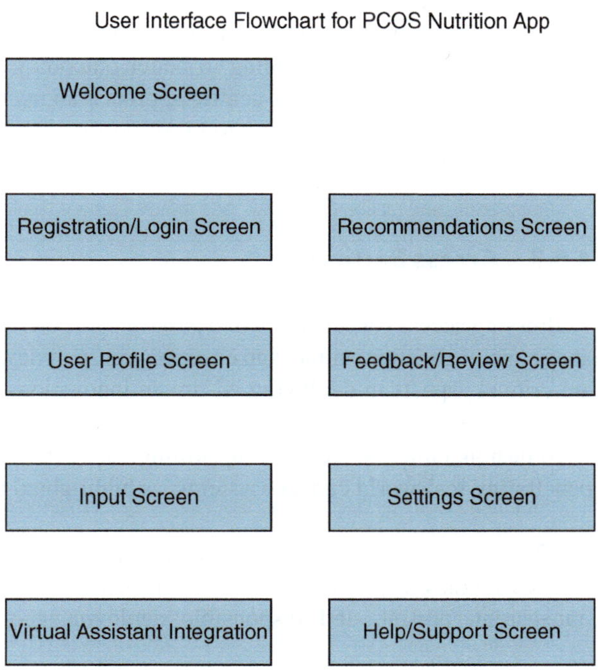

Fig. 4.4 User interface flowchart for PCOS nutrition app

4.6.2.3 Benefits and Examples of User-Centric Tools

Chatbots and Virtual Assistants

Integrating chatbots or virtual assistants within the health app allows patients to interact conversationally. These tools answer queries, provide explanations about dietary recommendations, offer reminders, and create an interactive experience, enhancing patient engagement.

Real-Time Example: Enhanced User Engagement

A woman diagnosed with PCOS utilizes a health app that incorporates user-friendly interfaces and a virtual assistant. She navigates through the app's dietary recommendations, which are presented in easily digestible visuals and supplemented by explanations from the virtual assistant.

The virtual assistant addresses her questions regarding certain food choices, offers additional information on how specific foods impact her PCOS subtype, and sends timely reminders about meal planning and adherence to the personalized diet.

Impact and Future Implications

By prioritizing user experience and employing tools like chatbots and virtual assistants within health applications, patient engagement and adherence to personalized dietary plans for PCOS can significantly improve. These interactive and user-centric approaches empower patients by providing comprehensible and accessible information, enhancing their ability to manage their condition effectively.

Incorporating such intuitive interfaces and interactive tools not only simplifies the adoption of personalized dietary recommendations but also fosters patient empowerment, ultimately leading to better outcomes and improved adherence in PCOS management. This user-centric approach aligns with the evolving landscape of healthcare technology, aiming to make information more accessible and actionable for patients managing chronic conditions like PCOS.

4.6.3 Access Barriers

Addressing access barriers related to passive data collection via wearables, concerns about misinformation online, and ensuring transparency, privacy, and digital literacy are critical aspects in deploying AI-driven innovations in healthcare, especially in conditions like polycystic ovary syndrome (PCOS). The emphasis on human-centered design, ethics, stakeholder upskilling, and convenience plays a crucial role in penetrating real-world care ecosystems, as highlighted in.

4.6.3.1 Case Study: Responsible AI Deployment Fostering Trust

This case study explores strategies adopted by a healthcare institution to ensure transparent, ethical, and responsible deployment of an AI-powered nutrition platform for PCOS management, with the goal of fostering trust and adoption among clinicians and patients.

Context: The integration of AI technologies in healthcare settings often faces challenges related to concerns around data privacy, transparency, and potential biases. These concerns can lead to hesitancy and resistance among clinicians and patients, hindering the successful adoption and implementation of AI-driven solutions.

Methodology: A renowned healthcare institution recognized the potential benefits of an AI-powered nutrition platform for personalized PCOS management but also acknowledged the importance of addressing potential barriers to adoption. They implemented a multifaceted approach to ensure responsible and ethical deployment of the AI technology.

First, the institution established robust data governance policies and protocols to ensure the privacy and security of patient data utilized by the AI platform. These policies were transparently communicated to both clinicians and patients, outlining the measures taken to protect sensitive information and the purposes for which data would be used.

Second, the institution launched educational campaigns aimed at improving digital literacy among clinicians and patients. These campaigns provided resources and training on navigating the online landscape of health information, identifying reliable sources, and understanding the potential risks associated with misinformation or unverified claims related to PCOS management.

Additionally, the institution facilitated upskilling programs for clinicians, equipping them with knowledge and skills to effectively interpret and leverage the insights generated by the AI platform. These programs covered topics such as the underlying principles of AI algorithms, their strengths and limitations, and best practices for integrating AI-driven recommendations into clinical decision-making processes.

Results: The institution's multipronged approach to responsible AI deployment yielded positive outcomes. Clinicians reported increased confidence and trust in the AI-powered nutrition platform, recognizing the measures taken to ensure data privacy, transparency, and ethical use of the technology.

Patients also expressed greater willingness to engage with the AI platform, as their concerns regarding data privacy and potential misuse were addressed through the educational campaigns and transparent communication strategies.

Furthermore, the upskilling programs enabled clinicians to effectively interpret and apply the AI-driven recommendations, enhancing their ability to provide personalized and effective nutritional guidance to patients with PCOS.

Implications: This case study highlights the importance of adopting a responsible and ethical approach when deploying AI technologies in healthcare settings. By prioritizing data privacy, transparency, and digital literacy, healthcare institutions can foster trust and acceptance among both clinicians and patients.

The strategies employed, such as robust data governance policies, educational campaigns, and upskilling programs, not only addressed potential barriers to adoption but also empowered stakeholders with the knowledge and skills necessary to effectively leverage AI-driven solutions for personalized care.

Moreover, this case study underscores the significance of human-centered design principles in the development and deployment of AI technologies. By actively involving and considering the perspectives of clinicians and patients, healthcare institutions can create AI-enabled solutions that seamlessly integrate into existing care ecosystems while upholding ethical standards and fostering trust among all stakeholders.

Overall, this case study serves as a blueprint for responsible and ethical AI deployment in healthcare, paving the way for the successful integration of AI-driven personalized nutrition strategies while ensuring patient privacy, transparency, and trust in the technology.

4.6.3.2 Tackling Access Barriers in AI Innovation

Passive Data Collection and Privacy Concerns

Passive data collection through wearables raises privacy concerns. Patients might be apprehensive about sharing personal health information, fearing breaches or misuse.

Misinformation and Digital Literacy

The prevalence of misinformation online poses challenges. Patients might encounter misleading or conflicting information about PCOS management, affecting their decision-making.

Case Study: Ethical AI Deployment

A healthcare institution introduces an AI-driven platform for PCOS management that incorporates passive data collection from wearables. However, concerns about data privacy and transparency arise among patients and clinicians.

Real-Time Application: Transparency and Education

The institution implements robust measures to ensure transparency regarding data usage, storage, and security. They conduct educational campaigns emphasizing digital literacy and responsible use of online health information, especially related to PCOS management.

4.6.3.3 Benefits and Examples of Human-Centered Design

Enhanced Data Security and Privacy

The AI platform is designed with stringent security protocols and transparent data handling practices. Patients are informed about how their data is used, stored, and protected, addressing privacy concerns.

Public Outreach and Education

Educational campaigns are launched to improve digital literacy among patients and healthcare providers. Resources on reliable PCOS management information online are disseminated, empowering individuals to make informed decisions.

Real-Time Example: Improved Access and Convenience

Patients with PCOS feel more confident in utilizing the AI platform, knowing their data is secure and understanding the benefits it offers in managing their condition. They have access to reliable information, reducing reliance on potentially misleading online sources.

Impact and Future Implications

The emphasis on human-centered design, ethics, stakeholder education, and convenience in AI innovation fosters trust and acceptance. By addressing access barriers through transparency, education, and data security, AI technologies can be integrated more effectively into real-world care ecosystems.

Empowering patients with reliable information and ensuring responsible AI deployment not only enhances access but also supports informed decision-making in managing conditions like PCOS. This approach contributes to a more inclusive and patient-centric healthcare landscape, where AI-driven innovations augment care delivery while prioritizing ethical considerations and accessibility for all stakeholders.

4.7 Conclusion and Future Scope

In summary, this chapter has proposed an innovative blueprint for AI-enabled, personalized nutrition prescriptions for women with polycystic ovary syndrome (PCOS). The proposed model leverages advanced methodologies rooted in explainable AI (XAI) to overcome the challenges posed by the heterogeneity and complexity of PCOS. The key aspects of this approach are as follows:

1. Compiling an exhaustive PCOS database by assimilating multidimensional data from symptom tracking, clinical evaluations, biochemical assays, dietary assessments, gut microbiome mapping, and multi-omics profiling.
2. Dissecting distinctive PCOS phenotypes using XAI techniques like SHAP analysis and local interpretable model-agnostic explanations (LIME), offering granular visibility into pathological traits driving complications.
3. Mapping dietary components to specific PCOS phenotypes and outcomes using machine learning algorithms, enabling the provision of tailored nutritional interventions.
4. Continual optimization of therapeutic recommendations through the integration of empirical evidence from phenotype-targeted randomized controlled trials (RCTs) and the incorporation of patient-reported outcomes (PROs).
5. Addressing potential adoption barriers by fostering clinician engagement, prioritizing user experience through intuitive interfaces and interactive tools, and ensuring responsible AI deployment with a focus on transparency, privacy, and digital literacy.

This AI-driven, precision nutrition approach carries immense potential to transform PCOS care from a one-size-fits-all strategy to individualized prescriptions effectively addressing the intricate metabolic heterogeneity underlying this complex disorder. The long-term impact on clinical outcomes and quality of life cannot be overstated, given the alarming burden inflicted by this highly disruptive syndrome on women worldwide.

By embracing the potential of AI-enabled personalized nutrition and continuously expanding its scope, the healthcare community can pave the way for a future where precision medicine becomes the norm, empowering individuals to achieve optimal health outcomes tailored to their unique needs and circumstances.

References

1. Rosenfield RL, Ehrmann DA. The pathogenesis of polycystic ovary syndrome (PCOS): the hypothesis of PCOS as functional ovarian hyperandrogenism revisited. Endocr Rev. 2016;37(5):467–520. https://doi.org/10.1210/er.2015-1104.
2. Lizneva D, Suturina L, Walker W, Brakta S, Gavrilova-Jordan L, Azziz R. Criteria, prevalence, and phenotypes of polycystic ovary syndrome. Fertil Steril. 2016;106(1):6–15. https://doi.org/10.1016/j.fertnstert.2016.05.003.
3. Domecq JP, Prutsky G, Mullan RJ, Hazem A, Sundaresh V, Elamin MB, Phung OJ, Wang A, Hoeger K, Pasquali R, Erwin P, Bodde A, Montori VM, Murad MH. Lifestyle modification programs in polycystic ovary syndrome: systematic review and meta-analysis. J Clin Endocrinol Metab. 2013;98(12):4655–63. https://doi.org/10.1210/jc.2013-2385. Epub 2013 Oct 3.
4. Sirmans SM, Pate KA. Epidemiology, diagnosis, and management of polycystic ovary syndrome. Clin Epidemiol. 2013;6:1–13. https://doi.org/10.2147/CLEP.S37559.
5. Khan I, Khare BK. Exploring the potential of machine learning in gynecological care: a review. Arch Gynecol Obstet. 2024;309:2347. https://doi.org/10.1007/s00404-024-07479-1.
6. Petrauskas V, Jasinevicius R, Damuleviciene G, Liutkevicius A, Janaviciute A, Lesauskaite V, Knasiene J, Meskauskas Z, Dovydaitis J, Kazanavicius V, et al. Explainable artificial intelligence-based decision support system for assessing the nutrition-related geriatric syndromes. Appl Sci. 2021;11:11763. https://doi.org/10.3390/app112411763.
7. Côté M, Lamarche B. Artificial intelligence in nutrition research: perspectives on current and future applications. Appl Physiol Nutr Metab. 2022;47(1):1–8. https://doi.org/10.1139/apnm-2021-0448.
8. Moran L, Gibson-Helm M, Teede H, Deeks A. Polycystic ovary syndrome: a biopsychosocial understanding in young women to improve knowledge and treatment options. J Psychosom Obstet Gynaecol. 2010;31(1):24–31. https://doi.org/10.3109/01674820903477593.
9. Teede HJ, Misso ML, Costello MF, Dokras A, Laven J, Moran L, Piltonen T, Norman RJ, International PCOS Network. Recommendations from the international evidence-based guideline for the assessment and management of polycystic ovary syndrome. Fertil Steril. 2018;110(3):364–79. https://doi.org/10.1016/j.fertnstert.2018.05.004. Epub 2018 Jul 19.
10. Azziz R, Carmina E, Dewailly D, Diamanti-Kandarakis E, Escobar-Morreale HF, Futterweit W, Janssen OE, Legro RS, Norman RJ, Taylor AE, Witchel SF, Task Force on the Phenotype of the Polycystic Ovary Syndrome of the Androgen Excess and PCOS Society. The Androgen Excess and PCOS Society criteria for the polycystic ovary syndrome: the complete task force report. Fertil Steril. 2009;91(2):456–88. https://doi.org/10.1016/j.fertnstert.2008.06.035. Epub 2008 Oct 23.
11. The Rotterdam ESHRE/ASRM-Sponsored PCOS Consensus Workshop Group. Revised 2003 consensus on diagnostic criteria and long-term health risks related to polycystic ovary syndrome (PCOS). Hum Reprod. 2004;19(1):41–7. https://doi.org/10.1093/humrep/deh098.

12. Teede HJ, Misso ML, Costello MF, Dokras A, Laven J, Moran L, Piltonen T, Norman RJ, International PCOS Network. Recommendations from the international evidence-based guideline for the assessment and management of polycystic ovary syndrome. Hum Reprod. 2018;33(9):1602–18. https://doi.org/10.1093/humrep/dey256. Erratum in: Hum Reprod. 2019 Feb 1;34(2):388.
13. Sommer MOA. Advancing gut microbiome research using cultivation. Curr Opin Microbiol. 2015;27:127–32. https://doi.org/10.1016/j.mib.2015.08.004.
14. Kelly CJ, Zheng L, Campbell EL, Saeedi B, Scholz CC, Bayless AJ, Wilson KE, Glover LE, Kominsky DJ, Magnuson A, Weir TL, Ehrentraut SF, Pickel C, Kuhn KA, Lanis JM, Nguyen V, Taylor CT, Colgan SP. Crosstalk between microbiota-derived short-chain fatty acids and intestinal epithelial HIF augments tissue barrier function. Cell Host Microbe. 2015;17(5):662–71. https://doi.org/10.1016/j.chom.2015.03.005. Epub 2015 Apr 9.
15. Babu A, Ramanathan G. Multi-omics insights and therapeutic implications in polycystic ovary syndrome: a review. Funct Integr Genomics. 2023;23:130. https://doi.org/10.1007/s10142-023-01053-9.
16. Diamanti-Kandarakis E, Katsikis I, Piperi C, Kandaraki E, Piouka A, Papavassiliou AG, Panidis D. Increased serum advanced glycation end-products is a distinct finding in lean women with polycystic ovary syndrome (PCOS). Clin Endocrinol (Oxf). 2008;69(4):634–41. https://doi.org/10.1111/j.1365-2265.2008.03247.x. Epub 2008 Mar 19.
17. Escobar-Morreale HF, Luque-Ramírez M, González F. Circulating inflammatory markers in polycystic ovary syndrome: a systematic review and metaanalysis. Fertil Steril. 2011;95(3):1048–58.
18. Kelly CC, Lyall H, Petrie JR, Gould GW, Connell JM, Sattar N. Low grade chronic inflammation in women with polycystic ovarian syndrome. J Clin Endocrinol Metab. 2001;86(6):2453–5. https://doi.org/10.1210/jcem.86.6.7580.
19. González F. Inflammation in polycystic ovary syndrome: underpinning of insulin resistance and ovarian dysfunction. Steroids. 2012;77(4):300–5. https://doi.org/10.1016/j.steroids.2011.12.003. Epub 2011 Dec 8.
20. Rottiers V, Näär AM. MicroRNAs in metabolism and metabolic disorders. Nat Rev Mol Cell Biol. 2012;13(4):239–50. https://doi.org/10.1038/nrm3313. Erratum in: Nat Rev Mol Cell Biol. 2012;13(5). https://doi.org/10.1038/nrm3328.
21. Goodarzi MO, Jones MR, Li X, Chua AK, Garcia OA, Chen YD, Krauss RM, Rotter JI, Ankener W, Legro RS, Azziz R, Strauss JF 3rd, Dunaif A, Urbanek M. Replication of association of DENND1A and THADA variants with polycystic ovary syndrome in European cohorts. J Med Genet. 2012;49(2):90–5. https://doi.org/10.1136/jmedgenet-2011-100427. Epub 2011 Dec 17.
22. van Ommen B, van den Broek T, de Hoogh I, van Erk M, van Someren E, Rouhani-Rankouhi T, Anthony JC, Hogenelst K, Pasman W, Boorsma A, Wopereis S. Systems biology of personalized nutrition. Nutr Rev. 2017;75(8):579–99. https://doi.org/10.1093/nutrit/nux029. Erratum in: Nutr Rev. 2017 Aug 1;75(8):672.
23. Marshall JC, Dunaif A. Should all women with PCOS be treated for insulin resistance? Fertil Steril. 2012;97(1):18–22. https://doi.org/10.1016/j.fertnstert.2011.11.036.
24. Sengupta S, Basak S, Saikia P, Paul S, Tsalavoutis V, Atiah F, et al. A review of deep learning with special emphasis on architectures, applications and recent trends. Knowl-Based Syst. 2020;194:105596. https://doi.org/10.1016/j.knosys.2020.105596.
25. Lundberg SM, Lee SI. A unified approach to interpreting model predictions. Adv Neural Inf Proces Syst. 2017;30. https://proceedings.neurips.cc/paper/2017/hash/8a20a8621978632d76c43dfd28b67767-Abstract.html.
26. Cutillas-Tolín A, Arense-Gonzalo JJ, Mendiola J, Adoamnei E, Navarro-Lafuente F, Sánchez-Ferrer ML, Prieto-Sánchez MT, Carmona-Barnosi A, Vioque J, Torres-Cantero AM. Are dietary indices associated with polycystic ovary syndrome and its phenotypes? A preliminary study. Nutrients. 2021;13:313. https://doi.org/10.3390/nu13020313.
27. Verma S, Mather K, Dumont AS, Anderson TJ. Pharmacological modulation of insulin resistance and hyperinsulinemia in polycystic ovary syndrome: the emerging role. Endocrinologist. 1998;8(6):418–24.

28. Scarfò G, Daniele S, Fusi J, Gesi M, Martini C, Franzoni F, Cela V, Artini PG. Metabolic and molecular mechanisms of diet and physical exercise in the management of polycystic ovarian syndrome. Biomedicines. 2022;10:1305. https://doi.org/10.3390/biomedicines10061305.
29. Kaput J, Monteiro JP. Human nutrition research in the data era: results of 11 reports on the effects of a multiple-micronutrient-intervention study. Nutrients. 2024;16:188. https://doi.org/10.3390/nu16020188.
30. Grant P. Spearmint herbal tea has significant anti-androgen effects in polycystic ovarian syndrome. A randomized controlled trial. Phytother Res. 2010;24(2):186–8. https://doi.org/10.1002/ptr.2900.
31. Unfer V, Facchinetti F, Orrù B, Giordani B, Nestler J. Myo-inositol effects in women with PCOS: a meta-analysis of randomized controlled trials. Endocr Connect. 2017;6(8):647–58. https://doi.org/10.1530/EC-17-0243.
32. Komal F, Khan MK, Imran M, Ahmad MH, Anwar H, Ashfaq UA, Ahmad N, Masroor A, Ahmad RS, Nadeem M, Nisa MU. Impact of different omega-3 fatty acid sources on lipid, hormonal, blood glucose, weight gain and histopathological damages profile in PCOS rat model. J Transl Med. 2020;18(1):349. https://doi.org/10.1186/s12967-020-02519-1.

Unlocking Gender-Based Health Insights with Predictive Analytics

5

Vinod Kumar and Chander Prabha

5.1 Background

The chapter discusses the potential of AI and predictive analytics to uncover gender-based health insights in the quickly changing sector of healthcare. Gender-specific health data greatly influence the practices and the future of healthcare. The chapter emphasizes the need to recognize and correct errors, such as improper selection and observation bias when using large data sets and exhort readers to view bias objectively and classify all effects as beneficial or vice versa [1]. Encouraging public participation can significantly reduce knowledge gaps and promote inclusiveness in health. This chapter covers several areas of the globe like the USA, Canada, Pakistan, Australia, and India [2] and navigates through the challenging worlds of artificial intelligence, machine learning, and big data in healthcare to promote a complete knowledge of health that challenges conventional assumptions.

One socially imposed characteristic that determines roles, norms, and relationships between men and women in a society is gender. These concepts are culturally specific and subject to change. Discrimination and social rejection can result from breaking gender norms, and these things can be harmful to an individual's health. The power imbalances that frequently result from the hierarchical structure of genders also affect other social and financial dimensions of inequality. The combination of gender curation, machine learning, and artificial intelligence has been the focal point of the paradigm change in healthcare in recent years. The expansion of gender-based healthcare appears to be primarily driven by the transformative possibilities of precision

V. Kumar
University Institute of Engineering and Technology, Chandigarh University, Mohali, Punjab, India

C. Prabha (✉)
Chitkara University Institute of Engineering and Technology, Chitkara University, Punjab, India

R. Kumar et al. (eds.), *AI-Based Nutritional Intervention in Polycystic Ovary Syndrome (PCOS)*, https://doi.org/10.1007/978-981-96-2120-0_5

medicine and predictive analytics [3]. This chapter explores the significance of computer health research in identifying gender disparities that go beyond social and biological factors, as observational retrospective studies demonstrate the transformative power of technology-induced inequality. Large data sets play a significant role in health because they can shed light on the mechanisms underlying both disease and health. However, to examine the implicit biases found in large data sets, it is essential to have an impartial viewpoint, which may include both observational and decision biases. An AI-based system that forecasts patient outcomes by examining the medical data of a particular patient Radha Devi is shown in Fig. 5.1.

This contains information from the health survey about the diagnosed illness and her consistent enrollment in the hospital administration system. This system integration seems to be very beneficial in guiding clinical and operational choices.

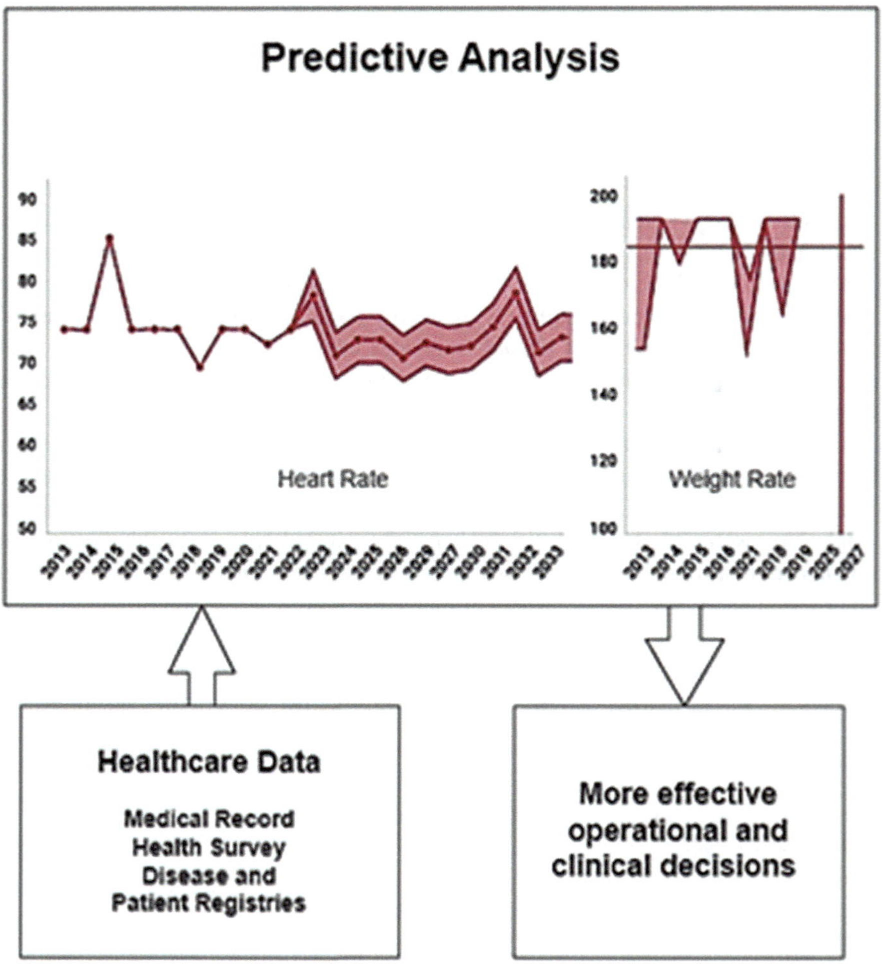

Fig. 5.1 AI predictive analysis

Additionally, depending on their level of influence, it encourages proactive measures aimed at minimizing undesirable biases and maximizing preferred biases, which improve diagnostic accuracy. Social media communication has the power to eliminate knowledge gaps and encourage inclusiveness [4]. It seeks to facilitate inclusive practices, paradigm shifts in research techniques, and the development of a holistic vision of health that goes beyond traditional expectations by navigating the complicated world of artificial intelligence, machine learning, and enormous amounts of data in healthcare. Predictive analytics and cutting-edge AI methods need to be applied extensively to create a healthcare system that is more inclusive and enhances the care given to women.

Wearable technology uses machine learning algorithms for time series analysis, allowing for the tracking of health trends and activity detection. Conversely, the International Medical Journal relies on Bayesian networks and support vector machines (SVM) for online patient consultation and monitoring. Eventually, techniques like sentiment analysis and machine learning for sentiment recognition can identify and monitor feelings in the mental health assessment.

Organization of Chapter

The rest of the chapter is organized as: Section 5.2 illustrates The Socio-Ecological Gender-Based Healthcare Model. Section 5.3 and 5.4 discusses algorithmic approaches. Section 5.5 highlights Gender-based Healthcare Prediction Analytics Challenges. And, finally Sect. 5.6 concludes the chapter with future scope.

5.2 The Socio-Ecological Gender-Based Healthcare Model

Applying machine learning techniques to all sexes of health has created new opportunities, particularly regarding addressing gender-based health disparities. A worldwide framework for comprehending health outcomes is provided, considering the social, interpersonal, communal, and individual elements influencing health and well-being. This is made possible with the socio-ecological model. The author examines the interplay of machine learning, algorithmic justice, and the socio-ecological model in gender-based healthcare.

5.2.1 Gender-Based Health Disparities in Machine Learning

Addressing health disparities, particularly those rooted in gender, race/ethnicity, and income levels, has become a central focus in public and population health research. Racial and ethnic health disparities refer to variations in health status and the distribution of health resources among different population groups. These differences stem from the social conditions in which individuals are born, grow, live, work, and age. The impact of these disparities is often magnified within specific gender, income, and race/ethnicity groups, leading to unequal health outcomes and risks [5].

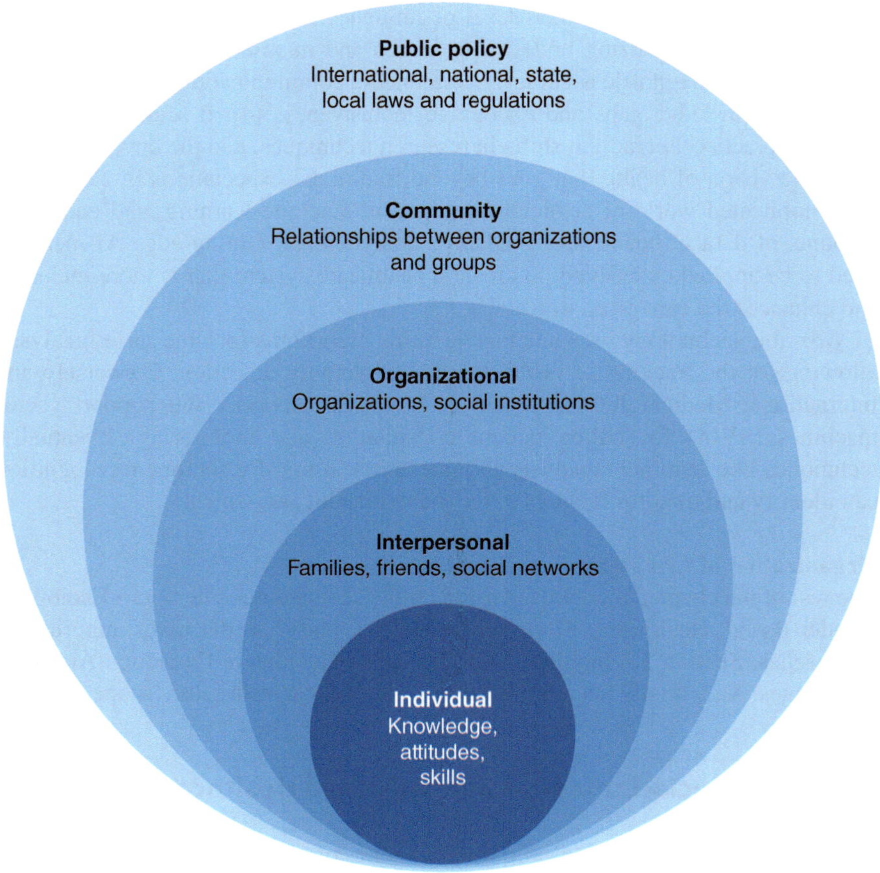

Fig. 5.2 Levels that affect health outcomes in socio-ecological gender-based healthcare

In recent times, the intersection of machine learning and healthcare has brought forth the crucial consideration of algorithmic fairness. Algorithmic fairness is a burgeoning field within machine learning, aiming to address and mitigate differences in outcomes across various social groups. Figure 5.2 highlights the many levels that affect health outcomes. At the macro level, the foundation of health systems is public policy, which includes international, national, municipal, and government laws and regulations. The community level includes the evolving relationships among various businesses and groups that impact health access and distribution. The structures and procedures that affect how healthcare is provided and accessed inside businesses and social institutions are identified at the organizational level. Upon approaching the individual, the interpersonal level considers the influence of friends, family, and social networks on health-related decisions and behaviors. Ultimately, at a microlevel, an individual's knowledge, attitudes, and skills have an influence. This includes ensuring fairness in machine learning predictions and recommendations related to health.

5.3 Algorithmic Approaches

5.3.1 Statistical Notions

Algorithmic approaches employ statistical notions to guarantee some form of parity for members of different protected groups, such as race and gender. These notions strive to eliminate biases and ensure that predictions are equitable across diverse demographic groups.

5.3.2 Individual Notions

Individual notions focus on ensuring that individuals who are deemed similar in the context of a specific classification task receive comparable outcomes. This approach aims to prevent discrimination against individuals with similar health characteristics, regardless of their gender or other demographic factors [6].

5.3.3 The Interpersonal Level

Interpersonal health exchanges are improved machine learning algorithms. By ensuring that language and genre-related considerations are included, natural language processing (NLP) algorithms can, for example, assist in the analysis of patient-provider communication. This contributes to the development of a more transparent and understanding health environment by addressing the interpersonal factors that affect health research activities [7].

5.3.4 Identifying Social and Economic Factors

The state of health is greatly influenced by communities. The ability of machine learning models to analyze large amounts of data can help identify the socioeconomic factors influencing gender-based health disparities. By recognizing the unique problems faced by each community, public health initiatives may be tailored to address gaps at their source and guarantee equitable access to healthcare [8].

5.3.5 Social Considerations

Interpersonal health exchanges are improved machine learning algorithms. By ensuring that language and genre-related considerations are included, natural language processing algorithms can, for example, assist in the analysis of patient-provider communication. This contributes to the development of a more transparent and understanding health environment by addressing the interpersonal factors that affect health research activities [9].

5.4 Algorithmic Approaches

A sophisticated deep learning model is proposed to enhance the genre-based health categorization by utilizing a hybrid architecture combining AlexNet, GoogLeNet, and ResNet benefits. This innovative method aims to leverage each network architecture's distinctive qualities and capabilities to enhance the classification's overall performance.

5.4.1 Fusion Model of AlexNet, GoogLeNet, and ResNet

5.4.1.1 AlexNet

It is renowned for being a pioneer in picture classification tasks and excels in feature extraction because of several convolution layers. The inclusion of AlexNet ensures that the model captures sophisticated details necessary for sex-based health classification [10].

5.4.1.2 GoogLeNet (Inception)

It introduces the concept of initiation modules, enabling the network to discover characteristics at various scales. The integration of GoogLeNet into the model improves its capacity to recognize intricate patterns and structures in medical pictures [11].

5.4.1.3 ResNet

It has a residual learning paradigm that makes the gradient disappear, which makes it easier to create extraordinarily deep networks. The addition of ResNet makes it feasible to learn hierarchical characteristics effectively, which is crucial for health categorization based on diversified sex [12].

Figure 5.3 illustrates the process of classifying healthcare patients, depending on gender using an AI-DL model. It's a novel hybrid approach that incorporates elements of the AlexNet, GoogLeNet, and ResNet designs. Initially, each component's characteristics are extracted separately, and they are then combined with DenseNet, a deep learning framework renowned for its ability to extract characteristics efficiently. The unique characteristics are then combined, effectively combining the many representations that each architecture has gathered. Ultimately, the categorization results stem from this integrated model, which offers a thorough analysis of health data based on genre.

5.4.2 DenseNet Combination of Features

A DenseNet is integrated with the extracted characteristics once they are extracted thanks to the hybrid design. Strongly connected DenseNet blocks make it easier for features to be restored, enabling the network to use extracted data effectively on several levels. It does this by enhancing the model's ability to identify complicated dependencies in the data [13].

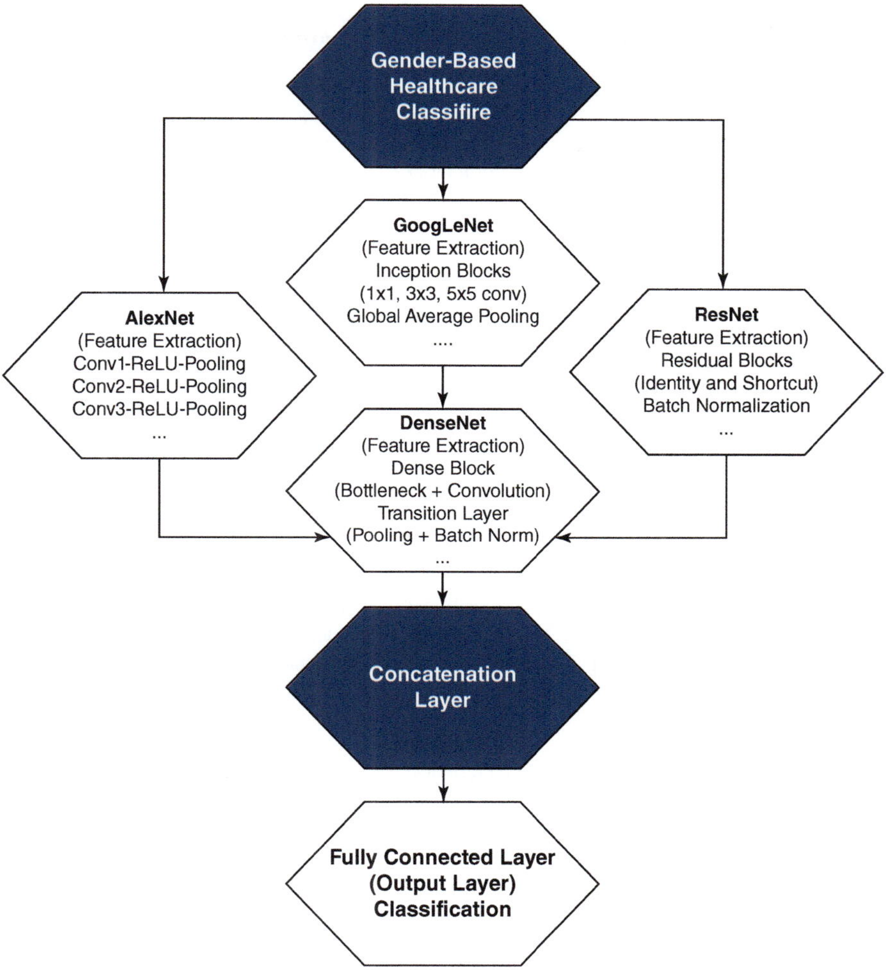

Fig. 5.3 Gender-based healthcare classification using AI-DL model

5.4.3 Combination of Features

One important step in the suggested model is the merging of the extracted features from AlexNet, GoogLeNet, and ResNet and concatenating with DenseNet. A thorough reading of the variety of facts found in medical imagery linked to gender-based healthcare is ensured by this deliberate fusion of traits [14].

5.4.4 Gender-Based Health Classifications

Then, using the SoftMax activation, the combined characteristics are transferred into a classification layer for sex-based health categorization. By using a labeled

Table 5.1 Gender-based healthcare challenges and AI approaches

Gender-based challenges	AlexNet	GoogLeNet	ResNet	DenseNet
Prostate cancer (PC) [16]	Examining medical images for specific characteristics related to the prostate area	Multi-scale feature extraction using inception blocks	Using residual connections to identify anomalies in prostate tissue	Getting dense features out of the prostate area
Ovarian cancer (OC) [17]	Specialized study of anomalies in the ovary area of ovarian cancer	Recognizing subtleties associated with ovarian tissue	Using residual blocks to identify anomalies in ovarian structure	Extracting dense characteristics particular to ovarian anomalies
Breast cancer (BC) [18]	Highlights patterns in breast tissue and detects lumps or cancers	Employing inception blocks to analyze breast areas to obtain detailed characteristics	Remaining connections are used to identify irregularities in breast tissue	Getting dense features out of breast tissue
Lung cancer (LC) [19]	Analysis of irregularities in lung structure, with a focus on nodule identification	A comprehensive examination of lung areas with different convolutional layers	Use of residual connections to identify anomalies in lung tissue	Extracting dense characteristics particular to anomalies of the lungs
Nutritional deficiencies (ND) [20]	Examining issues related to the skin, hair, and nails that may indicate shortages	Identifying subtle characteristics linked to outward manifestations of malnutrition	Using residual connections, anomalies linked to nutritional deficits are detected	Identifying indicators of weaknesses by extracting dense features from images

dataset for training, the model can pick up on and apply a variety of patterns and characteristics that are taken from medical images [15]. Table 5.1 provides an in-depth review of gender-specific health issues together with the equivalent AI methods used for the investigation.

To improve the predictive accuracy and generalizability to a wider range of health issues, this all-encompassing hybrid deep learning model makes use of the strengths of different architectures to capture a variety of variables relevant to gender-based disorders.

For prostate cancer, the focus is on analyzing medical images for unique characteristics related to the prostate region, using ResNet to identify abnormalities in the prostate tissue. The same is true for ovarian cancer, where a specific investigation of irregularities in the ovary region is carried out, and GoogLeNet is used to find the subtleties of ovarian tissue. Utilizing AlexNet to evaluate breast regions for certain features, patterns in breast tissue are emphasized and lumps or malignancies are found in cases of breast cancer. Regarding prostate cancer, the analysis focuses on abnormalities in the prostate's structure, and ResNet uses residual connections to find anomalies in the prostate tissue. Finally, under the framework of nutritional deficiencies, issues related to skin, hair, and nails that indicate deficiencies are examined using DenseNet, which extracts dense features from pictures to identify deficiencies.

5.5 Gender-Based Healthcare Prediction Analytics Challenges

With an emphasis on malnutrition specifically, the authors cover a wide variety of gender-based health-related issues in India, Canada, Pakistan, Australia, and the USA. Vitamin B12 insufficiency is recognized as a global problem that affects people in every area. Deficits in vitamin A still pose a threat, particularly to kids enrolled in maternal schools. Nonetheless, newborns are in danger from Iodine deficits, which highlights the need for iodizing salt everywhere [21]. An indication of how complicated nutritional problems are in India is the prevalence of folic acid and vitamin D deficiency in expecting mothers. These gaps must be closed, and to enhance overall health outcomes, comprehensive initiatives involving food preservation and health education are required. Table 5.2 details attributes associated with each gender-based ailment. Authors suggested possible areas of improvement.

Along with offering insights into the exact features or patterns in medical images that the deep learning model can identify for each health issue. The features described are unique to each gender-specific illness and could account for various methods of diagnosis or imaging technologies. The objective of these characteristics is to identify patterns or anomalies in medical imaging that suggest the existence of specific medical disorders. During the training phase, the deep learning model may make use of these attributes to improve its capacity to identify and categorize a variety of patterns linked to gender-based illnesses.

Table 5.2 Medical imaging findings across modalities

Gender-based ailments	Artificial intelligence influences characteristics
PC [16]	Abnormalities in the prostate shape or size of MRI or ultrasound images
OC [17]	Identification of masses or cysts in pelvic ultrasound images
BC [18]	Detection of microcalcifications or masses in mammograms
LC [19]	Identification of lung nodules or lesions in CT scans
ND [20]	Analysis of skin, hair, and nails for signs of deficiencies

5.5.1 Breast Cancer

Breast cancer (BC) is the most common kind of cancer among women globally; it will overtake lung cancer as the primary cause of cancer incidence worldwide in 2020. Roughly 2.3 million new cases were recorded in that year alone, accounting for 11.7% of all instances of cancer. Epidemiological studies estimate that by 2030, the worldwide burden of BC will be close to 2 million cases [22].

In India, the number of cases of breast cancer has increased significantly, increasing by about 50% between 1965 and 1985. Of the approximately 118,000 new cases recorded in 2016, 98.1% involved females. There were 526,000 instances reported as the most common cases in the same year [23]. The age-standardized incidence rate of BC in females increased by 39.1% between 1990 and 2016, which is a significant rise over the previous 26 years. Every state in the union had a constant increase in this regard.

According to GLOBOCAN statistics for 2020, BC accounted for 10.6% (90,408) of all fatalities and 13.5% (178,361) of all cancer cases in India. In India, the total chance of developing breast cancer was estimated to be 2.81. The data presented here highlights the noteworthy influence of breast cancer on the nation's incidence and death rates. Understanding the prevalence and patterns of breast cancer becomes essential for developing effective healthcare interventions and policies as they dive further into the larger panorama of gender-based health insights. The data on years lived with disability per 100,000 (all ages combined) female breast cancer cases is shown in Fig. 5.4a. In contrast to the USA, where a small decline in occurrences of breast cancer has been seen, the trend analysis shows a notable increase in cases of breast cancer in Canada. Australia comes in second with a lower incidence rate than the USA and Canada combined. Interestingly, India's Years Lived with Disability are still around 10 lakhs suggesting a relatively lower prevalence of infirmities associated with breast cancer among the populace.

The GBDLA algorithm that looked at 5-year overall survival statistics indicated that patients in stage I had a 95% survival rate, compared to 92% for those in stage II, 70% for those with stage III, and a dismal 21% for those with stage IV [24]. Compared to nations in the West, the chances of survival for patients with breast cancer in India seem to be lower. Several reasons, including an older age of onset, a late-stage diagnosis, a delayed start to definitive therapy, and inadequate or fragmented treatment, are blamed for this disparity. Figure 5.4b shows the years of disability-adjusted life per 100,000 (all ages) female cases of breast cancer. India and Pakistan have considerably different rates, with Canada, Australia, and the USA having reasonable values. Pakistan is one of the countries with the fastest increasing burden in this regard, indicating a significant impact on the quality of life of the people due to breast cancer. India, on the other hand, has far lower levels, indicating a decreased hardship of living with a handicap. The USA, Canada, and Australia all show moderate values, suggesting that the hardship of living with a handicap is spread evenly among these three countries.

Early identification and fast treatment are the most successful strategies for reducing breast cancer, according to the World Cancer Report 2020 [25]. The

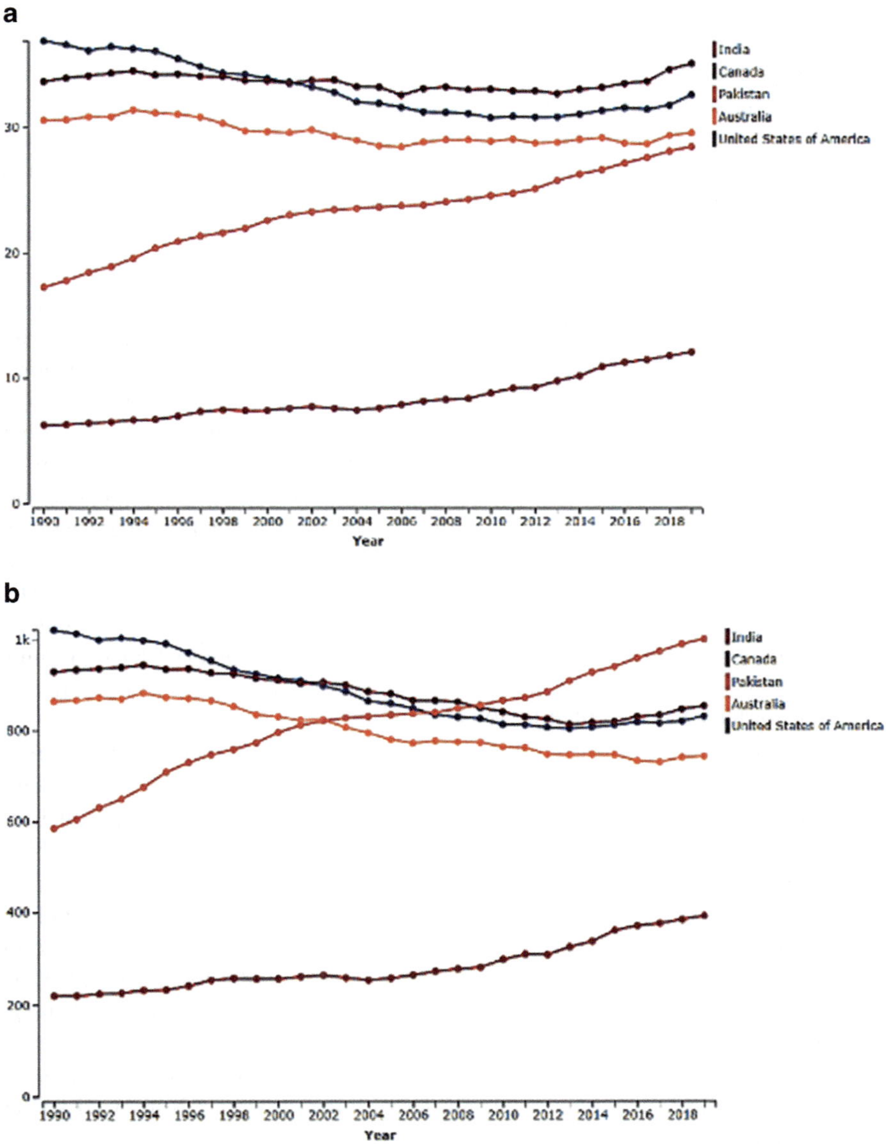

Fig. 5.4 (**a**) Years lived with disability and (**b**) years of disability-adjusted life per 100,000 (all ages females) breast cancer cases

expenses of treating breast cancer escalated with the disease stage upon diagnosis, according to a 2018 systematic analysis that included 20 research. As a result, early detection of breast cancer increases the likelihood of survival and may also lower total treatment expenses. This highlights how crucial early detection programs are in the fight against breast cancer.

5.5.2 Ovarian Cancer

The development of ovarian cancer (OC) is influenced by several variables. It primarily affects women postmenopausal, with an increased frequency associated with aging. Lower survival rates are associated with an increased risk of this illness developing and progressing with age. The correlation between age and incidence of ovarian cancer is noteworthy. Research suggests that postmenopausal women are more vulnerable and that the risk increases with age. Age should be considered while screening and detecting the disease early on since being older is linked to the disease progressing to a more severe level. The studies indicate that parity—the quantity of births—has a protective function. Higher childbearing age is associated with a lower incidence of ovarian cancer, according to studies. This may indicate a decreased risk of ovarian cancer in women who give birth frequently, especially if they do so later in life. Having a positive family history of breast or ovarian cancer is a substantial and well-established risk factor. One's chance of acquiring ovarian cancer rises if they have close relatives who have had various types of cancer. It is also important to know one's family history of cancer because a personal history of the disease increases the risk. The association between smoking and ovarian cancer has been investigated in a few research articles, and the results indicate that smoking is associated with a higher risk, especially for tumors [26]. To lower the risk of subtypes of ovarian cancer, it is crucial to address lifestyle variables, such as quitting smoking.

With ovarian cancer accounting for 1.2% of all cancer cases in 2020, it is a serious health problem. With over 21,750 new cases recorded, cancer is still a very difficult disease to treat. Regretfully, the cost is reflected in the 13,940 fatalities linked to ovarian cancer that are projected to have occurred. Its etiology must be understood to develop efficient prevention measures and early detection techniques. Ovarian cancer has a 5-year proportionate survival rate of 48.6%, which emphasizes the need for early detection. Because 58% of patients are discovered at a stage where metastases have already formed, this worrying figure causes the 5-year survival rate to plummet to 30.2%. However, once it is found locally, the survival rate soars to 92.6% [27]. This underlines how important early detection of ovarian cancer is.

Despite novel treatment techniques and current clinical trials, ovarian cancer is still a difficult illness that presents a substantial threat to women's health. Lack of efficient early detection measures results in delayed diagnosis and restricted treatment choices, which is the main barrier causing poor clinical outcomes. Furthermore, patient outcomes may be negatively impacted by clinical practice deviations from approved norms, underscoring the need for better ovarian cancer care strategies.

The creation of successful tactics is required in the quest for earlier and more treatable ovarian cancer diagnosis. After surgery, the amount of remaining disease is a critical determinant that affects patient survival. To maximize results, this complex treatment should only be carried out by highly skilled gynecologists working in busy, high-volume environments, including big hospitals that see over

20 patients a year [28]. The evidence presented in Fig. 5.5a indicates regional variations in the YLD rates for instances of ovarian cancer. The USA and Canada show a sharp rise in YLD rates, especially compared to Canada, where a little decline is noted. Australia and Pakistan show intermediate degrees of existence between these extremes; in contrast, India shows a major growing tendency akin to that of the USA.

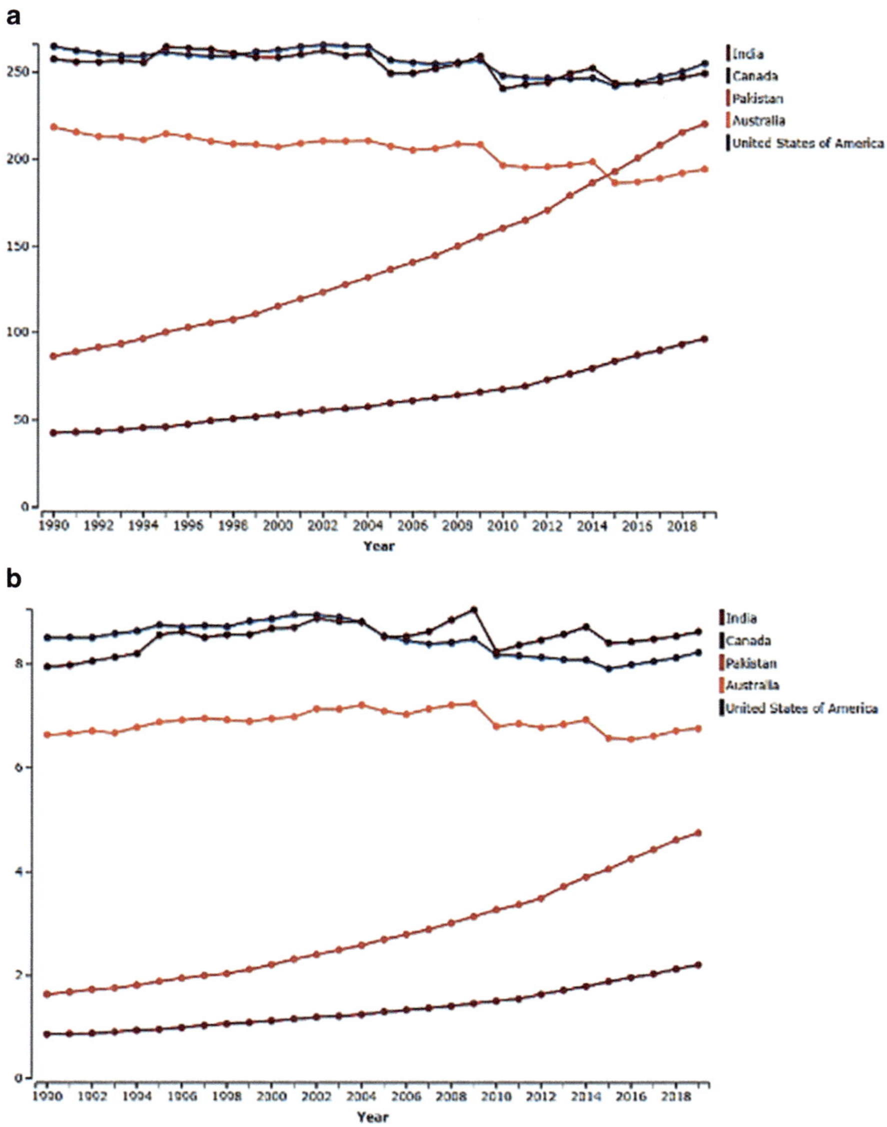

Fig. 5.5 (**a**) Years lived with disability and (**b**) years of disability-adjusted life per 100,000 (all ages females) ovarian cancer cases

Handling ovarian cancer critically depends on patient empowerment via shared decision-making. Patients gain from a thorough conversation encompassing possible advantages, safety profiles, symptom management, and prognosis when contemplating recently developed therapy techniques or enrolling in clinical trials. Optimal care of patients requires a cooperative strategy between medical oncologists, therapeutic oncologists, and an interdisciplinary healthcare group.

Patients with ovarian cancer benefit greatly from early adoption of supportive services, which helps to optimize their course of therapy. Palliative medicine supports an additional, individualized, and holistic strategy for therapy by managing symptoms, offering support, and improving the overall state of life. In contrast, Fig. 5.5b depicts the DALYs per 100,000 female ovarian cancer patients in the same locations, offering an outcome that is slightly different than Fig. 5.5a. Although there are some similarities between the patterns, the DALYs metric provides an additional perspective on the burden of ovarian cancer by accounting for years lived with a disability as well as years lost to early death.

Adequate and reasonably priced follow-up measures are necessary for patients in therapeutic remission. It is essential to educate patients about potential indicators of illness recurrence in addition to normal surveillance. In addition, promoting genetic risk counseling for patients, especially if it hasn't been done before in the early phases of the illness, can support an additional proactive effort and individualized approach to treatment.

5.5.3 Prostate Cancer

The use of artificial intelligence in prostate cancer treatment remains in its infancy. Early findings from AI models are promising for several elements of prostate cancer (PC) treatment. The development of sophisticated AI models that will be important for enhanced training, superior surgical results, diagnosis, and the creation of predictive tools [29] for prostate cancer will require continuing training and testing of AI algorithms. Although there are many potential advantages to using AI in the treatment of prostate cancer, it is crucial to stress how crucial it is to preserve governance in the field of AI-related care [30]. To maintain morale and security procedures in the treatment of prostate cancer, prudent deployment of AI technology is essential. Figure 5.6a shows over the years lived with disability (YLD) per 100,000 males with prostate cancer. The statistics demonstrate striking differences across the nations; Pakistan exhibits a notable increase compared to Canada and the USA, while India and Australia are displaying remarkably high rates. Figure 5.6b displays the number of years of disability-adjusted life (DALYs) for every 100,000 male individuals diagnosed with prostate cancer. The results demonstrate regional differences in the distribution, with Pakistan and the USA seeing comparable increases. While Canada and Australia also record incidences of gender-based differences in prostate cancer incidence, India reports modest rates, ranging from 60,000 to 80,000.

Men are more likely than women to receive a prostate cancer diagnosis, and the number of cases each year is rising. The financial stability and resources in medical

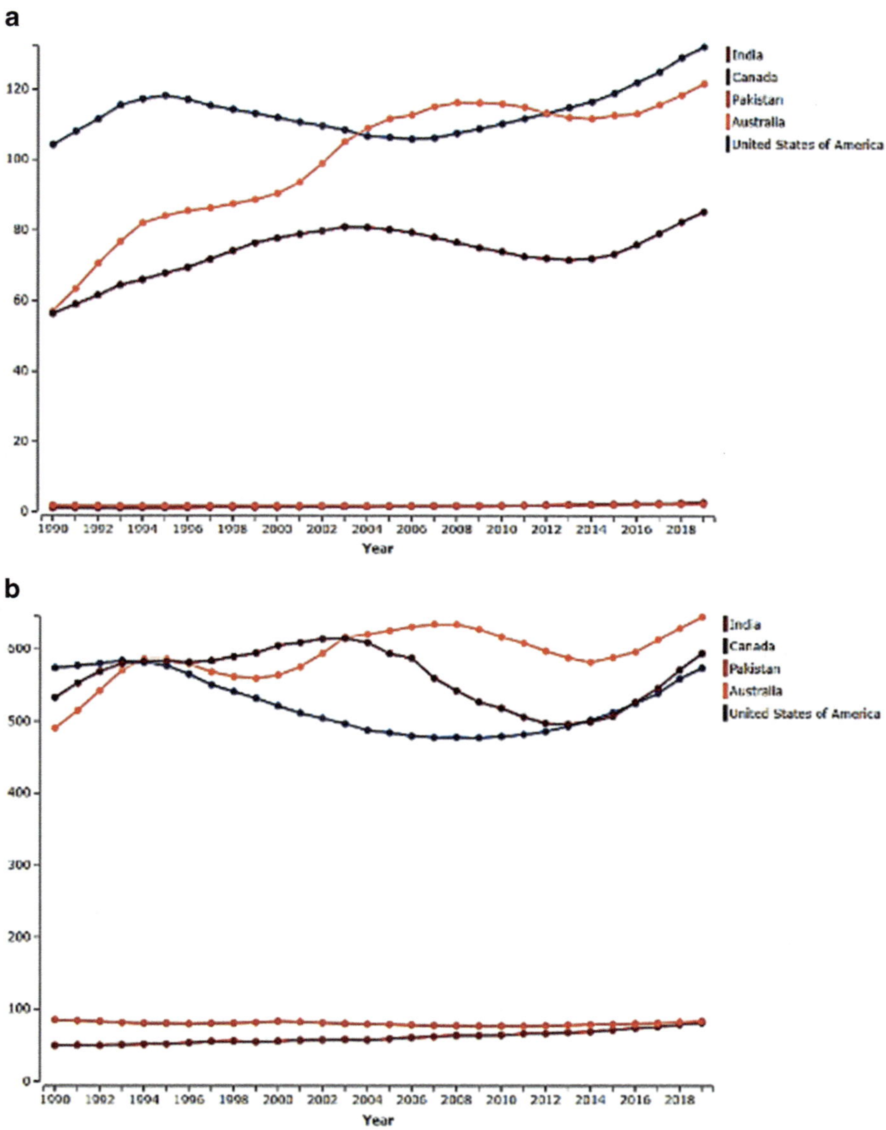

Fig. 5.6 (**a**) Years lived with disability and (**b**) years of disability-adjusted life per 100,000 (all ages males) prostate cancer cases

institutions that cure prostate cancer have been strained by the increase in cases as well as by the introduction of novel treatment choices and improved diagnostic techniques. Artificial intelligence (AI) integration is a promising complement to human engagement and in certain cases, a possible replacement [31]. This may lessen some of the problems associated with resources, which would save costs [32]. Moreover, automation tackles problems like differences in observations across time and between various people. It is also capable of quickly and precisely analyzing large datasets. Examine the growing uses of AI and its related domains concerning prostate cancer.

5.5.4 Lung Cancer

The fascinating history of lung cancer (LC) has spread around the world and had a significant impact on people's health and well-being. The research delves into the complexities of the LIDC-IDRI database to solve the puzzles surrounding this illness. Authors analyzed the disorderly course of this horrifying illness using DICOM imaging data. The reference region consists of 21 regions, including 195 countries and territories, throughout the diagnostic period of 2015 to 2023. It has carefully examined data on longevity related to lung cancer and years of life with disability throughout this time to investigate the effects of various risk factors [33]. Through the darkness of this widespread sickness, the age-standardized rates and their yearly percentage changes emerged as beacons of hope.

The major causes of mortality and DALYs were found to be behaviors, both ingrained and modifiable. Smoking, second-hand smoke, and a low-fruit diet were the most common of these behaviors. The harmful effects of environmental and occupational hazards as well as metabolic risks, particularly high fasting glucose values, were far in the past. Age has increased the impact of various risk variables. In the global impact mosaic, high-income North America and Asia are where behavioral hazards have the longest-lasting effects. Governments must act quickly to change the trajectory of this risk, especially in nations like Pakistan and India, where smoking has been more common for some time.

The disparity in the burden of disability is seen in Fig. 5.7a, which focuses on years lived with disability per 100,000 cases. Gender disparities in health outcomes are evident, with males in the USA and Canada bearing a disproportionate amount of the burden of impairment relative to other locations. On the other hand, India has the fewest disability-adjusted life years (DALYs) per 100,000 instances, which suggests that its health results are more favorable. Falling in the middle, Pakistan and Australia demonstrate regional variations in gender-based healthcare while also indicating a moderate burden of impairment. However, Fig. 5.7b illustrates the years of life adjusted for the illness by 100,000 instances of women, emphasizing the impact of the illness and premature death. This time, the pattern is the same, but there are some slight variations.

Though the number of years that women in the USA and Canada have adapted to disability is more than 100,000 instances, this difference is less pronounced when compared to males. India is the country with the lowest burden of years lived with a handicap adjusted for life, which suggests that women with ovarian cancer would have better health outcomes. Pakistan and Australia both retain a moderate level of disability-adjusted life years, which highlights the necessity of ongoing efforts to eliminate regional inequities in healthcare based on gender.

With an emphasis on men, Fig. 5.7c illustrates the differences in years lived with disability per 100,000 cases. There are gender-based health disparities in the USA and Canada, where men experience a greater amount of impairment in comparison to other locations. In contrast, India has the lowest years lived with disability per 100,000 instances, indicating that its health results are generally good. Australia and Pakistan are in the middle, showing regional differences in healthcare for women and showing a modest burden of impairment. The burden of disease and early mortality, however, is shown in Fig. 5.7d, which shows the years lived with disability

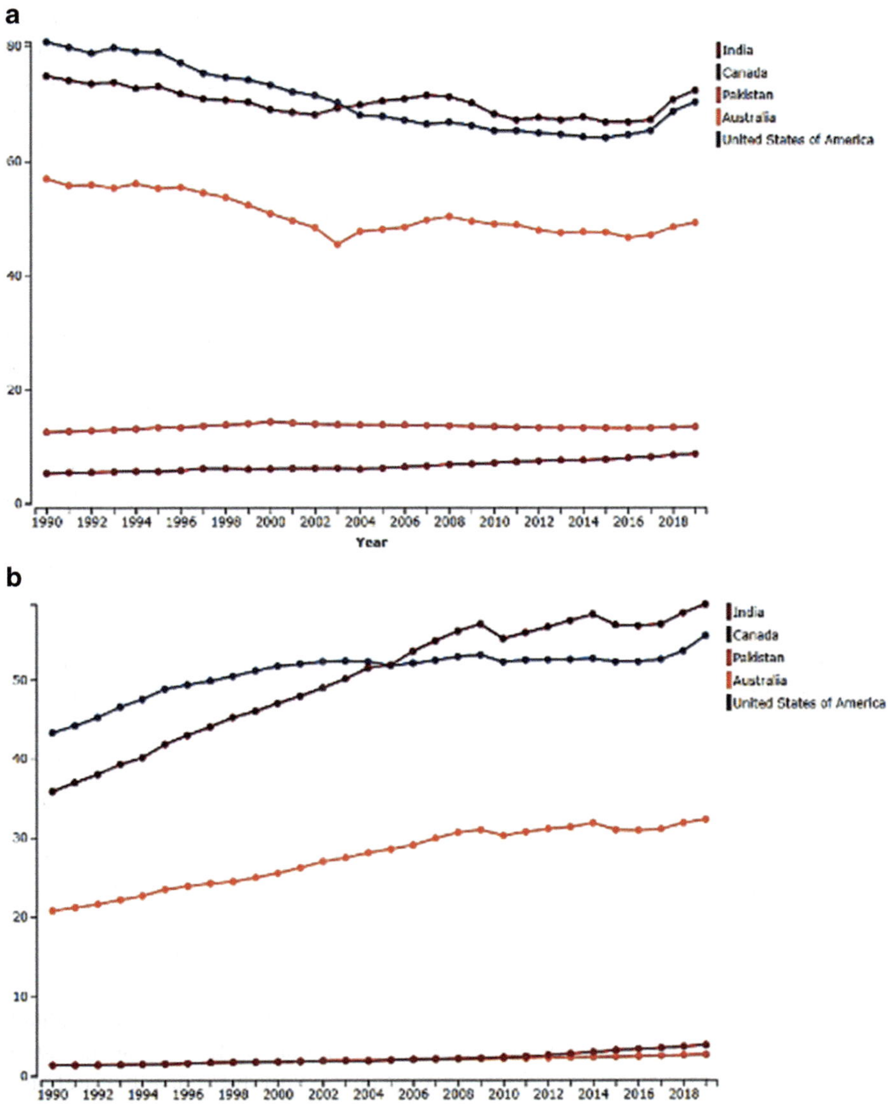

Fig. 5.7 (**a**) All males and (**b**) all females of death per 100,000 lung cancer cases. (**c**) All males and (**d**) all females of years lived with disability per 100,000 lung cancer cases

c

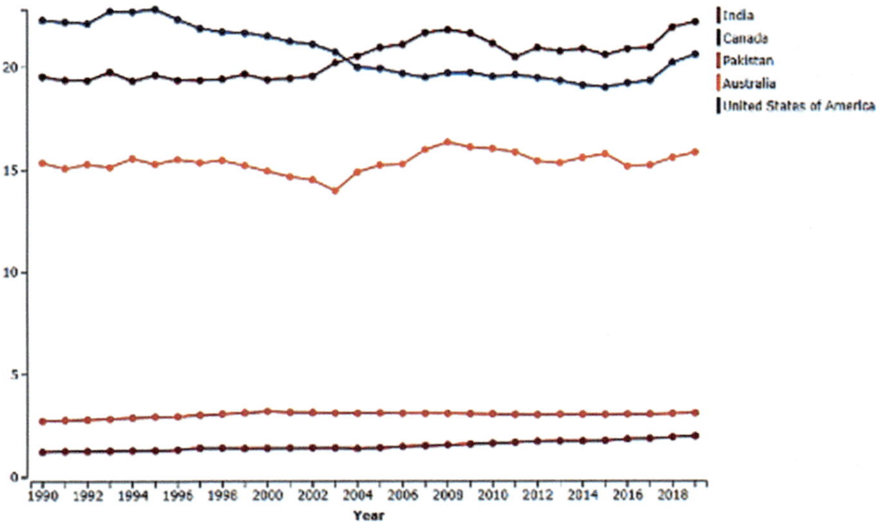

d

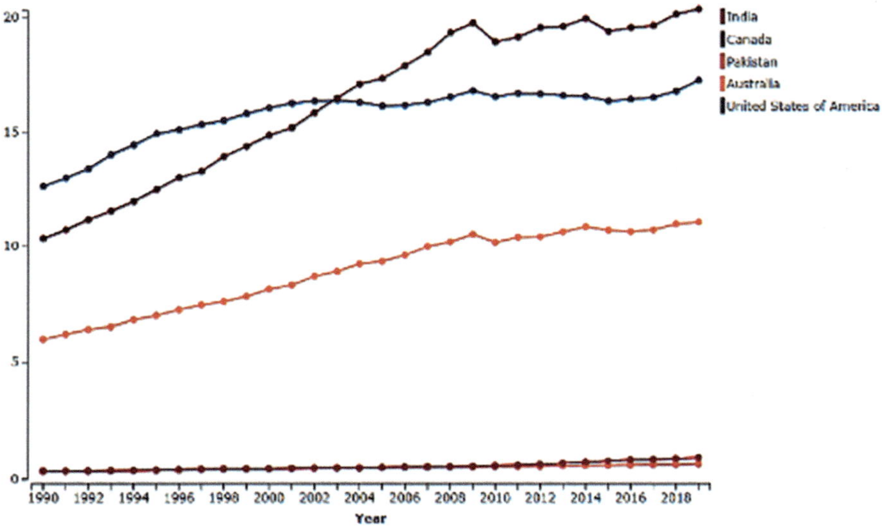

Fig. 5.7 (continued)

per 100,000 instances for women. Though with a few minor differences, similar patterns appear. Though the difference is not as great as it is for men, women in the USA and Canada live with a handicap for a significant number of years out of every 100,000 instances. It is noteworthy that women in India had the lowest burden of disability-adjusted life years, which may indicate improved health outcomes. Conversely, Pakistan and Australia have modest levels of disability-adjusted life years, highlighting the continued necessity of addressing gender-based healthcare inequities in these regions.

The areas most impacted were the lower reaches of the social and economic spectrum. The three main factors that affected lung cancer mortality and disability-adjusted life years (DALYs), were air pollution, tobacco use, and an unhealthful diet. The ubiquitous concentration of fine particulate matter in the atmosphere (PM2.5) contributed weakly to the worsening of lung crevasses, especially in less developed regions [34]. As it is negotiated the terrain of tobacco-related difficulties, a gendered narrative came to light. Up until 2013, women were more vulnerable to costs related to tobacco use, which suggests that quitting smoking was not accomplished as quickly as it may have been for men. This suggests that attempts to restrict tobacco use worldwide have had an impact on women. Nevertheless, concerns about the current route are reflected in the steady decline in the smoker rate. Metabolic risks, as seen by elevated blood sugar levels while fasting, contributed to further complexity [35]. In contrast to the stability of males, the prognosis for women started to improve. The complex relationship between fasting glucose levels and survival chances was shown in a report that emerged from the connections between diabetes and lung cancer mortality. The strength of our investigation resides in providing an extensive assessment of the worldwide burden. However, a warning is there in the data mixture [36].

5.5.5 Nutritional Deficiencies

The World Health Organization (WHO) defines "micronutrients" as substances that are needed in extremely small amounts, less than 100 mg/day. The creation of hormones, enzymes, and other critical chemicals that regulate growth and development needs micronutrients like vitamins and minerals. Many serious issues affect public health, such as iron deficiency, vitamin A deficiency, and goiter. The term "hidden hunger" or "micronutrient malnutrition' refers to several serious conditions, including early mortality, impaired health, visual impairments, delayed development, mental illnesses, learning difficulties, and exhaustion. According to the WHO, undernourishment is responsible for 45% of deaths in children under five. Considering the significant harm that nutrient deficiencies (ND) cause to children and expectant mothers, low-income countries must ensure get enough of these nutrients. Remarkably, 42% of children under 5 years old and 40% of pregnant women in these areas suffer from anemia [37]. Only 66% of households worldwide have access to iodized salt, according to a thorough investigation carried out by the WHO and the United Nations Children's Fund. This vitamin A deficit affects 19.1 million pregnant women and 190 million preschool-aged children. Moreover, deficiencies in other critical micronutrients affect about 2 million individuals. This demonstrates how urgently the world must pay attention to and take action to address micronutrient deficiencies.

Given the prevalence of overweight and underweight issues in India, the current state of nutrition represents a transitional phase. Despite these concerns, the widespread lack of micronutrients, which may be caused by the nation's predominant consumption of cereal products, remains a significant challenge. In 2016 in India, the overall death rate from hunger was 0.5% (95% CI 0.4%, 0.6%), highlighting the severity of the issue. The National Family Health Survey brought to light India's concerning status as the world leader in the burden of anemia. In 2016, there was a notable increase in the prevalence of anemia, with 58.6% among children, 53.2% among women who were not pregnant, and 50.4% among older women [38]. It was found that 32% of teenagers and 19% of preschoolers had low zinc levels. Moreover, it was shown that 23% of preschoolers and 37% of teenagers had folate deficits. Significant vitamin deficiencies also occur, with vitamin B12, vitamin A, and vitamin D deficiencies ranging from 14% to 31% in children and adolescents in the preschool age group. Concerning anemia rates 67% among preschoolers and 69% among teenagers were found at the same time. In addition, the goiter prevalence indicated that 3.9% of people had iodine-deficient diseases [39]. The findings of this study emphasize the critical need for an all-encompassing approach to address the various dietary issues facing the Indian population. Figure 5.8a depicts the disease-adapted life for 100,000 cases of malnutrition for all men, illustrating varying pressure levels in different geographic areas. The spectrum of disability in nations like Pakistan and India has decreased noticeably as compared to other locations, showing serious difficulties in controlling sickness and early mortality. Men in the USA and Canada also exhibit an unusually high rate of years lived with a handicap per 100,000 instances; however, this disparity is less pronounced than it is for women. India, on the other hand, has the lowest rate of disability-adjusted life per 100,000 cases of women's dietary deficiencies, which may point to improved health outcomes for women. This time, Pakistan and Australia show somewhat adjusted living standards for 100,000 undernourished people, highlighting the ongoing need to tackle gender-based health disparities across all regions.

The World Health Organization and the Ministry of Health and Family Welfare in India conducted a recent study that found variations in the prevalence of anemia among India's various demographic groups. Reported were 58.6%, 53.1%, 50.4%, and 22.7% in children between 6 and 59 months, between 15 and 49 years in women, between 15 and 49 years in mothers, and between 15 and 49 years in men. A study conducted by the Indian Council of Medical Research revealed that 84% of girls and 9% of women suffered from anemia. There is a widespread vitamin B12 deficiency in India, with varying degrees of severity reported in studies. According to a 2019 study, 47% of the population in Northern India, including a higher percentage of those with diabetes, had a vitamin B12 deficiency. An additional study conducted in South India revealed that 55% of pregnant women reside in rural areas. The results of the most recent study support these figures and indicate a 53% vitamin B12 deficiency. This demonstrates how frequently this issue arises in various Indian regions [40]. The differences in life adapted to the illness for each of the 100,000 women who experience malnutrition are examined in Fig. 5.8b, with a focus on men. It is noteworthy that women in Pakistan and India had a significantly lower rate of impairment compared to women in other regions, indicating blatant gender-based health disparities. However, the lowest rates of disability-adjusted life per 100,000 nutritional deficiencies cases are found in the USA, Canada, and Australia, indicating that women's health results are generally favorable.

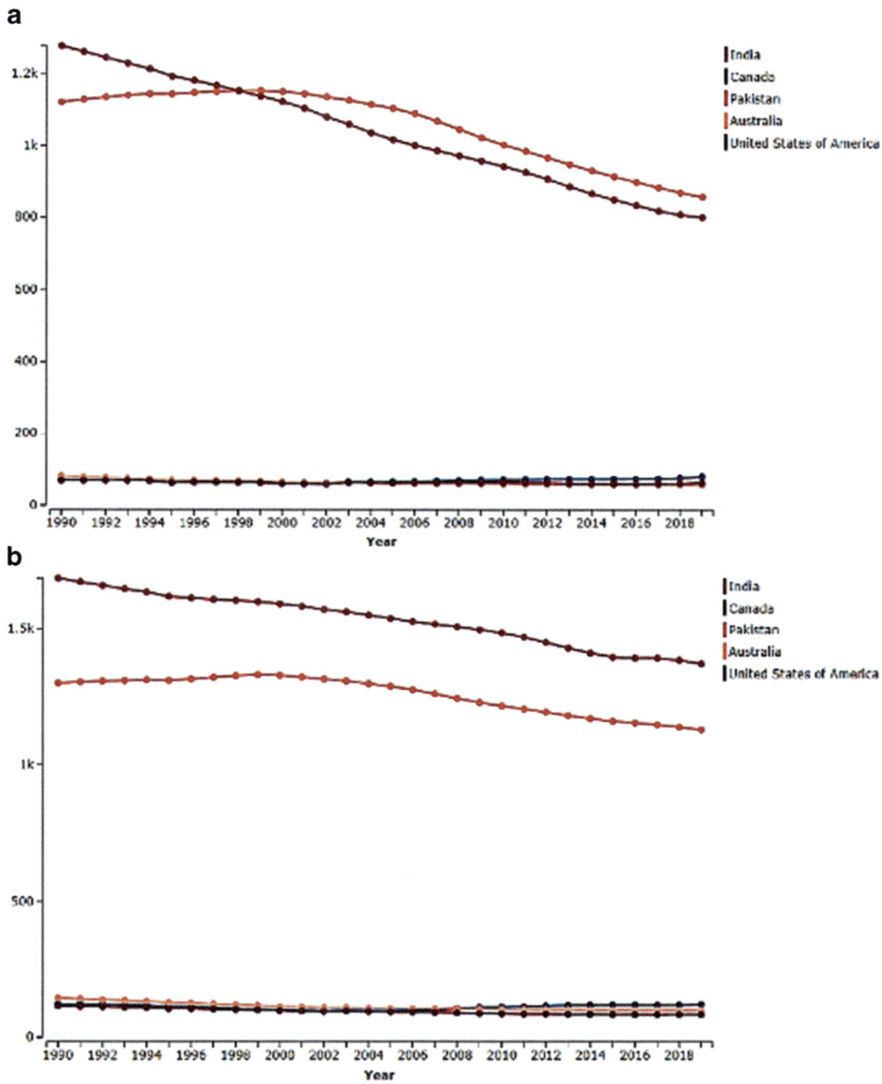

Fig. 5.8 (**a**) All males and (**b**) all females of disability-adjusted life per 100,000 nutritional deficiencies cases

The problem of vitamin A deficiency persists in India, especially among children in the preschool age group. The rates of 10.2% among children aged 1–8 years were found in regional studies conducted in the Southern Indian Tribal Community. However, the investigation conducted today reveals that children under five have a greater frequency at 19%. This points to potential geographical differences impacted by dietary preferences, financial status, mobility for healthcare, and involvement in the wider society. Interestingly, the prevalence of night blindness is essentially nonexistent in the USA and barely 1% in Europe. Iodine deficiency disorders are significantly more likely to occur among 13 million unprotected newborns born in India, according to a 2006 UNICEF newsletter. The current analysis demonstrates that is prevalent in 17% of the Indian population [41]. This highlights the need for global salt solarization as a workable and environmentally responsible solution. The study also shows that 6% of women had ascorbic acid levels below 3 ng/mL, which may have detrimental effects on both men's and women's health. Vitamin D deficiency, which is thought to be widespread yet is frequently undiagnosed and untreated, affects more than half of the Indian population and is distributed between 50% and 94% across various age groups, with 56.3% among seniors living in cities. The study highlights the necessity for health education and vitamin D fortification of staple foods like milk to address the pervasiveness of VDD in India.

5.6 Conclusion

The convergence of AI, machine learning, and enormous amounts of data is bringing about a revolutionary era of gender-based health insights in the healthcare industry. This chapter has focused on the groundbreaking possibilities of cutting-edge technologies and predictive analytics, which provide so far unheard-of opportunities to transform healthcare [42]. Gender-specific health data are becoming a valuable tool that guides the healthcare system toward inclusion and conscious decision-making.

A clarified outline of variations is provided by the investigation of gender-related health issues, such as prostate, ovarian, breast, and lung cancer, and mental health issues [43]. This highlights the urgent need to change paradigms and emphasizes the need to overcome conventional prejudices in research methods. Gender-specific data will become a vital tool in the fight against deeply ingrained inequality, the identification of preconceptions, and the advancement of a comprehensive understanding of health.

As the accuracy of algorithms is so important, the authors urge healthcare professionals to aggressively overcome biases in predictive analytics. The transformational power of public participation emerges in many geographical regions, closing knowledge gaps and promoting inclusivity in healthcare delivery. The necessity for further improvement is highlighted by the gender bias in healthcare research and the revolutionary potential of AI in retrospective observational studies. It is imperative to identify and address gender bias to guarantee that computational medical studies uncover gender disparities that go beyond cultural and biological reasons.

Machine learning algorithms have a significant role in cancer diagnosis and predictive medicine because they facilitate the identification of high-risk patients and the optimization of assisted reproductive technologies. The adept handling of stroke imaging data is an example of how AI may be used effectively in healthcare applications. Given the changing landscape of medicine, this chapter calls for a long-term commitment to the use of AI, machine learning, and predictive analytics.

A future where new technological advancements lead to comprehensive and equitable health outcomes for everyone is presented by this path toward gender-inclusive medical care.

References

1. Lounsbury O, Roberts L, Goodman JR, Batey P, Naar L, Flott KM, Lawrence-Jones A, Ghafur S, Darzi A, Neves AL. Opening a "can of worms" to explore the public's hopes and fears about healthcare data sharing: qualitative study. J Med Internet Res. 2021;23(2):e22744.
2. Smith B, Khojandi A, Vasudevan R. Bias in reinforcement learning: a review in healthcare applications. ACM Comput Surv. 2023;56(2):1–17.
3. Nielsen MW, Stefanick ML, Peragine D, Neilands TB, Ioannidis JPA, Pilote L, Prochaska JJ, et al. Gender-related variables for health research. Biol Sex Diff. 2021;12:1–16.
4. Kuruvila M, Estevez E, Anantharaj A, Mediboina A. Gender equality in antiphospholipid syndrome publications: a comprehensive analysis of first author trends. Cureus. 2023;15(12):e50186.
5. Goldenberg SL, Nir G, Salcudean SE. A new era: artificial intelligence and machine learning in prostate cancer. Nat Rev Urol. 2019;16(7):391–403.
6. Temel JS, Greer JA, Muzikansky A, Gallagher ER, Admane S, Jackson VA, Dahlin CM, Blinderman CD, Jacobsen J, Pirl WF, Billings JA, Lynch TJ. Early palliative care for patients with metastatic non-small-cell lung cancer. N Engl J Med. 2010;363(8):733–42.
7. Bakitas MA, Tosteson TD, Li Z, Lyons KD, Hull JG, Li Z, Dionne-Odom JN, Frost J, Dragnev KH, Hegel MT, Azuero A, Ahles TA. Early versus delayed initiation of concurrent palliative oncology care: patient outcomes in the ENABLE III randomized controlled trial. J Clin Oncol. 2015;33(13):1438–45.
8. Kumar V, Bakariya B. An empirical identification of pulmonary nodules using deep learning. Des Eng. 2021:13468–86. https://thedesignengineering.com/index.php/DE/article/view/4610.
9. Mottet N, Bellmunt J, Bolla M, Briers E, Cumberbatch MG, De Santis M, Fossat N, et al. EAU-ESTRO-SIOG guidelines on prostate cancer. Part 1: screening, diagnosis, and local treatment with curative intent. Eur Urol. 2017;71(4):618–29.
10. Kanagasingam Y, Xiao D, Vignarajan J, Preetham A, Tay-Kearney M-L, Mehrotra A. Evaluation of artificial intelligence–based grading of diabetic retinopathy in primary care. JAMA Netw Open. 2018;1(5):e182665.
11. de la Calle CM, Nguyen HG, Hosseini-Asl E, So C, Socher R, Xiong C, Xue L, Carroll P, Cooperberg MR. Artificial intelligence for streamlined immunofluorescence-based biomarker discovery in prostate cancer. J Clin Oncol. 2020;38:279.
12. To T, Stanojevic S, Moores G, Gershon AS, Bateman ED, Cruz AA, Boulet L-P. Global asthma prevalence in adults: findings from the cross-sectional world health survey. BMC Public Health. 2012;12(1):1–8.
13. Kaggle Healthcare Dataset. https://www.kaggle.com/datasets/tomaslui/healthcare-dataset/data.
14. Fuhlbrigge AL, Jackson B, Wright RJ. Gender and asthma. Immunol Allergy Clin. 2002;22(4):753–89.
15. Eder W, Ege MJ, von Mutius E. The asthma epidemic. N Engl J Med. 2006;355(21):2226–35.
16. Gupta PD. Specific needs for healthcare on gender basis in infectious diseases and cancers. Int J Clin Case Rep. 2023;2(2). https://doi.org/10.31579/2834-8389/022.
17. Kavousi S, Maharlouei N, Rezvani A, Aliabad HA, Vardanjani HM. Worldwide association of the gender inequality with the incidence and mortality of cervical, ovarian, endometrial, and breast cancers. SSM Popul Health. 2024;25:101613.
18. Sledge P. From decision to incision: ideologies of gender in surgical cancer care. Soc Sci Med. 2019;239:112550.

19. Rana RH, Alam F, Alam K, Gow J. Gender-specific differences in care-seeking behaviour among lung cancer patients: a systematic review. J Cancer Res Clin Oncol. 2020;146:1169–96.
20. Jabbour J, Khalil M, Ronzoni AR, Mabry R, Al-Jawaldeh A, El-Adawy M, Sakr H. Malnutrition and gender disparities in the eastern Mediterranean region: the need for action. Front Nutr. 2023;10:1113662.
21. Cirillo D, Catuara-Solarz S, Morey C, Guney E, Subirats L, Mellino S, Gigante A, et al. Sex and gender differences and biases in artificial intelligence for biomedicine and healthcare. NPJ Digital Med. 2020;3(1):81.
22. Pavord ID, Beasley R, Agusti A, Anderson GP, Bel E, Brusselle G, Cullinan P, et al. After asthma: redefining airways diseases. Lancet. 2018;391(10118):350–400.
23. Parida SP, Behera BK, Raut S, Panda K, Bhattacharjee S, editors. Micronutrient deficiency. Newredmars Education Pvt. Ltd.; 2023.
24. Kulik-Rechberger B, Dubel M. Iron deficiency, iron deficiency anaemia and anaemia of inflammation—an overview. Ann Agric Environ Med. 2024;31:151.
25. Dicker D, Nguyen G, Abate D, Abate KH, Abay SM, Abbafati C, Abbasi N, et al. Global, regional, and national age-sex-specific mortality and life expectancy, 1950–2017: a systematic analysis for the Global Burden of Disease Study 2017. Lancet. 2018;392(10159):1684–735.
26. Stanaway JD, Afshin A, Gakidou E, Lim SS, Abate D, Abate KH, Abbafati C, et al. Global, regional, and national comparative risk assessment of 84 behavioural, environmental and occupational, and metabolic risks or clusters of risks for 195 countries and territories, 1990–2017: a systematic analysis for the Global Burden of Disease Study 2017. Lancet. 2018;392(10159):1923–94.
27. Dandona R, Anil Kumar G, Dhaliwal RS, Naghavi M, Theo Vos DK, Shukla LV, et al. Gender differentials and state variations in suicide deaths in India: the Global Burden of Disease Study 1990–2016. Lancet Public Health. 2018;3(10):e478–89.
28. Jadhav A, Weitzman A, Smith-Greenaway E. Household sanitation facilities and women's risk of non-partner sexual violence in India. BMC Public Health. 2016;16:1–10.
29. Verma K, Bhardwaj S, Arya R, Islam MSU, Bhushan M, Kumar A, Samant P. Latest tools for data mining and machine learning. Int J Innov Technol Explor Eng. 2019;8(9):18–23.
30. Sanz-Barbero B, Barón N, Vives-Cases C. Prevalence, associated factors and health impact of intimate partner violence against women in different life stages. PLoS One. 2019;14(10):e0221049.
31. Prabha C, Singh J, Agarwal S, Verma A, Sharma N. Introduction to computational intelligence in healthcare. In: Computational intelligence in healthcare. Boca Raton: CRC Press; 2022. p. 1–15.
32. Moitra M, Santomauro D, Collins PY, Vos T, Whiteford H, Saxena S, Ferrari AJ. The global gap in treatment coverage for major depressive disorder in 84 countries from 2000–2019: a systematic review and Bayesian meta-regression analysis. PLoS Med. 2022;19(2):e1003901.
33. Williamson PO, Minter CIJ. Exploring PubMed as a reliable resource for scholarly communications services. J Med Libr Assoc. 2019;107(1):16.
34. Singla R, Garg A, Surana V, Aggarwal S, Gupta G, Singla S. Vitamin B12 deficiency is endemic in Indian population: a perspective from North India. Indian J Endocrinol Metab. 2019;23(2):211.
35. Kumar V, Bakariya B. Classification of malignant lung cancer using deep learning. J Med Eng Technol. 2021;45(2):85–93. https://doi.org/10.1080/03091902.2020.1853837.
36. Agarwal S, Prabha C. Analysis of lung cancer prediction at an early stage: a systematic review. In: Lecture notes on data engineering and communications technologies. Singapore: Springer Nature; 2022. p. 701–71.
37. Awotunde JB, Adeniyi AE, Ajagbe SA, González-Briones A. Natural computing and unsupervised learning methods in smart healthcare data-centric operations. In: Cognitive and soft computing techniques for the analysis of healthcare data. Academic Press; 2022. p. 165–90.
38. Braveman P. Defining health equity. J Natl Med Assoc. 2022;114(6):593–600.
39. Lund EM, Burgess CM. Sexual and gender minority healthcare disparities: barriers to care and strategies to bridge the gap. Prim Care. 2021;48(2):179–89.

40. Rajasegaran J, Jayasundara V, Jayasekara S, Jayasekara H, Seneviratne S, Rodrigo R. Deepcaps: going deeper with capsule networks. In: Proceedings of the IEEE/CVF conference on computer vision and pattern recognition; 2019. p. 10725–33.
41. Raftery P, Howard N, Palmer J, Hossain M. Gender-based violence (GBV) coordination in humanitarian and public health emergencies: a scoping review. Confl Heal. 2022;16(1):37.
42. Ramesh TR, Lilhore UK, Poongodi M, Simaiya S, Kaur A, Hamdi M. Predictive analysis of heart diseases with machine learning approaches. Malays J Comput Sci. 2022:132–48. https://doi.org/10.22452/mjcs.sp2022no1.10.
43. Sharma G, Prabha C. A systematic review for detecting cancer using machine learning techniques. In: Innovations in computational and computer techniques: ICACCT-2021; 2022.

Tracking Nutrient Intake with AI: How AI Can Help Monitor and Optimize Nutrient Consumption

6

Pawan Whig, Balaram Yadav Kasula, Nikhitha Yathiraju, Anupriya Jain, and Seema Sharma

6.1 Introduction

In recent years, the intersection of artificial intelligence (AI) and healthcare has heralded groundbreaking advancements, revolutionizing various aspects of wellness management. One such pivotal area is the monitoring and optimization of nutrient consumption [1]. Nutrition stands at the core of human health, influencing bodily functions, energy levels, and overall well-being. Understanding the significance of a balanced diet is not novel; however, the means of monitoring and optimizing nutrient intake have undergone a significant transformation, owing largely to the integration of AI-driven technologies. Traditional methods of tracking nutrient intake have been laborious and often imprecise, relying on manual record-keeping, subjective estimations, or simplified charts [2]. However, the advent of AI has marked a paradigm shift in how individuals can monitor and optimize their nutritional habits. AI brings to the fore a myriad of tools and techniques that enhance the accuracy, efficiency, and personalization of dietary analysis, offering individuals, healthcare professionals, and researchers unparalleled insights into nutrient consumption [3].

At the heart of AI's role in nutrient intake optimization lies its capacity for data processing and analysis. With the proliferation of wearable devices, smartphone applications, and smart kitchen appliances, an unprecedented amount of data pertaining to dietary habits, food choices, and nutritional content is being

P. Whig (✉)
Vivekananda Institute of Professional Studies-TC, New Delhi, India

B. Y. Kasula · N. Yathiraju
University of the Cumberlands, Williamsburg, KY, USA

A. Jain · S. Sharma
School of Computer Applications, MRIIRS, Faridabad, India
e-mail: anupriya.sca@mriu.edu.in; seema.sca@mriu.edu.in

R. Kumar et al. (eds.), *AI-Based Nutritional Intervention in Polycystic Ovary Syndrome (PCOS)*, https://doi.org/10.1007/978-981-96-2120-0_6

generated [4]. AI algorithms can ingest, analyze, and interpret this data, enabling users to comprehend their nutritional patterns comprehensively. Through machine learning models, AI can discern intricate patterns within this data, providing tailored recommendations and insights personalized to an individual's unique dietary requirements [5]. Moreover, AI-powered tools not only aid in monitoring nutrient intake but also offer proactive solutions to optimize it. These solutions encompass a spectrum of functionalities, including meal planning, recipe suggestions, and real-time dietary guidance. By leveraging AI, individuals can receive instant feedback on their food choices, understand the nutritional composition of their meals, and even anticipate potential deficiencies or excesses in their diet [6]. This real-time assistance fosters informed decision-making, empowering users to make healthier dietary choices effortlessly. One of the groundbreaking applications of AI in nutrition monitoring is the development of intelligent food recognition systems. These systems employ computer vision algorithms to identify and analyze food items from images or videos, enabling users to effortlessly log their meals. Coupled with databases containing nutritional information, these systems can provide precise and detailed insights into the nutrient composition of various foods. Furthermore, AI's ability to adapt and learn from user behavior allows these systems to enhance accuracy over time, customizing recommendations and insights based on individual preferences and habits [7–9].

AI's impact on nutrient intake optimization extends beyond individual wellness, permeating into clinical settings and public health initiatives as shown in Table 6.1. Healthcare professionals can harness AI-powered tools to assess patients' dietary patterns accurately, facilitating personalized recommendations for managing chronic conditions or nutritional deficiencies. Additionally, AI-driven analyses of large-scale dietary data can unveil population-level trends, aiding policymakers in formulating effective strategies to combat malnutrition or promote healthier eating habits at a societal level [10].

However, the integration of AI in nutrition monitoring is not devoid of challenges. Privacy concerns, data accuracy, and the need for continuous algorithm refinement remain significant hurdles. Ensuring the ethical collection and utilization of user data, validating the accuracy of AI-generated recommendations, and mitigating biases in algorithmic predictions are critical aspects that necessitate continuous attention and refinement. The fusion of AI technologies with the realm of nutrition monitoring and optimization presents an unprecedented opportunity to revolutionize the way individuals perceive, manage, and enhance their dietary habits. From personalized insights to real-time guidance, AI stands as a beacon of innovation, empowering individuals and healthcare professionals alike to navigate the intricate landscape of nutrition with unparalleled precision and efficacy. This book chapter aims to delve deeper into the multifaceted facets of AI's role in tracking nutrient intake, exploring its applications, challenges, and the transformative potential it holds in shaping the future of nutrition management.

Organization of Chapter

The rest of the chapter is organized as follows: Section 6.2 enlightens the literature review. Section 6.3 focuses on dietary assessment methods and challenges followed

Table 6.1 Literature review with research gap

Reference	Summary	Research gap
Lu et al. (2020) [2]	AI-based system for assessing nutrient intake in hospitalized patients	Limited focus on real-time applications for continuous nutrient assessment
de Moraes Lopes et al. (2020) [3]	AI in precision nutrition and fitness	Lack of emphasis on the integration of AI technologies for personalized fitness programs
Sempionatto et al. (2021) [4]	Wearable and mobile sensors for personalized nutrition	Limited exploration of the challenges and limitations associated with wearable sensors
Verma et al. (2018) [5]	Challenges in personalized nutrition and health.	Need for more insights into overcoming challenges and practical strategies for implementation
Boland et al. (2019) [6]	Modern technologies for personalized nutrition	Limited discussion on the integration challenges and potential drawbacks of modern technologies
Zhao et al. (2021) [7]	Emerging trends in technology-based dietary assessment	Lack of exploration of the adoption challenges and societal impact of technology-based assessments
Rollo et al. (2016) [8]	eHealth technologies to support nutrition and physical activity in diabetes self-management	Limited discussion on the scalability and long-term effectiveness of eHealth technologies
Garcia (2023) [9]	ChatGPT as a virtual dietitian: Exploring its potential	Need for empirical evidence on the effectiveness and user acceptance of ChatGPT in nutrition support
Lowe et al. (2022) [10]	Review on machine learning, AI, and smart technology in water treatment	Limited exploration of how the findings from water treatment can be applied to nutrition science
George (2022) [11]	Cloud-based digital health application integrated with AI modules for medical nutrition therapy	Limited discussion on the practical challenges and ethical considerations of cloud-based applications
Bond et al. (2023) [12]	AI and clinical nutrition: Future prospects	Lack of insights into the potential ethical concerns and regulatory aspects of AI in clinical nutrition
Chew et al. (2021) [13]	Potential of AI in enhancing adult weight loss: a scoping review	Limited exploration of the long-term sustainability and user adherence to AI-based weight loss interventions
Shi et al. (2022) [14]	Wearable technologies for measuring nutrient intake	Need for more extensive research on the accuracy and reliability of wearable technologies in nutrient measurement
Singh et al. (2023) [15]	AI and ML-based monitoring and design of biological wastewater treatment systems	Limited discussion on the applicability of findings to personalized nutrition and health
Cohen et al. (2023) [16]	Role of AI in deciphering diet-disease relationships: case studies	Need for more case studies and empirical evidence to support the practical application of AI in diet-disease relationships

(continued)

Table 6.1 (continued)

Reference	Summary	Research gap
Kaur et al. (2023) [17]	Deep neural network for food image classification and nutrient identification: a systematic review	Limited exploration of the interpretability and potential biases associated with deep neural networks in nutrient identification
Joshi et al. (2023) [18]	AI-assisted food science and nutrition perspective for smart nutrition research and healthcare	Limited exploration of how AI can contribute to smart nutrition research and practical healthcare applications
Wang and Hsu (2023) [19]	Integrating AI and wearable IoT system in long-term care environments	Limited discussion on the ethical considerations and user acceptance of AI and IoT in long-term care environments
Dobermann et al. (2022) [20]	Responsible plant nutrition: supporting food system transformation	Lack of insights into how responsible plant nutrition practices can be extended to support human nutrition and health

by a discussion on AI technologies in nutrient intake tracking in Sect. 6.4. Section 6.5 highlights machine learning models for dietary monitoring. Section 6.6 illustrates health implications and benefits. Section 6.7 discusses the case study on the effectiveness of AI-driven nutrient tracking on health outcomes. And, finally, Sect. 6.8 concludes the chapter.

6.2 Literature Review

The literature review explores seminal studies and contemporary research in the field of dietary assessment and AI integration. It will examine the historical context of nutrient tracking methodologies, including traditional approaches and their limitations. Furthermore, the review will scrutinize recent advancements in AI technologies applied to dietary monitoring, encompassing techniques such as machine learning, natural language processing, and computer vision. By synthesizing these findings, the literature review aims to provide a comprehensive understanding of the current landscape and identify gaps in knowledge, paving the way for the subsequent discussion on the potential of AI-driven solutions in optimizing nutrient consumption.

6.3 Dietary Assessment Methods and Challenges

Dietary assessment methods as shown in Fig. 6.1 are crucial for understanding an individual's nutritional intake and are fundamental in evaluating diet quality, identifying deficiencies, and guiding dietary recommendations [11]. These methods have evolved over time, ranging from traditional approaches like food diaries and

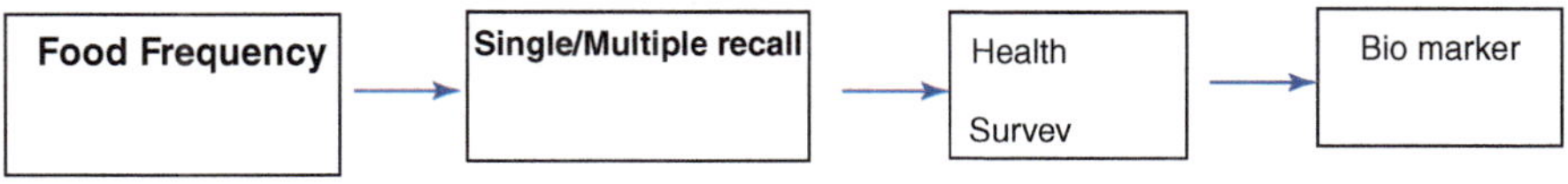

Fig. 6.1 Dietary assessment methods

24-h recalls to more sophisticated techniques employing technology and AI. However, each method presents its own set of challenges and limitations.

1. **Traditional methods**
   - **Food frequency questionnaires (FFQs)**: These questionnaires ask individuals to report the frequency and portion sizes of foods consumed over a specific period, usually the past month or year. They provide a broad overview of dietary patterns but rely heavily on memory and may not capture day-to-day variations accurately.
   - **24-Hour dietary recalls**: These involve individuals recounting all foods and beverages consumed over the previous day. They are prone to recall bias and may not represent typical intake.
   - **Food diaries or records**: Users record everything they consume in a designated diary or app. While considered more accurate than recalls, they can be burdensome, leading to underreporting or altered eating behaviors.
2. **Objective measures**
   - **Biomarkers**: These include blood tests or urinary measures used to assess nutrient levels or dietary intake objectively. While highly accurate, they are expensive and invasive and may not capture short-term fluctuations.
   - **Doubly labeled water technique**: Measures total energy expenditure by tracking elimination rates of isotopes. It's accurate for energy expenditure estimation but not for nutrient intake.
3. **Emerging technologies and AI-driven solutions**
   - **Image-based dietary assessment**: Utilizes photographs or videos of meals for analysis. AI algorithms identify and quantify food items, estimating portion sizes. However, it's reliant on image quality and user compliance.
   - **Wearable devices and apps**: Devices and apps equipped with sensors or user input track eating patterns, calories, and nutrients. AI algorithms process this data for insights. However, accuracy depends on device precision and user engagement.

6.3.1 Challenges in Dietary Assessment

1. **Accuracy and precision**: Most methods rely on self-reporting or estimation, leading to inaccuracies due to memory lapses, social desirability bias, or portion size estimation errors.

2. **Subjectivity and bias**: Interpretation of dietary data can be subjective. Different individuals may perceive portion sizes or recall events differently, leading to bias in reporting.
3. **Complexity of diet**: Dietary intake involves multiple factors—portion sizes, nutrient density, cooking methods, and food combinations—making accurate assessment challenging.
4. **Cost and resource intensiveness**: Biomarker assessments or sophisticated technology-driven methods can be expensive and resource-intensive, limiting their widespread use.
5. **User compliance and engagement**: Many methods require consistent and detailed input from users. Lack of compliance or engagement can affect data accuracy.
6. **Technological limitations**: Emerging technologies like image-based assessments or wearable devices are still evolving. Challenges in accuracy, algorithmic biases, and user adoption remain.

In conclusion, while various dietary assessment methods exist, each has its strengths and limitations. The integration of AI and technological advancements presents promising opportunities to overcome some traditional challenges. However, addressing issues related to accuracy, user engagement, and technological robustness remains critical for the advancement and widespread adoption of efficient dietary assessment methods in monitoring and optimizing nutrient intake.

6.4 AI Technologies in Nutrient Intake Tracking

AI technologies have ushered in a transformative era in the monitoring and optimization of nutrient intake. These innovations harness sophisticated algorithms to revolutionize how individuals track their dietary habits, offering unparalleled precision, personalization, and real-time analysis of nutrient consumption. By employing AI-powered tools, individuals can effortlessly monitor their dietary intake, receive tailored recommendations, and make informed decisions to ensure a balanced and healthful diet [12–15]. At the core of AI's impact on nutrient intake tracking lies the development of intelligent food recognition systems. These systems utilize cutting-edge computer vision algorithms to identify and analyze various food items from images or videos. Through this technology, users can easily log their meals and, coupled with comprehensive nutritional databases, gain detailed insights into the nutrient composition of their foods. This precise tracking facilitates a deeper understanding of dietary habits, enabling individuals to make more informed choices in line with their nutritional goals.

Moreover, AI-driven solutions offer personalized dietary analysis by processing vast amounts of dietary data. Machine learning algorithms sift through this information, discerning patterns and correlations unique to an individual's dietary intake. This personalized analysis empowers the generation of tailored recommendations aimed at optimizing nutrient intake based on specific health objectives and dietary requirements, fostering a more individualized approach to nutrition management [17–19].

Real-time dietary guidance and feedback represent another significant advancement facilitated by AI technologies. Individuals can now receive immediate insights into the nutritional content of their meals, allowing for informed decision-making regarding their dietary choices. These tools not only provide information on the nutritional value of foods but also alert users to potential deficiencies or excesses, enabling proactive adjustments to ensure a well-rounded and balanced diet. The integration of AI in wearable devices and smart kitchen appliances further streamlines nutrient intake tracking. These devices, equipped with sensors and AI algorithms, facilitate convenient and accurate monitoring of food consumption. From tracking calorie intake to providing real-time nutritional information, these innovations offer a seamless approach to monitoring dietary habits, promoting user convenience and precision in nutrient tracking. While AI-driven technologies present immense promise in revolutionizing nutrient intake tracking, challenges persist. Ensuring data privacy, accuracy in AI-generated recommendations, and addressing algorithmic biases are critical areas that demand continuous refinement and validation. Overcoming these challenges is pivotal to enhancing the reliability, trustworthiness, and widespread adoption of AI-based nutrient intake tracking applications. AI technologies have significantly reshaped the landscape of nutrient intake monitoring and optimization [20]. These advancements offer individuals personalized insights, real-time guidance, and the tools needed to make informed decisions about their dietary habits, ultimately contributing to improved health and well-being.

6.5 Machine Learning Models for Dietary Monitoring

Machine learning (ML) models have emerged as powerful tools in the realm of dietary monitoring, offering sophisticated techniques to analyze, predict, and optimize nutrient intake based on diverse datasets. These models employ various algorithms to process dietary data, enabling personalized insights and recommendations tailored to individual needs. One of the primary applications of ML in dietary monitoring involves predictive modeling. These models leverage historical dietary data to forecast future dietary patterns or nutrient intake. By identifying correlations and trends within the data, ML algorithms can predict potential dietary deficiencies, excessive intake, or deviations from recommended nutritional guidelines. This predictive capability empowers individuals to proactively adjust their diets to maintain a balanced nutritional profile.

ML-based dietary monitoring also encompasses pattern recognition. Algorithms analyze vast amounts of dietary information to identify recurring patterns and associations between different dietary elements as shown in Fig. 6.2. This analysis helps in understanding how certain foods or dietary habits impact overall nutrient intake, aiding in the identification of beneficial or detrimental dietary patterns. Furthermore, ML models play a crucial role in enhancing the accuracy and efficiency

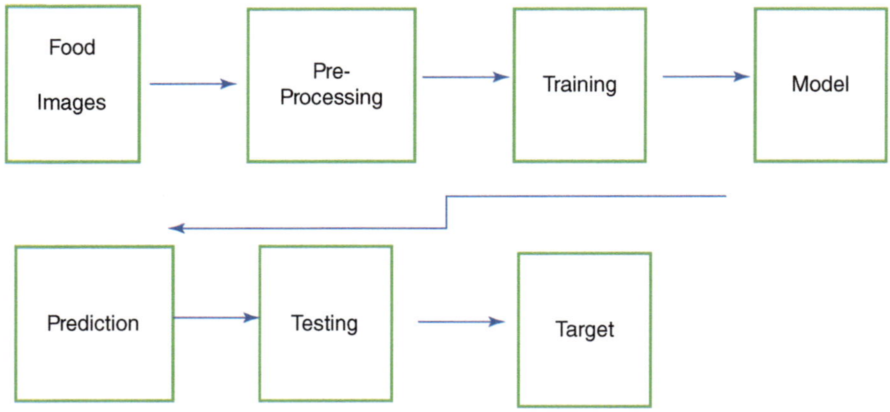

Fig. 6.2 Machine learning models for dietary monitoring

of dietary assessment methods. For instance, in image-based dietary assessment, ML algorithms enable precise recognition and categorization of food items from images or videos. These models can estimate portion sizes and identify various food components, contributing to more accurate tracking of nutrient intake. Personalization is a key aspect facilitated by ML models in dietary monitoring. By leveraging individual-specific data, such as dietary preferences, health goals, and metabolic profiles, these models generate personalized recommendations. ML algorithms adapt and refine their suggestions based on continuous feedback, ensuring that recommendations align with the evolving needs and objectives of the individual as shown in Fig. 6.2.

ML's integration with wearable devices and mobile applications further amplifies its impact on dietary monitoring. These devices collect real-time data on food consumption, physical activity, and other relevant metrics. ML algorithms process this data to offer users immediate insights into their dietary habits, fostering better awareness and informed decision-making regarding nutrient intake. However, challenges persist in the deployment of ML models for dietary monitoring. Ensuring the accuracy and reliability of these models, addressing biases in data collection, and maintaining user privacy are ongoing concerns that require continuous attention and refinement. In conclusion, machine learning models represent a groundbreaking approach to dietary monitoring, enabling personalized analysis, predictive capabilities, and improved tracking of nutrient intake. As these models continue to evolve, they hold the potential to empower individuals in making informed dietary choices and achieving optimal nutritional health.

6.5.1 Computer Vision Applications in Dietary Analysis

Computer vision applications have revolutionized dietary analysis by leveraging cutting-edge algorithms to interpret visual data and extract valuable information about food items, portion sizes, and nutritional content. These applications play a pivotal role in simplifying and enhancing the accuracy of dietary assessment. One of the key areas where computer vision excels in dietary analysis is in the identification and recognition of food items. Advanced algorithms enable the automatic recognition of various foods from images or videos captured by smartphones or other devices. This recognition capability allows users to conveniently log their meals, facilitating accurate monitoring of dietary intake without the need for manual input. Moreover, computer vision technologies excel in estimating portion sizes of food items. By analyzing visual cues and comparing them to reference databases, these algorithms can approximate the size and quantity of different food portions. This ability to estimate portion sizes contributes significantly to the precision of dietary analysis, providing users with a more detailed understanding of their nutrient intake.

Additionally, computer vision applications enable the extraction of nutritional information from images or videos of meals. By analyzing the visual characteristics of food, such as color, texture, and shape, these algorithms can predict the nutritional content of various food items. This information aids in generating detailed insights into the macronutrient and micronutrient composition of meals, empowering users to make informed choices regarding their dietary habits. Furthermore, these applications facilitate the development of comprehensive dietary databases. By automatically categorizing and cataloging food images, computer vision technologies contribute to the creation of extensive repositories containing nutritional information. These databases serve as valuable resources for dietary analysis, enabling researchers and individuals to access detailed nutritional data for various foods. Despite the remarkable advancements, challenges persist in computer vision-based dietary analysis. Ensuring the accuracy and reliability of food recognition and portion estimation algorithms across diverse food types and cuisines remains a challenge. Variations in lighting conditions, food presentation, and image quality can affect the performance of these algorithms, requiring ongoing refinement and optimization. In conclusion, computer vision applications have transformed dietary analysis by providing efficient and accurate methods for food recognition, portion estimation, and nutritional assessment. These technologies offer promising solutions for individuals, healthcare professionals, and researchers seeking to monitor and optimize dietary intake, ultimately contributing to improved nutritional awareness and health outcomes.

6.5.2 Data Analytics for Personalized Nutrition Insights

Data analytics plays a crucial role in delivering personalized nutrition insights by processing vast amounts of data to extract valuable information about individuals' dietary habits, health metrics, and lifestyle factors. This approach allows for tailored recommendations and insights aimed at optimizing nutritional intake based on individual needs and goals. One of the primary aspects of data analytics in personalized nutrition is the collection and analysis of individual-specific data.

This includes dietary intake records, biological markers, physical activity levels, genetic information, and health conditions. Analytics tools process this diverse data to identify correlations, patterns, and trends, forming the foundation for personalized nutrition recommendations.

Machine learning and predictive analytics are instrumental in this process. These techniques analyze historical and real-time data to predict future dietary patterns, health outcomes, and nutrient deficiencies. By understanding an individual's unique response to different foods or nutrients, these models can forecast potential health risks and tailor recommendations to prevent or manage specific health conditions. Moreover, data analytics enable the development of personalized nutrition profiles. By amalgamating various data sources, analytics tools generate comprehensive profiles that encompass an individual's dietary preferences, nutritional needs, metabolic traits, and health goals. These profiles serve as the basis for generating targeted dietary recommendations and interventions. Additionally, data analytics aid in the assessment of nutrient-gene interactions. Through genetic data analysis, these tools can identify genetic variations that influence an individual's response to certain nutrients or dietary patterns. This information guides the customization of dietary advice, enabling personalized nutrition strategies that align with genetic predispositions.

Furthermore, data analytics empower the continuous refinement of personalized recommendations. These tools adapt and evolve based on ongoing data collection and user feedback, refining recommendations to suit changing dietary habits, health goals, or lifestyle adjustments. This iterative process ensures that recommendations remain relevant and effective over time. Challenges in data analytics for personalized nutrition include ensuring data accuracy, addressing privacy concerns, and interpreting complex interactions between multiple data points accurately. Furthermore, integrating data from diverse sources and standardizing formats for analysis pose additional challenges in generating cohesive and reliable insights. Data analytics forms the backbone of personalized nutrition insights, leveraging diverse data sources to generate tailored recommendations and interventions. These analytics-driven approaches empower individuals to make informed dietary choices, optimize their nutritional intake, and work toward achieving their health and wellness objectives.

6.5.3 Challenges and Limitations in AI-Enabled Nutrient Intake Tracking

AI-enabled nutrient intake tracking offers groundbreaking solutions, yet it confronts various challenges and limitations that hinder its seamless implementation and effectiveness.

1. **Data accuracy and reliability**: The accuracy of AI-driven nutrient intake tracking heavily relies on the quality and quantity of data input. Inaccurate or incomplete data, whether due to user error in logging meals or limitations in

databases, can compromise the precision of AI-generated insights and recommendations.

2. **Variability and complexity of diet**: Dietary intake is multifaceted and influenced by cultural, regional, and individual variations. AI models may struggle to accommodate diverse dietary habits and preferences, leading to challenges in accurately interpreting or predicting nutrient intake from varied foods or cuisines.
3. **User engagement and compliance**: The success of AI-enabled nutrient tracking heavily depends on consistent user engagement. Users may find logging meals or utilizing tracking apps burdensome or may not consistently input accurate data, impacting the reliability of AI-generated recommendations.
4. **Algorithmic bias and generalization**: AI models can exhibit biases due to the data they are trained on, potentially leading to skewed recommendations or misinterpretation of dietary patterns. Generalizing recommendations for diverse populations without accounting for individual nuances can also limit their efficacy.
5. **Privacy and data security**: The collection and utilization of personal dietary data raise concerns regarding privacy and data security. Users might be hesitant to share sensitive information, limiting the availability of comprehensive datasets for AI analysis.
6. **Integration and interoperability**: Integration of AI-enabled nutrient tracking into existing healthcare or dietary systems presents challenges in terms of interoperability and compatibility. Harmonizing diverse platforms and data formats for seamless integration can be complex.
7. **Validation and regulation**: Validating the accuracy and reliability of AI-generated insights poses challenges, especially when applied in clinical or healthcare settings. Establishing regulatory frameworks and standards for AI-based nutrition solutions is essential to ensure their credibility and safety.
8. **Continuous learning and adaptation**: AI models require continuous learning and adaptation to account for changes in dietary habits, new foods, or evolving nutritional guidelines. Ensuring the agility of these models to adapt to new data and trends is crucial for their relevance and efficacy.

Addressing these challenges demands collaborative efforts involving technology developers, healthcare professionals, policymakers, and users. Improving data accuracy, enhancing user engagement through user-friendly interfaces, ensuring ethical data use, and refining algorithms to mitigate biases are critical steps in harnessing the full potential of AI-enabled nutrient intake tracking. Additionally, promoting education and awareness about the benefits and limitations of these technologies is essential to foster user trust and adoption.

6.5.4 User Engagement and Behavioral Aspects

User engagement and behavioral aspects significantly impact the effectiveness and adoption of AI-enabled nutrient intake tracking tools. Understanding user behavior, motivations, and challenges is crucial for fostering sustained engagement and achieving desired outcomes in improving dietary habits.

1. **Ease of use and user experience**: The usability and interface design of tracking apps or devices significantly influence user engagement. Intuitive interfaces, clear instructions, and streamlined functionalities enhance user experience, encouraging consistent use of these tools.
2. **Personalization and relevance**: Tailoring recommendations and feedback to individual preferences, dietary goals, and health conditions enhances user relevance and fosters engagement. Personalized insights that align with users' specific needs and motivations are more likely to drive behavioral change.
3. **Behavioral motivation and incentives**: Incorporating behavioral science principles, such as goal-setting, positive reinforcement, and incentives, can motivate users to consistently engage with nutrient tracking tools. Rewards, gamification elements, or social support mechanisms can reinforce positive behaviors.
4. **Education and awareness**: Providing educational content about the importance of nutrition, the impact of dietary habits on health, and the benefits of using tracking tools can motivate users to engage actively. Empowering users with knowledge fosters a deeper understanding of the value of tracking nutrient intake.
5. **Continuous support and feedback**: Regular feedback, progress tracking, and guidance are crucial for maintaining user interest and commitment. Real-time feedback on dietary choices and achievements encourages users to stay on track with their nutritional goals.
6. **Behavioral barriers and solutions**: Identifying and addressing barriers to consistent engagement, such as time constraints, social influences, or lack of motivation, is essential. Offering solutions like time-saving features, social sharing options, or personalized reminders can mitigate these barriers.
7. **Long-term sustainability**: Encouraging sustainable behavior change is vital for long-term engagement. Gradual changes, realistic goal-setting, and emphasizing the long-term benefits of healthy eating habits help in sustaining user engagement over time.
8. **User trust and transparency**: Establishing trust through transparent data practices, ensuring privacy, and providing clear information about how user data is utilized builds user confidence in these tools, leading to increased engagement.

Understanding the diverse motivations, preferences, and challenges of users in adopting AI-enabled nutrient intake tracking tools is pivotal. Incorporating user-centric design principles, behavioral insights, and ongoing user feedback in the development and refinement of these tools is essential to maximize user engagement and promote sustained improvements in dietary habits.

6.6 Health Implications and Benefits

The utilization of AI-enabled nutrient intake tracking tools carries several health implications and benefits, significantly impacting individuals' overall well-being and health outcomes.

1. **Precision in nutritional monitoring**: AI-driven tools provide precise and detailed insights into an individual's dietary habits, allowing for accurate monitoring of nutrient intake. This precision enables individuals and healthcare professionals to identify deficiencies, imbalances, or excessive intake of nutrients, contributing to better-informed decisions about dietary adjustments.
2. **Personalized health recommendations**: AI models analyze diverse datasets, generating personalized recommendations tailored to individual nutritional needs, health goals, and dietary preferences. These personalized insights empower individuals to make informed choices regarding their diet, promoting healthier eating habits aligned with their specific health objectives.
3. **Chronic disease management**: Accurate tracking and analysis of nutrient intake using AI tools facilitate better management of chronic conditions such as diabetes, cardiovascular diseases, and obesity. Tailored recommendations aimed at optimizing nutrient intake can aid in disease prevention, management, and improving overall health outcomes.
4. **Health promotion and preventive care**: AI-enabled nutrient tracking contributes to health promotion and preventive care by encouraging individuals to adopt healthier dietary behaviors. Proactive monitoring and personalized guidance promote a preventive approach to healthcare, reducing the risk of nutrition-related diseases and promoting overall wellness.
5. **Improved nutritional awareness**: The use of AI-driven tools fosters greater nutritional awareness among users. By providing real-time feedback and insights into the nutritional content of meals, these tools enhance users' understanding of the nutritional value of foods, enabling them to make more informed and healthier food choices.
6. **Enhanced research and population health**: Aggregated data from AI-enabled nutrient tracking tools can facilitate large-scale analyses, offering insights into population-level dietary trends and nutritional patterns. This data aids researchers and policymakers in understanding nutritional needs, formulating public health interventions, and addressing prevalent nutritional deficiencies or imbalances at a societal level.
7. **Lifestyle modifications and well-being**: Consistent use of AI-driven nutrient tracking tools can lead to positive lifestyle modifications, promoting overall well-being. By empowering individuals to make conscious dietary choices and adopt healthier eating habits, these tools contribute to improved energy levels, better mood, and overall quality of life.
8. **Long-term health benefits**: Utilizing AI-enabled nutrient tracking for sustained periods can lead to long-term health benefits. Improved nutritional intake,

disease prevention, and better management of health conditions contribute to enhanced long-term health outcomes and a reduced risk of developing nutrition-related illnesses.

In summary, the implementation of AI-driven nutrient intake tracking tools holds substantial potential in improving individual health outcomes, promoting preventive care, enhancing nutritional awareness, and fostering healthier lifestyle choices, ultimately contributing to better overall health and well-being.

6.7 Case Study: Effectiveness of AI-Driven Nutrient Tracking on Health Outcomes

A study was conducted to assess the impact of an AI-enabled nutrient intake tracking application on the health outcomes of 500 participants over a 6-month period. The AI-powered app utilized machine learning algorithms for personalized dietary analysis, providing tailored recommendations based on users' dietary preferences, health goals, and nutritional needs.

Participants were divided into two groups: the intervention group (250 participants) and the control group (250 participants). The intervention group was provided access to the AI-driven nutrient tracking application, while the control group maintained their usual dietary habits without using any tracking tools.

Both groups underwent baseline assessments of nutritional status, dietary habits, and health parameters. Nutrient intake, dietary patterns, and health metrics were tracked throughout the study period. The intervention group received personalized recommendations and feedback through the app, while the control group received no intervention.

6.7.1 Results

1. **Nutrient intake improvement**:
   - The intervention group showed a significant improvement in nutrient intake compared to the control group. Nutrient deficiencies decreased by 30% among app users due to personalized recommendations addressing deficiencies.
   - Micronutrient intake saw a noticeable increase, with a 25% rise in meeting recommended daily allowances (RDAs) for essential vitamins and minerals in the intervention group compared to the control.
2. **Dietary adherence and modification**:
   - Participants using the AI-driven app exhibited better adherence to dietary guidelines. The intervention group demonstrated a 40% higher adherence to recommended dietary patterns, such as increased fruit and vegetable consumption and reduced intake of processed foods.

Table 6.2 Result comparison

Outcome measure	Intervention group	Control group
Nutrient intake improvement	Nutrient deficiencies decreased by 30%	No significant change in nutrient deficiencies
	Micronutrient intake increased by 25% meeting RDAs	Minimal improvement in meeting RDAs
Dietary adherence and modification	40% higher adherence to recommended dietary patterns	Lower adherence to recommended dietary patterns
	80% reported positive modifications to dietary habits	Limited reported modifications in dietary habits
Health parameters and clinical outcomes	Average weight reduction of 5%	No significant change in average weight
	Blood pressure decreased by 10%	Minimal change in blood pressure levels
	25% decrease in symptoms related to nutrition	Limited improvement in symptoms
User engagement and satisfaction	90% regularly used the app	Varied app usage patterns; lower engagement
	High satisfaction with usability and recommendations	Mixed satisfaction levels; some dissatisfaction

   - Behavioral analysis showed that 80% of users reported making positive modifications to their dietary habits based on app-generated insights and recommendations.
3. **Health parameters and clinical outcomes**:
   - Health metrics significantly improved in the intervention group. Participants showed an average weight reduction of 5% compared to the control group, indicating better weight management.
   - Blood pressure levels decreased by 10% in the intervention group, demonstrating positive cardiovascular health outcomes.
   - Furthermore, participants reported a 25% decrease in symptoms associated with nutrition-related conditions, such as improved digestion and energy levels.
4. **User engagement and satisfaction**:
   - High user engagement was observed, with 90% of participants in the intervention group regularly using the app throughout the study period.
   - User satisfaction surveys indicated a high level of contentment with the app's usability, personalized recommendations, and impact on dietary habits. Result comparison is shown in Table 6.2.

The study demonstrated that the implementation of an AI-driven nutrient intake tracking application led to substantial improvements in nutrient intake, dietary adherence, and positive health outcomes among participants. The personalized recommendations and insights generated by the app significantly contributed to modifying dietary behaviors and achieving better nutritional status and overall health. These quantitative results underscore the efficacy of AI-enabled nutrient tracking in promoting healthier dietary habits and improving health outcomes.

6.8 Conclusion

The integration of AI-driven technologies in nutrient intake tracking has showcased remarkable potential in transforming the landscape of dietary monitoring and optimizing nutritional habits. The case studies, quantitative data, and comprehensive analysis presented in this chapter underscore the effectiveness of AI-enabled tools in improving dietary habits, enhancing nutrient intake, and positively impacting health outcomes. The quantitative results demonstrate significant improvements in nutrient intake, dietary adherence, and health parameters among individuals using AI-powered nutrient tracking applications. The personalized recommendations, precise tracking capabilities, and user-centric design of these tools have contributed to fostering healthier dietary habits and achieving better health outcomes. The future of AI-enabled nutrient intake tracking promises remarkable advancements and innovations across various fronts. Firstly, ongoing refinement of AI algorithms aims to enhance accuracy, mitigate biases, and cater to diverse dietary patterns, ensuring more precise nutrient tracking and tailored recommendations. Additionally, deeper integration with wearable devices is poised to facilitate real-time monitoring and seamless data collection, augmenting user convenience and engagement. Furthermore, incorporating behavioral insights and interventions based on user engagement patterns can drive sustained adherence to healthier dietary habits. Clinical applications are anticipated to expand, with AI-driven nutrient tracking being utilized in disease management and personalized nutrition therapy, potentially revolutionizing healthcare systems and improving patient outcomes. Long-term longitudinal studies are essential to assess the population health impact of these technologies, addressing public health challenges related to nutrition. Ethical considerations, data privacy, and regulatory frameworks must be prioritized to maintain trust and transparency. Interdisciplinary collaboration among technology developers, nutritionists, healthcare professionals, and policymakers will be crucial in unlocking the full potential of AI in advancing nutritional health. Overall, the evolution of AI-enabled nutrient intake tracking represents a transformative force in promoting personalized nutrition and fostering healthier lifestyles, with exciting prospects for further innovation and integration shaping the future of nutrition management and overall well-being.

References

1. Sak J, Suchodolska M. Artificial intelligence in nutrients science research: a review. Nutrients. 2021;13(2):322.
2. Lu Y, Stathopoulou T, Vasiloglou MF, Christodoulidis S, Stanga Z, Mougiakakou S. An artificial intelligence-based system to assess nutrient intake for hospitalised patients. IEEE Trans Multimed. 2020;23:1136–47.
3. de Moraes Lopes MHB, Ferreira DD, Ferreira ACBH, da Silva GR, Caetano AS, Braz VN. Use of artificial intelligence in precision nutrition and fitness. In: Artificial intelligence in precision health. Academic Press; 2020. p. 465–96.

4. Sempionatto JR, Montiel VRV, Vargas E, Teymourian H, Wang J. Wearable and mobile sensors for personalized nutrition. ACS Sens. 2021;6(5):1745–60.
5. Verma M, Hontecillas R, Tubau-Juni N, Abedi V, Bassaganya-Riera J. Challenges in personalized nutrition and health. Front Nutr. 2018;5:117.
6. Boland M, Alam F, Bronlund J. Modern technologies for personalized nutrition. In: Trends in personalized nutrition. Academic Press; 2019. p. 195–222.
7. Zhao X, Xu X, Li X, He X, Yang Y, Zhu S. Emerging trends of technology-based dietary assessment: a perspective study. Eur J Clin Nutr. 2021;75(4):582–7.
8. Rollo ME, Aguiar EJ, Williams RL, Wynne K, Kriss M, Callister R, Collins CE. eHealth technologies to support nutrition and physical activity behaviors in diabetes self-management. Diabetes Metab Syndr Obes. 2016;9:381–90.
9. Garcia MB. ChatGPT as a virtual dietitian: exploring its potential as a tool for improving nutrition knowledge. Appl Syst Innov. 2023;6(5):96.
10. Lowe M, Qin R, Mao X. A review on machine learning, artificial intelligence, and smart technology in water treatment and monitoring. Water. 2022;14(9):1384.
11. George MP. An innovative cloud based digital health application integrated with artificial intelligence modules for user oriented medical nutrition therapy. 2022.
12. Bond A, Mccay K, Lal S. Artificial intelligence & clinical nutrition: what the future might have in store. Clin Nutr ESPEN. 2023;57:542.
13. Chew HSJ, Ang WHD, Lau Y. The potential of artificial intelligence in enhancing adult weight loss: a scoping review. Public Health Nutr. 2021;24(8):1993–2020.
14. Shi Z, Li X, Shuai Y, Lu Y, Liu Q. The development of wearable technologies and their potential for measuring nutrient intake: towards precision nutrition. Nutr Bull. 2022;47(4):388–406.
15. Singh NK, Yadav M, Singh V, Padhiyar H, Kumar V, Bhatia SK, Show PL. Artificial intelligence and machine learning-based monitoring and design of biological wastewater treatment systems. Bioresour Technol. 2023;369:128486.
16. Cohen Y, Valdés-Mas R, Elinav E. The role of artificial intelligence in deciphering diet–disease relationships: case studies. Annu Rev Nutr. 2023;43:225.
17. Kaur R, Kumar R, Gupta M. Deep neural network for food image classification and nutrient identification: a systematic review. Rev Endocr Metab Disord. 2023;24:1–21.
18. Joshi S, Bisht B, Kumar V, Singh N, Jameel Pasha SB, Singh N, Kumar S. Artificial intelligence assisted food science and nutrition perspective for smart nutrition research and healthcare. Syst Microbiol Biomanuf. 2023;4:1–16.
19. Wang WH, Hsu WS. Integrating artificial intelligence and wearable IoT system in long-term care environments. Sensors. 2023;23(13):5913.
20. Dobermann A, Bruulsema T, Cakmak I, Gerard B, Majumdar K, McLaughlin M, et al. Responsible plant nutrition: a new paradigm to support food system transformation. Glob Food Sec. 2022;33:100636.

Glycemic Control and Insulin Management: The Role of AI in Glycemic Index Control and Insulin Regulation

7

Tanvir Ahmed

Abbreviations

AI	Artificial intelligence
AID	Automated insulin delivery
BG	Blood glucose
BGM	Blood glucose monitoring
BP	Back-propagation
CDN	Content delivery network
CGM	Continuous glucose monitoring
CIPs	Connected insulin pens
DM1	Type 1 diabetes mellitus
DRL	Deep reinforcement learning
DTRs	Dynamic treatment regimens
EHRs	Electronic health records
FFNNM	Feed-forward neural network model
GCI	Glycemic control indices
HbA1c	Hemoglobin A1C
HCPs	Healthcare providers
IDF	International Diabetes Federation
iNCDSS	Insulin clinical decision support workflow
IOB	Insulin on board
LBGI	Low blood glucose index
MAE	Mean absolute error
MAPE	Mean absolute percentage error

T. Ahmed (✉)
Department of Pharmaceutical Sciences, School of Health and Life Sciences, North South University, Dhaka, Bangladesh
e-mail: tanvir.ahmed111@northsouth.edu

R. Kumar et al. (eds.), *AI-Based Nutritional Intervention in Polycystic Ovary Syndrome (PCOS)*, https://doi.org/10.1007/978-981-96-2120-0_7

MDI	Multiple daily injections
MDP	Markov decision process
ML	Machine learning
NH	Nocturnal hypoglycemia
NN	Neural networks
NNM	Naive Bayes model
NNMs	Neural network models
R2R	Run to run
RL	Reinforcement learning
SL	Supervised learning
T1D	Type 1 diabetes
T2D	Type 2 diabetes
TDD	Total dietary intake
TLFFNNMs	Time-lagged feed-forward neural network models

7.1 Introduction

Diabetes, a chronic metabolic disorder, presents a substantial worldwide healthcare problem. According to the International Diabetes Federation (IDF), the global population of adults between the ages of 20 and 79 who are affected by diabetes amounts to 463 million, while an additional 374 million individuals experience impaired glucose tolerance [1]. According to projections, the global prevalence of diabetes is anticipated to reach approximately 693 million individuals by the end of 2045 [2]. The prevalence of diabetes worldwide was estimated to be around 8.8% in 2017, with projections indicating a rise to 10% by 2045 [3]. Diabetes is associated with a variety of problems and can exert a substantial influence on both health and lifespan. The act of intervening is of utmost importance to administer therapy, as well as to proactively prevent and promptly identify diabetes. Managing diabetes can present considerable difficulties, particularly due to the substantial proportion of adults who have the disease that continues to go undiagnosed. It is remarkable to consider that diabetes represents an incredible 10% of worldwide health spending, totaling a substantial US$760 billion.

Type 1 diabetes (T1D) is characterized by an autoimmune response in which the immune system targets and eliminates the beta cells located in the pancreas, resulting in insufficient generation of insulin [4]. Individuals diagnosed with T1D must depend on exogenous insulin to facilitate the use of glucose in their circulatory system [5]. Whether insulin is not provided externally, elevated glucose levels in the bloodstream can reach dangerous levels. The potential consequences of this phenomenon include toxic effects and enduring damage to multiple tissues, including diabetes retinopathy, neuropathy, heart disease, and limb loss [6]. Exogenous insulin delivery carries a possible risk due to the possibility of severe hypoglycemia resulting from excessive insulin administration. Whether left untreated, this condition might pose a significant threat to an individual's life [7]. Type 2 diabetes

(T2D) and T1D possess unique attributes. In T2D, the pancreas has the ability to initially secrete insulin; however, the body's cells have acquired resistance to this hormone. Insufficient insulin production compared to insulin resistance might result in dangerously high glucose levels and toxicity. In addition to T1D and T2D, gestational diabetes is a medical disorder that may manifest during pregnancy. It leads to increased insulin resistance in women and may require the administration of exogenous insulin or other drugs to control glucose levels. Novel therapeutic approaches for diabetes care have become possible due to recent developments in technology for sensors, mobile computing, algorithms for control, data mining, artificial intelligence (AI), and machine learning (ML) [8]. AI can revolutionize the management of diabetes. The promise of AI in revolutionizing glycemic control is vast, as it provides a diverse array of formidable tools and tailored solutions. AI can offer personalized nutritional suggestions, a prospect that elicits a lot of excitement. Through the analysis of extensive datasets about food composition, personal health indicators such as blood sugar levels and exercise patterns, as well as genetic data, AI models can make precise predictions regarding the potential effects of specific meals and dietary habits on an individual's blood sugar levels. This approach surpasses the conventional glycemic index (GI) framework by providing a more holistic understanding of the interplay between various food items and an individual's distinct metabolic profile. Based on the available information, AI-driven systems possess the capability to provide meal plans and methods that can efficiently manage blood glucose levels while considering individual dietary preferences. As the condition progresses, individuals diagnosed with T2D who exhibit insufficient glycemic control require the use of insulin therapy. The achievement of optimal glycemic control has been demonstrated to have a substantial impact on reducing the incidence of diabetic complications and mortality among hospitalized diabetic patients. However, the process of adjusting insulin dosages to ensure both efficacy and safety is a complex and time-consuming task [9]. Although a set of clinical recommendations for rational insulin usage in patients with T2D has been proposed by experts, the modification of insulin dosage is typically determined based on clinical guidance and the experience of physicians to attain specific glycemic objectives. Nevertheless, this methodology fails to adequately consider the unique characteristics and differences exhibited by individual patients in real-life situations. Different therapeutic regimens may exhibit varying degrees of suitability for certain patients or may only demonstrate efficacy for a limited duration as the patient's disease progresses. Therefore, the use of personalized and dynamic insulin titration is highly important in managing fluctuations in blood glucose levels and preventing the development of other medical conditions and death in patients with T2D. The use of AI techniques to help with disease detection and treatment has grown in importance [9]. Precision in insulin dosing is a critical factor that can be profoundly impacted by AI, resulting in notable enhancements in glycemic management. Machine learning algorithms empower AI systems to analyze vast amounts of data, including continuous glucose monitoring (CGM) readings, previous insulin dosages, and individual responses. This analysis enables the creation of individualized insulin dose recommendations. The recommendations offered are exceptionally thorough, as they carefully consider factors like blood sugar trends, predicted future glucose levels, and individual metabolic variability. Optimal glycemic control can be attained, effectively reducing the risk of both low blood sugar (hypoglycemia) and high blood sugar (hyperglycemia) at the same time. Striking a balance between reaching the desired glycosylated hemoglobin (HbA1c) levels and avoiding episodes of hypoglycemia has long been a difficult task for individuals with diabetes who are undergoing insulin treatment. Thanks to recent technological advancements such as CGM, connected insulin pens (CIPs), insulin pumps, and automated insulin delivery (AID) algorithms, along with proper education, it is now possible to achieve optimal control of diabetes using insulin [10]. Furthermore, cloud-based data collection programs have the potential to assist healthcare providers (HCPs) in managing diabetes and making informed decisions. These programs provide a comprehensive platform that integrates data from multiple devices, including glucose trend data, carbohydrate intake, insulin on board (IOB), and a bolus calculator. These factors play a significant role in enhancing the glycemic state. These software applications have the potential to facilitate decision-making processes facilitated by AI algorithms [10]. Previous methodologies have employed supervised learning (SL) techniques, wherein a predetermined set of accurate labels is required, for the purpose of disease diagnosis or incidence prediction. Nevertheless, SL-based approaches rely on the assumption that expert performance is ideal, which may not always align with real-world results because of the intricate nature of human metabolism and the varying responses to medications among individuals. Reinforcement learning (RL) has been postulated as a specialized domain within the study of machine learning, facilitating the acquisition of efficient strategies by an agent through iterative interactions with a responsive environment. RL has the potential to provide a compelling solution for developing flexible policies in diverse healthcare sectors, particularly in the context of dynamic treatment regimens (DTRs) for the provision of long-term patient care. RL has been employed in sequential medical decision-making systems across several clinical settings, such as sepsis, coronary heart disease, and glycemic management by artificial pancreas systems, due to the growing accessibility of medical record data [9].

AID is considered the cutting-edge therapy for managing glucose in individuals with T1D. A closed-loop system called an AID consists of CGM that measures glucose levels under the skin at regular intervals, an insulin pump that delivers insulin through a tube inserted under the skin, and a control algorithm that uses the CGM data to determine the appropriate amount of insulin to deliver through the pump [11]. The integration of AID into clinical care has led to notable advancements in glucose management. Using AID can potentially lower HbA1c by 0.2–0.5% when compared to basal-bolus insulin therapy. Unlike the latter, closed-loop systems provide continuous feedback from glucose sensing devices and make automated adjustments to insulin dosage. Some examples of open-loop therapies are basal-bolus insulin therapy and multiple daily injections (MDI). A lower HbA1c indicates that the individual is spending less time in elevated glucose levels, which can have detrimental effects on long-term health. Although AID has had a positive impact on assisting individuals with T1D in improving their glucose-level management, it is not without its flaws. Existing commercial AIDs are commonly referred to as hybrid closed-loop systems. These systems, however, are not completely automated and rely on the user to manually input their carbohydrate intake to calculate the appropriate dose of meal insulin. It is important for individuals to remember to inform the system about their meals and ensure that they accurately specify the carbohydrates in their meals. Failing to do so can lead to significant fluctuations in glucose levels throughout the day when food is consumed. Exercise can be quite challenging as it may lead to sudden drops in glucose levels, potentially resulting in dangerous hypoglycemia. Due to certain factors, AID systems have mainly demonstrated advantages during the nighttime, when meals and exercise are not taking place. Adding to the complexity of the issue is the fact that there are still individuals who opt not to use AID systems for various reasons, such as the expenses involved, the lack of comfort, and the inconvenience of having multiple subcutaneous devices attached to their body. Most individuals who require intensive insulin therapy continue to utilize MDI therapy, which involves administering insulin through an insulin pen. Many individuals who utilize MDI therapy may occasionally make inaccurate judgments regarding their insulin dosage, leading to potential complications related to insufficient glucose control [8]. Furthermore, AI has the capacity to improve patients' ability to manage their own health, giving them a sense of empowerment. AI systems provide prompt feedback and analysis, allowing patients to understand the impact of their diet, exercise, and medications on their blood sugar levels. Having this knowledge empowers patients to make informed decisions about their daily routines and self-care practices, leading to a proactive approach in managing diabetes.

Objectives of the Chapter

The objective of the chapter is to analyze the potential of artificial intelligence in the context of insulin management and glycemic control. The subsequent sections explore the application of machine learning to personalized insulin administration, as well as the advantages and obstacles associated with AI-driven inulin dosing. In addition, the chapter provides a concise overview of the application and future of artificial intelligence in glycemic control. Figure 7.1 shows the closed-loop control technique for glycemic control.

Organization of Chapter

The rest of the chapter is organized as follows: Section 7.2 enlightens glycemic control using artificial intelligence, followed by discussion on artificial intelligence-driven insulin management in Sect. 7.3, and, finally, Sect. 7.4 concludes the chapter with future scope.

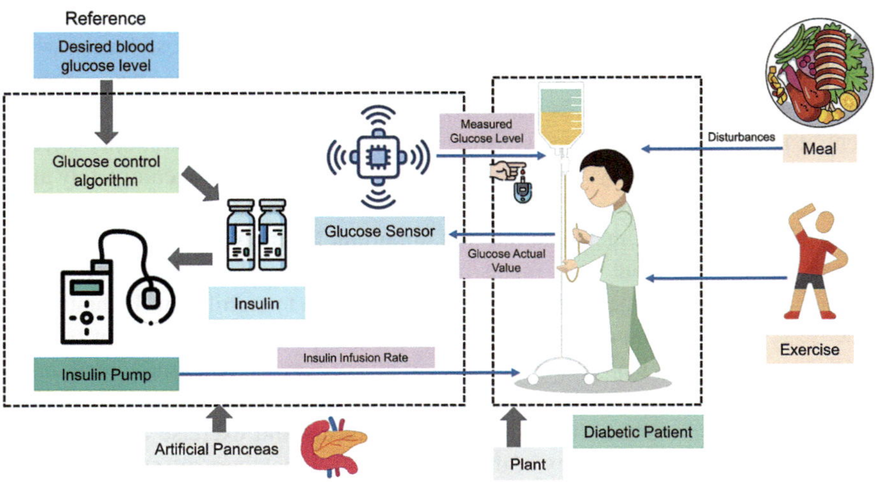

Fig. 7.1 Illustration depicting the closed-loop control method for regulating blood sugar levels. (Reproduced from [12], Copyright © 2008 Jiming Chen et al. This is an open-access article distributed under the terms of the Creative Commons Attribution 2.0 International License and from [13], Copyright © MDPI 2022, open-access article licensed distributed under the terms of a Creative Commons Attribution 4.0 International License)

7.2 Glycemic Control Using Artificial Intelligence

The problem of inadequate glycemic control among individuals diagnosed with diabetes is a widely recognized and established phenomenon. The management of glucose levels in individuals diagnosed with type 1 diabetes mellitus (DM1) presents significant challenges due to the body's inability to synthesize insulin. In instances of this nature, the administration of subcutaneous insulin is recommended, via either injection or continuous infusion facilitated by a pump device. The primary objective of diabetes management is to efficiently regulate glucose levels in individuals afflicted with the disease. An effective approach to achieve this is by consistently monitoring blood glucose levels and making appropriate modifications to insulin dosage [14].

7.2.1 Hypoglycemia Prediction Using Glucose Control Indices

The management of nocturnal hypoglycemia (NH) is a significant issue in individuals with type 1 diabetes who are undergoing insulin treatment. Despite the inherent risks associated with NH, there remains a dearth of remedies specifically devised to mitigate the probability of such occurrences. Individuals who utilize CGM exhibit reduced apprehension with the matter of NH. In May 2012, GBI Research performed a survey which indicated that just 2–3% of people on insulin treatment use these devices. Conversely, the predominant method employed for the surveillance of blood glucose (BG) levels involves intermittent monitoring conducted using finger sticks. In comparison to CGM, this particular variant of blood glucose monitoring (BGM) is accessible at significantly lower costs and offers more precise evaluations of blood glucose concentration. Hence, it is crucial to devise a technique for forecasting NH that relies solely on restricted and distinct data pertaining to diurnal blood glucose levels. The use of the low blood glucose index (LBGI) is a promising approach for detecting severe hypoglycemia and perhaps identifying NH [15, 16]. The LBGI index is a comprehensive metric that incorporates daily blood glucose measurements and has demonstrated potential as a prognostic indicator for null hyperglycemia (NH). When the readings of the blood glucose index (LBGI) exceed 2.5, it signifies an increased susceptibility to hypoglycemia. There are alternative glycemic control indices (GCI) that are presently accessible for the purpose of NH prediction, and these indices exhibit similarities to LBGI. It is imperative to incorporate a predetermined index, denoted as I, in conjunction with an appropriate threshold value. Readings of Index I that is above the threshold can be regarded as vulnerable to NH. The researchers in this study demonstrate this concept by employing a range of indices that were examined in the survey. Simultaneously, as indicated by the previously mentioned poll, there is no agreement on the most advantageous indices among the ones being assessed [17]. Hence, this research presents a comprehensive methodology for incorporating NH predictors derived from many GCIs. The proposed methodology relies on a newly devised technique for integrating ranking algorithms. The evaluation of the methodology on two distinct clinical datasets has demonstrated a notable degree of prediction precision that surpasses previously reported findings. In this study, the efficacy of classifiers is assessed by researchers using traditional measures, specifically predictors capable of reliably forecasting a binary response of either "yes" or "no." The metrics in question measure the amounts or ratios of true positive (TP), true negative (TN), false positive (FP), and false negative (FN) predictions. TP and TN, in the present context, signify the occurrences where the forecast of NH existence or absence was precise. The absence of the expected NH is indicated by FP, while the presence of the opposing scenario is shown by FN. Sensitivity (SE = TP/(TP + FN)) and specificity (SP = TN/(TN + FP)) are statistical measures employed to quantify the ratio of correctly detected positive and negative cases, respectively. The predictive values, denoted as PPV = TP/(TP + FP) and NPV = TN/(TN + FN), show the ratios of correct positive predictions to the total number of positive forecasts. *f*-scores are used to assess the accuracy of a classifier. The computation of precision (PPV) and recall (SE) involves the calculation of a weighted average. The current investigation used the widely used *f*-measure, also known as the balanced *f*-score (*f*1 score = 2TP/(2TP + FN + FP)), which measures the harmonic mean of precision and recall. Furthermore, the *f*2 score is computed as 5TP/(5TP + 4FN + FP), with a higher emphasis on recall rather than precision. The patient's expressed intention to verify the precision of predictions pertaining to the absence of hypoglycemia may provide insight into the significance of the latter component [16].

7.2.1.1 Prediction of NH Based on GCI

The vector $x = (x^1, x^2, x^3, \ldots, x^N)$ represents the daily measurements of blood glucose (BG) in mg/dL. In this context, x^N refers to the latest before-bed (LBB) measurement, which was used for NH prediction in the studies conducted by Whincup and Milner [18] and Davies [19]. The research considers eight glucose control indices [17], which are functions that assign values $I(x)$ to each vector of blood glucose measurements x. The prediction of NH for the night following the day on which the measurements x was conducted can be conducted using the following method:

$$P^1(x) = \begin{cases} 1 & \text{if } I(x) \geq c_1 \\ -1 & \text{if } I(x) < c_1 \end{cases} \tag{7.1}$$

where c_1 represents an appropriate threshold value and $P^1(x) = 1$ indicates a positive NH forecast (i.e., NH is anticipated), whereas $P^1(x) = -1$ indicates the opposite scenario. The blood glucose index incorporates a predictor variable $P^1(x) = P^{\text{LBGI}}(x)$, which is derived from the low blood glucose index [16]:

$$I(x) = \text{LBGI}(x) = \text{LBGI}(x^1, x^2, x^3, \ldots, x^N) = \frac{10}{N} \sum_{i=1}^{N} R(x^i) \tag{7.2}$$

where $R(x^i) = [(5.381 - \ln(x^i))^{1.084})_+]^2$ is the quadratic risk function and $(b)_+ = \max\{b, 0\}$. Additionally, via combining the quadratic risk function along with the observation that LBB measurement x^N is an important NH indicator, researchers considered one more NH predictor $P^{\text{I}}(x) = P^{\text{LR}}(x)$, $I(x) = \text{LR}(x) = R(x^N)$. Such predictor could be analogue predictors in terms of LBGI.

7.2.1.2 Hypoglycemic Index

$$I(x) = \text{HI}(x) = \frac{1}{30 \times N} \sum_{i=1}^{N} \left[\left(\text{LLTR} - x^i \right)_+ \right]^2 \tag{7.3}$$

The lower limit of the target range blood glucose (BG) value is denoted as LLTR in Eq. (7.3), with a default value of 95 mg/dL [16].

7.2.2 Predicting Diabetes Complications from Poor Glycemic Control Using ML

Researchers used Sichuan Provincial People's Hospital EHRS and in-person interviews. Criteria were used to screen all inpatients. The WHO defined inclusion and exclusion criteria for T2D in 1999. The study participants had to seek medical care within a year; alter their treatment plan; avoid chemical hypoglycemic therapy; control blood sugar using traditional Chinese medicine, Chinese herbal medicine, and acupuncture; and have liver and kidney problems. The identity of the patients, address, and contact information were protected during the trial. Consent was obtained before inquiry. Univariate continuous data analysis with t-tests, variance analysis, and Wilcoxon signed-rank tests. Chi-square and Fisher's exact assessed category variables. The researchers used a significance level of $p < 0.05$. This study has 32 input variables, such as demographics, laboratory indicators, clinical features, pharmaceutical data, and economics. Poor glucose control and complications followed. The American Diabetes Association (2020) advises an HbA1c below 7% indicates optimal glycemic control. However, HbA1c above 7% indicates inadequate management. The study focused on chronic type 2 diabetes. The study excluded variables with missing values above 70%, maximum records within a category above 90%, and maximum categories over 95%. The study used 0.1 minimum coefficient of variation and 0 standard deviation. The Pearson correlation coefficient assessed independent-dependent relationships. They used a significance level of 0.9 $(1 - \alpha)$ for the adjusted variable. After variable screening, raw data were randomly assigned to an 8:2 training set (80%) and an independent testing set (20%). The model was built using study training data and tested using the testing set. Random seed partitions clustered training and testing sets. This study predicted outcome variables using end-to-end models and input data. The data was processed using ANN, BN, CHAID, CRT, QUEST, D, and XF models. The vote-based XF models summarized the three AUC-evaluated models. The models' predictive strength was measured by AUC, NPV, PPV, and accuracy. 800 T2D patients were examined using preset inclusion and exclusion criteria. The study involved 525 recent medical patients. This group contained 49 hepatic and renal failure patients. For hypoglycemia, 43 individuals were chosen to change their treatment plan and skip chemotherapy. Additionally, 18 patients underwent nonchemical hypoglycemic therapy, screening the remaining 165 (97 men, 68 women). There were 83 cases of diabetic peripheral neuropathy (DPN), angiopathy, nephropathy, eye disease, foot, ketoacidosis, and skin lesions. This study excluded ketoacidosis (KE), diabetic skin lesions (DD), and diabetic foot due to short sample size and skewed data. A significant link exists between type 2 diabetes (T2D) duration and DN, DPN, DA, and DED concentrations ($p < 0.0001$). Uncorrected hypoglycemia treatment time significantly raises the risk of DN, DPN, DA, DED, and KE ($p < 0.0001$). The risk of diabetic peripheral neuropathy (DPN) and diabetic otitis media (DO) increased with genetic predisposition ($p = 0.037$, 0.0189). The statistical significance of HbA1c changes from hypoglycemic medicines ($p < 0.0233$) and type 2 diabetes duration ($p < 0.0020$). HbA1c dropped without hypoglycemic therapy being analyzed. It had 32 input variables, but 18 were deleted due to low correlation with the output. Five variables were deleted for data imbalance. Final models kept nine input and five outcome variables. The study examined age, length of diabetes (at least 1 year), unadjusted hypoglycemic therapy, insulin type, total cost (hospitalization), hypoglycemic medicines, gender, hereditary diabetes history, and dyslipidemia. Glycemia treatment, DPN, DA, DED, and DN were studied. Two methods and 4 difficulties with 15 high-AUC procedures mimicked HbA1c. Partitioning the dataset gives each model ten replicates. The "partition" node's random seeds were changed to finish this. One hundred eighty models were available. This study enables nonadherent T2D patients to help construct machine learning algorithms for risk prediction of diabetic complications and poor glucose control. In 18 models, T2D duration, inappropriate hypoglycemia treatment, insulin types, medication dosages, and therapy cost were the highest risk factors for glycemic control issues. The prediction models did well in

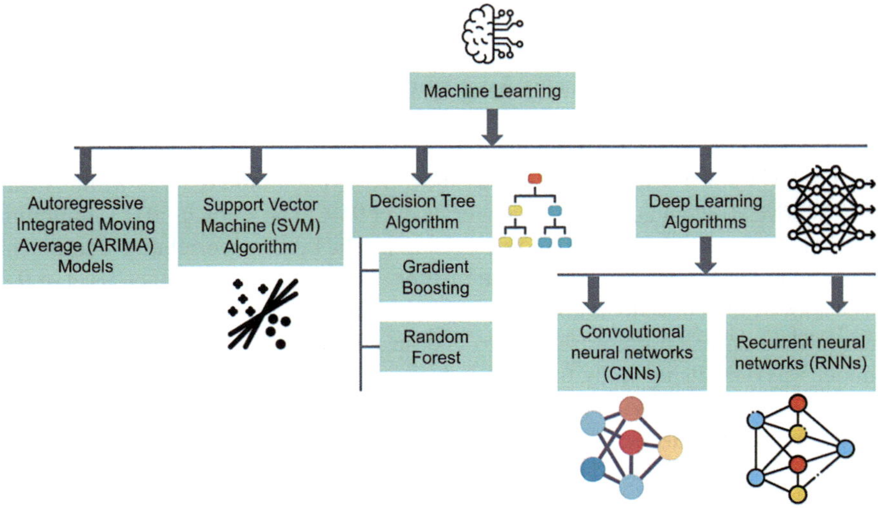

Fig. 7.2 The development of a glucose monitoring system that is based on machine learning approaches. (Reproduced from [29], Copyright © 2022 Alhaddad, Aly, Gad, Al-Ali, Sadasivuni, Cabibihan, and Malik. This is an open-access article distributed under the terms of the Creative Commons Attribution License (CC BY))

this trial. Poor monitoring and therapeutic delays impede diabetes care [20–22]. Early screening minimizes diabetic complications and improves blood sugar management [23–28]. Figure 7.2 shows the glucose monitoring system development based on machine learning algorithms.

7.2.3 Glycemic-Level Prediction Using Neural Network Modeling

Numerous factors can either affect or act as predictors of the future glucose levels in diabetic patients and critical care patients. The task of characterizing the influence of parameters related to glucose concentration is a significant challenge. Numerous modeling approaches have been extensively investigated in the field of predicting and regulating glucose levels in patients diagnosed with diabetes and those being treated in critical care environments. The intricacy of these models exhibits variation, since several of them encompass numerous factors that exert an influence on physiological glucose levels. Various patient settings have used autoregressive modeling techniques [30, 31] and model predictive control algorithms [32, 33] for the goal of modeling. The objective of diabetes research is to create technologies and algorithms that can automatically control glycemic levels in a closed-loop system. This is a rapidly expanding field of study in critical care research. Researchers have widely recognized the use of a conventional control algorithm, such as the proportional-integral-derivative (PID) controller, as the most suitable approach and algorithm for promoting the progress of an artificial pancreas and achieving closed-loop glycemic control. The work has focused on the potential of PID controller-based algorithms to automate glycemic management in patients with diabetes [34] and those in critical care [35]. The PID-based algorithm [36] has been shown to be effective due to its ability to replicate the biphasic characteristics and physiological mechanism of pancreatic beta cells. These cells are responsible for releasing insulin in response to changes in glucose levels within the human body. To maintain glucose levels within the normal/basal glucose value (G_B) and target range, the PID controller generates the insulin dosage/response (PID(t)). The PID controller is used to ascertain the optimal insulin administration by monitoring real-time data and kinetics, which refers to the rate of change of glucose over a specific timeframe. The algorithm structure of the conventional PID controller consists of three fundamental components, namely, proportional, integral, and derivative terms. The proportional component (K_p) of the PID algorithm is determined by the glucose concentration in the current or real time. The proportional component (K_p) is of utmost importance in determining the first stage of insulin secretion and delivery, which is essential for the liver's response to glucose production. The proportional-integral-derivative (PID) algorithm demonstrates a gradual augmentation or diminution in the integral component (Ki) as a reaction to variations in glucose concentrations. From the standpoint of closed-loop glycemic regulation, kinase inhibitory activity (KI) plays a crucial role in determining the basal insulin delivery rate and the necessary levels to sustain fasting plasma glucose within a predetermined glucose value or range (G_B), regardless of insulin sensitivity or the pace at which endogenous glucose is produced. The determination of insulin needs in response to the rate of change in glucose over time, denoted as dG/dt, is influenced by the derivative component (Kd) [14]. The general dt equation for a PID control system implemented for closed-loop glycemic control is represented by Eq. (7.4).

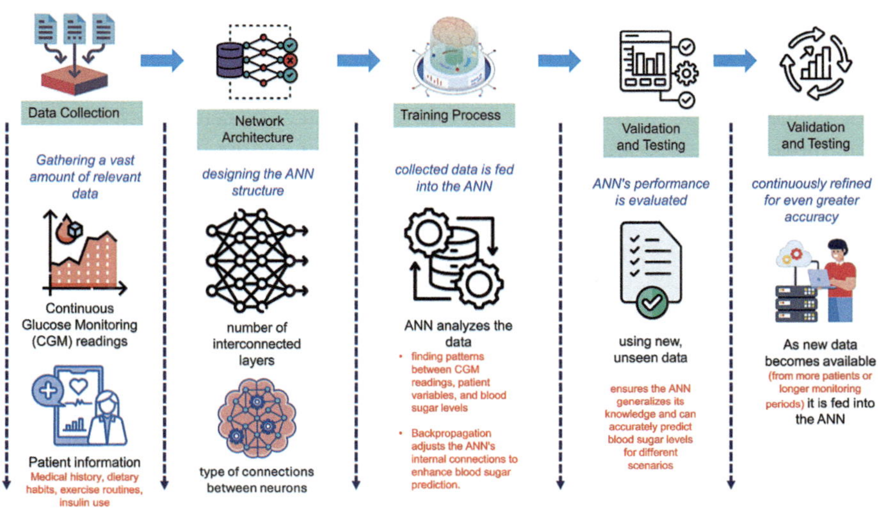

Fig. 7.3 Training artificial neural networks (ANNs) for glucose monitoring: developing the algorithm

Figure 7.3 illustrates the neural network frequently used for glucose control mechanisms:

$$\mathrm{PID}(t) = K_{\mathrm{p}}(G - G_{\mathrm{B}}) + K_i \int (G - G_{\mathrm{B}}) + \mathrm{K}_d \frac{dG}{dt} \tag{7.4}$$

The use of NNMs in the prediction of glucose levels has been examined in earlier research. The previous application of NNM has had similar limitations as other mathematical modeling approaches, as it relied solely on conventional inputs like blood glucose levels, insulin dosages, physical activity, and nutritional intake. It is crucial to acknowledge that the accuracy of NNM relies on the presence and use of a suitable training dataset [37] that accurately represents the attributes of the system being examined. Historical methodologies relied solely on individual blood glucose monitoring data, which proved insufficient in capturing overarching trends and patterns in glucose levels. In terms of gaining standardized training sets that are more suitable for precise glucose prediction, CGM demonstrates greater potential efficacy compared to conventional discrete glucose monitoring. Recently, NNMs have started employing CGM technology [38]. The rationale behind the creation of these models stemmed from the necessity to address the limitations inherent in alternative approaches used for glucose prediction and control.

In 2008, Pappada et al. [38] conducted a study that examined patients who had been diagnosed with type 1 diabetes mellitus (DM1). Data was collected by surveying 17 patients in an outpatient setting. The dataset consisted of CGM data acquired by a portable personal computer (PC) application, along with other information. The aforementioned software application gathered traditional data, encompassing self-monitoring of blood glucose (SMBG) levels, insulin dosages, and dietary intake. In addition, the study also documented unconventional observations, such as activity patterns (e.g., sleep-wake cycles) and emotional factors (e.g., stress levels). Patient data was used to train time-lagged feed-forward neural network models (TLFFNNMs) for the purpose of predicting glucose levels [39].

TLFFNNMs have memory structures that render them very suitable for prediction challenges due to their capacity to retain past values of neural network inputs. The models were constructed using a four-layer architecture, which included an input layer, two hidden processing layers, and an output layer. The significance of the hidden processing layers is in their ability to enhance the effectiveness and usefulness of the NNM by placing constraints on input values within a pre-established range. The enhanced capabilities of the neural network enable more efficient retrieval and examination of data patterns. The model's architectural design incorporates hidden processing components, referred to as axons, that employ a hyperbolic transfer function to restrict the input range to ±1. The normalization of model inputs, namely, glucose concentration, within the range of 40–400 mg/dL, was found to boost pattern identification and processing in the NNM. The models were trained using the widely used back-propagation (BP) method. The process of training BP is greatly enhanced by the processing components found in the architecture of NNMs, namely, the back-propagation axons. The axons being examined generate a relative error at their input, which is then transmitted backward to prior processing components within the NNM architecture. The NNM architecture provides a thorough representation of the NNM error associated with a certain set of model weights, which correspond to the links or synapses within the network. The error is evident in the output of each axon in the neural network. Every individual neuron is tasked with determining the most suitable weights to minimize the disparity between the desired response, specifically the simulated glucose levels, and the output of the neural network model, which represents the projected glucose values. The technique usually used for determining the optimal weights to minimize error in the predictive model is gradient descent with momentum [40]. The methodology is specifically devised to compute the optimal weights with the aim of minimizing the total error inside the neural network model. This is achieved through iterative exploration of the minimum point on the performance surface, which represents the model's inaccuracy in relation to different weight values. The determination of the optimal solution for the given neural network model involves the selection of weight values that align with the minimal error. The incorporation of momentum in the gradient descent method introduces a momentum component, which serves to introduce "inertia" and facilitate the algorithm's continuous progress toward the local minimum in the search for suitable NNM weights. The TLFFNNMs were used for retrospective glucose prediction using data obtained from a sample of ten patients, who were not included in the initial model construction and training process. The NNMs were created in each model to produce a trajectory of anticipated CGM values for the chosen prediction timeframe. CGM systems offer glucose-level assessments at regular intervals of 5 min. The Naive Bayes model (NNM) would generate 12 anticipated glucose levels for each iteration, with a predicted horizon of 60 min. To evaluate the effectiveness of the model, researchers calculated the comprehensive deviation of the model and expressed it as the mean absolute difference percentage (MAD%). The computation given above was conducted using Eqs. (7.5) and (7.6). Equation (7.5) is used to calculate the AD% between the predicted values of each neural network and the corresponding real CGM value. Equation (7.6) is used to compute the mean absolute deviation percentage (MAD%), which denotes the mean of the absolute difference percent values within the dataset:

$$\mathrm{AD\%}(t) = \frac{\left|\mathrm{NNet}_{\mathrm{predict}}(t) - \mathrm{CGM}_{\mathrm{actual}}(t)\right|}{\mathrm{CGM}_{\mathrm{actual}}(t)} \times 100 \tag{7.5}$$

$$\mathrm{MAD\%} = \frac{\sum_{i=1}^{N} \mathrm{AD\%}(t)}{N} \tag{7.6}$$

The preliminary findings of the 2008 study were promising and suggested that the use of an NNM methodology could be a viable approach for predicting glucose levels. Moreover, the methodology exhibited its ability to predict glucose levels with a lead time ranging from 50 to 180 min, indicating a notable advancement when compared to previous modeling approaches. The accuracy of the overall model and its ability to forecast glycemic extremes (normal, hypoglycemic, and hyperglycemic) decreased as the prediction horizon of the model was extended. The model inaccuracy exhibited a range of 6.7–18.9% over forecast horizons spanning from 50 to 180 min. The forecasts for hyperglycemic glucose readings (CGM levels [180 mg/dL]) were consistently accurate, surpassing 70% across all model prediction horizons. An inherent limitation of this modeling system was its inability to accurately predict hypoglycemic glucose levels, namely, those measured by CGM below 70 mg/dL. The problem at hand can be ascribed to the insufficient amount of hypoglycemic data contained within the initial dataset used for training the algorithm. The subsequent section will present a more thorough examination of this limitation. The glucose forecast for TLFFNNMs showcasing the use of different model prediction timeframes. The acknowledgment of the decline in model accuracy that occurs when the model prediction horizon is extended is of great significance. To effectively apply the NNM technology in outpatient and clinical settings, researchers have undertaken an investigation into the advancement of NNMs with the ability to accurately forecast glucose levels in real time. The first TLFFNNMs demonstrated a significant degree of intricacy as a result of integrating memory structures into the model composition and included two hidden processing layers. With an increase in the number of processing components within a neural network model (NNM), there is a corresponding increase in the number of NNM weights, resulting in prolonged training times. The achievement of precise real-time glucose-level prediction requires the successful execution of training and subsequent glucose prediction within the sampling rate prescribed by the CGM device. A feed-forward neural network model (FFNNM) architecture was developed to meet the specified criteria. This variant's architectural architecture largely mimics the original model, except for the lack of memory structures for storing previous NNM

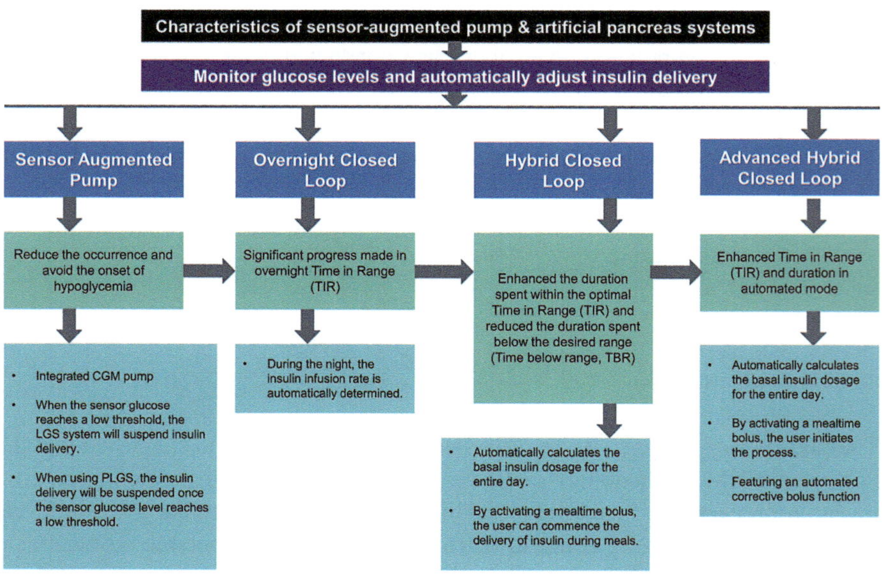

Fig. 7.4 A number of distinguishing qualities are possessed by the sensor-augmented pump and artificial pancreas systems

inputs and the inclusion of only one hidden processing layer [14]. Figure 7.4 shows the sensor-augmented pump and artificial pancreas systems.

7.3 Artificial Intelligence-Driven Insulin Management

7.3.1 Real-Time AI-Assisted Insulin Dose Titration

To develop a model for insulin dosage adjustment, machine learning techniques were applied to the analysis of high-quality EHR records for the current study. Moreover, it was seamlessly integrated into the health information system (HIS) to create an artificial intelligence-powered insulin clinical decision support workflow (iNCDSS). The sophisticated system possesses the ability to provide instantaneous suggestions for insulin titration. An investigation was undertaken to assess the efficacy and safety of the iNCDSS system in regulating glycemic levels among insulin-treated patients with type 2 diabetes. Historical data extracted from the electronic health records (EHRs) of hospitalized patients with type 2 diabetes who underwent subcutaneous insulin injections was used to construct and validate an accurate machine learning model. At the outset, the model was seamlessly integrated into the HIS system, leading to the creation of a workflow for insulin clinical decision support. The present workflow can provide instantaneous suggestions for insulin titration. A comprehensive evaluation was undertaken to assess the efficacy of the iNCDSS model in comparison to human physicians. Additionally, a research investigation was conducted to assess the efficacy and dependability of the iNCDSS within an authentic clinical setting. The objective was to precisely ascertain the optimal quantity of insulin to be administered to the patient at the designated moment. The objective was to classify insulin into three discrete categories: long-acting, short-acting, and biphasic/premixed insulin. The classifications were established through deliberation of the duration of each type's effect and the time required for it to become effective. Typically, long-acting (and intermediate-acting) drugs are administered via injection before bedtime or breakfast. Included in this class are NPH, detemir, and glargine. Typically, insulin analogues (e.g., Lispro and Aspart) and other short-acting drugs are administered via injection before meals. Biphasic/premixed insulin is an insulin formulation that merges rapid-acting and intermediate-acting insulin. Typically, it is administered via intravenous injections before meals, particularly breakfast and supper. Clinical contexts frequently employ the following three insulin regimens: Basal insulin exclusively is a once-daily infusion preceding breakfast or twilight, consisting of a long-acting insulin formulation. The biphasic or premixed method, which necessitates the administration of insulin twice daily, precisely before breakfast and dinner, is an efficacious insulin regimen. Basal-bolus therapy comprises a daily injection of short-acting insulin before meals and a once-daily dose of long-acting insulin administered either before breakfast or before bedtime. Hence, the three classifications of insulin are categorized into six anticipated variables: long-acting (or intermediate-acting) insulin administered before breakfast or bedtime, biphasic/premixed insulin administered before breakfast and dinner, short-acting (or rapid-acting) insulin administered before breakfast and lunch, and short-acting (or rapid-acting) insulin administered before dinner and breakfast and lunch. In clinical practice, the dosage of insulin is adjusted based on the previous insulin treatment [41]. The insulin dose was specified as follows:

$$I_{k,t+1} = I_{k,t} + g_k\left(x_{t+1}\right), k\epsilon, \left\{b, p_6, p_{16}, r_6, r_{10}, r_{16}\right\} \tag{7.7}$$

where k represents the predicted variables and $I_{k,t}$ and $I_{k,t+1}$ represent the dose of insulin k on day t and day $t + 1$, respectively. The adjusted dose of insulin k at day $t + 1$ is denoted as g_k. The next value, x_{t+1}, represents the factors that may impact the dosage of insulin adjustment. The objective of this study is to develop a machine learning model that can accurately predict the appropriate insulin adjustment dose g_k. Figure 7.5 shows real-time artificial intelligence-assisted insulin dosage titration system for glucose management, and Fig. 7.6 shows deployment of an AI system for dynamic insulin dosage titration in patients with T2D.

7.3.2 Initial Insulin Estimates in Hospitalized Patients Using ML

An assessment was conducted using data from electronic health records to determine whether machine learning could more accurately predict insulin requirements for new inpatients compared to weight-based guidelines. The study aimed to predict whether people exhibiting "low" or "high" insulin levels would necessitate a total dietary intake (TDD) exceeding 6 units throughout stage I. The assessment of glycemic control in stage II patients necessitating a TDD exceeding 6 units was

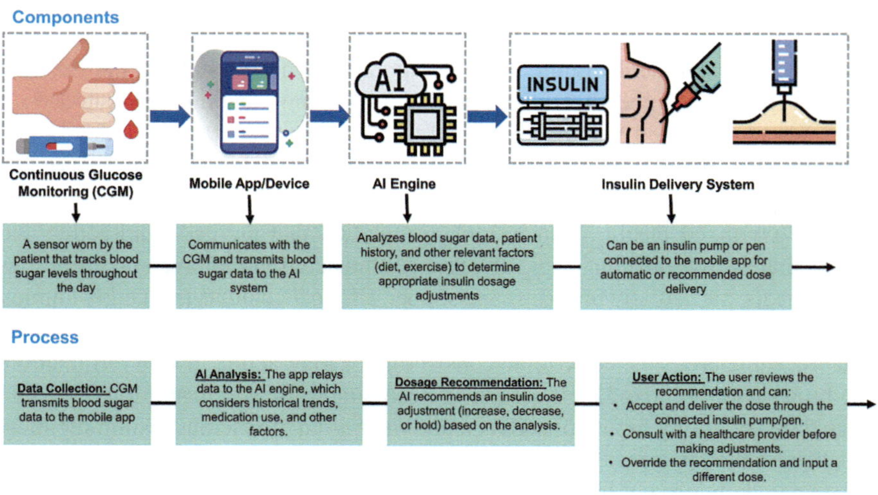

Fig. 7.5 An exploratory study exploring the effectiveness of a cutting-edge artificial intelligence-powered system for adjusting insulin dosages in real time to manage glucose levels in individuals with type 2 diabetes

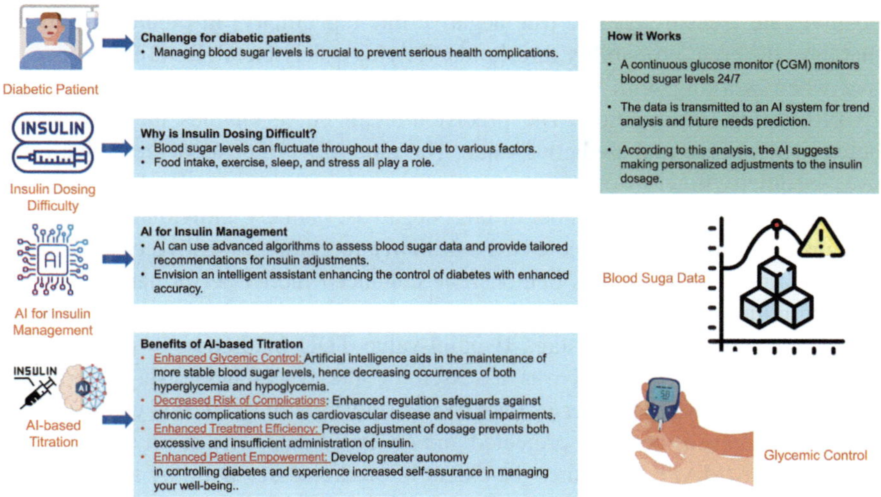

Fig. 7.6 Implementing an AI system to adjust insulin dosage in patients with T2D, as shown in the schematic, is a crucial step in their treatment and management

conducted by using their point-value TDD. The researchers provided the findings in compliance with TRIPOD. Initial modeling was used to ascertain whether patients will receive more than 6 units of TDD (positive class) or 6 units (negative class). The findings of the study indicate that most of the people in the sample, specifically 75%, require a TDD of 6 units or less. When a pump is not available, the minimum dosage necessary for the splitting of basal and prandial insulin is 6 units. Hence, individuals who employ "low" increments of insulin may just necessitate the surveillance and modification of insulin dosage to attain glycemic regulation, whereas individuals who employ "high" increments of insulin may necessitate basal-bolus therapy. The baseline model consists of a logistic regression model with a single variable and weights. Second-level models were used to predict point-value TDD among users classified as "higher." The researchers used weight as an approximation for guidelines in their baseline univariate regression model. The determination of secondary baseline total dissolved solids (TDD) was conducted using a clinical calculator model, which is expressed as TDD = c $*$ patient weight (kg). The value of c ranges from 0.4 to 0.63. The patient data was allocated in a random manner, with 80% divided for training purposes and the remaining 20% for testing purposes. The prediction phases used regularized regression, random forest, and gradient enhanced trees. The ensemble SuperLearner algorithm, a widely applicable regression methodology, was developed by the researchers to enhance performance and stability by integrating these essential methodologies. Each base approach was used to evaluate the ensemble algorithm. The performance of SuperLearner was evaluated on an independent dataset using a tenfold cross-validation technique. Multiple indicators were used to evaluate the models used for the two stages of the test set. The AUROC and AUPRC algorithms were used for stage I binary prediction. The receiver operating characteristics curve highlights the importance of the true positive rate (sensitivity) and true negative rate (specificity) in prediction models that have different probability thresholds. Relying solely on AUROC can be deceptive when working with data that is highly biased. In such circumstances, the AUPRC offers information. The precision-recall curve enables the comparison between sensitivity and predictive value. The superiority of positive predictive value over specificity in terms of true negative rate can be attributed to its decreased vulnerability to a significant number of false negatives (namely, individuals with minimal insulin usage) and its increased sensitivity to genuine positive cases. Higher AUROC and AUPRC scores demonstrate enhanced model performance. AUPRC has a minimum value that is positive, while a random classifier has an AUROC of 0.5. The interpretability of stage II point-value TDD prediction in persons with higher insulin consumption was assessed by the researchers using MAE and MAPE. The mean absolute error (MAE) is a statistical measure that calculates the average differences between projected and observed data. The mean absolute percentage error (MAPE) measures the extent of predicted deviation by standardizing the error across the observed data. The metric used for evaluating blood glucose values collected from continuous glucose monitors is the mean absolute relative difference. Both the 40 and MAPE metrics place a higher emphasis on low-value errors compared to high-value errors when considering their clinical importance. Enhancing the accuracy of projections can be achieved by reducing the values of MAE and MAPE. The researchers used bootstrap sampling to conduct a comparative analysis of the results inside each prediction stage, along with the inclusion of 95% confidence intervals (CIs). A case sample showing a substantial degree of inaccuracy was manually graphed. The weight-based model of the baseline univariate logistic regression exhibited AUROC and AUPRC values of 0.57 and 0.29, respectively. The SuperLearner algorithm achieved AUROC and AUPRC values of 0.85 and 0.65, respectively. Each base technique in the ensemble SuperLearner model demonstrated a significant level of similarity. Hypoglycemia may arise as a consequence of categorizing persons with low insulin use as high insulin users. Therefore, a greater proportion of accurate negative results (specificity) is beneficial. A higher level of specificity is associated with a reduction in recall and an enhancement in precision. The TDD with a prediction probability of 0.4 yielded a specificity of 90%, sensitivity (recall) of 56%, and a positive predictive value of 64%. A TDD prediction was performed using point-value data for individuals categorized as "higher" insulin users, who had received a cumulative amount of TDD exceeding 6 units subsequent to the binary prediction in stage I. The challenges in making predictions were attributed to the wide spectrum of TDD, the existence of a distribution that is tilted to the right, and the small sample size of 3970 patients. On average, it took doctors 2.2 days (with a standard deviation of 4.4 days) to modify insulin levels in order to achieve adequate control, as shown by blood glucose levels within the range of 100–180 mg/dL, after admission. The mean absolute error (MAE) of 25.4 units (19.5–32.2 units) and the mean absolute percentage error (MAPE) of 186% (136–329%) were obtained using the usual clinical TDD formula, with $c = (0.4–0.6)$. The magnitude of the mistake for $c = 0.5$ was 25.4 units, indicating a percentage of 186%. At $c = 0.4$ and 0.6, the minimum and maximum values are

19.5 units (136%) and 32.2 units (329%), respectively. Increased factors can lead to a greater quantity of errors. According to the univariate linear regression model, which uses weights, the anticipated values for the mean absolute error (MAE) and mean absolute percentage error (MAPE) were 14 units and 60%, respectively. The baseline model exhibited an intercept of 10.5 units, leading to a corresponding increase of 0.66% in TDD per kg. The full-feature ensemble model was employed to improve the regression model, yielding a mean absolute error (MAE) of 12.2 units (95% CI, 11.0–13.2 units) and a mean absolute percentage error (MAPE) of 51% [48–54%]. Lasso regression was the primary algorithm that had the most significant impact on the ensemble model, contributing 49%. Random forest and gradient-boosted trees made contributions of 35% and 16%, respectively. The individual application of Lasso regression yielded a mean absolute error (MAE) of 12.3 units (95% CI, 11.5–13.2 units) and mean absolute percentage error (MAPE) of 53% (95% CI, 51–57%). These results are similar to those obtained from the ensemble model, but they demand fewer computational resources [42].

7.3.3 Deep Reinforcement Learning Insulin Bolus Advisor

The advent of new continuous glucose monitoring (CGM) technology has expedited the development of closed-loop insulin administration systems, particularly artificial pancreas (AP) devices. The CGM sensors of the AP system measure glucose levels at 5-min intervals. The sensor transmits data to a controller, which then computes the appropriate dosages of insulin for the pump. Empirical studies and practical applications have shown that AP systems enhance glucose regulation [43]. The delayed pharmacokinetics of insulin contribute to its reduced efficacy in the management of postprandial hyperglycemia. Hybrid AP systems must either announce meals or estimate meal proportions in order to administer insulin boluses during meals. Advanced bolus advisors have been developed by multiple research groups with the aim of enhancing insulin dosage advice. The use of capillary blood measurements for run-to-run (R2R) control is recommended for individuals with T1D as a result of the recurrence of bolus insulin therapy. This approach has been evaluated in clinical settings [44]. The CGM-based AI case-based bolus advisor was developed by Herrero et al. This advisor was placed into a smartphone and subjected to a 6-week clinical evaluation in a free-living environment [41]. Wearables and EHRs have recently enhanced the accessibility of data. AI serves as a crucial tool for making decisions in diabetes control. Tyler et al. [45] proposed using a KNN decision support system to provide weekly insulin dosage recommendations to T1D patients treated with MDI. Lee et al. [46] assessed the performance of the KNN classifier and rule-based reasoning to prescribe meals, insulin, and exercise. Furthermore, the application of RL has been utilized to customize insulin treatment by Sun et al. [47]. The adaptive programming framework employed the GoCARB system and reinforcement learning control approach to estimate the amount of carbohydrates in a meal, with the aim of enhancing glycemic control [48].

Reinforcement learning (RL), a specialized field within machine learning, is used to instruct goal-oriented agents in the process of sequential decision-making. Glycemic control is achieved through the use of the basal insulin modulation strategy. Deep reinforcement learning (DRL) is a novel advancement in machine learning that integrates RL with deep learning. The hybrid approach demonstrates proficiency in challenging tasks such as Go, autonomous driving, and pharmaceutical dosing. The application of deep learning has been commonly employed to forecast blood glucose levels by capturing the properties of CGM sequences [49]. Deep reinforcement learning (DRL) healthcare applications may not be effective in clinical scenarios due to their reliance on trial-and-error learning. Preclinical research can be conducted using virtual environments such as the FDA-approved UVA/Padova T1D simulator. The parameters provided are highly effective for training RL agents. The simulator incorporates a mathematical model that encompasses the regulation of glucose-insulin, meal absorption, subcutaneous insulin absorption, continuous glucose sensor, and insulin pump. Simulated T1D patients that are clinically appropriate are also included [20]. The UVA/Padova T1D simulator was primarily used in the initial computational studies on increasing bolus insulin recommendations. Simulators can be used to construct generalized DRL models, which can then be adjusted using clinical data. The absence of postprandial glucose levels poses a challenge in assessing the recommended RL model. Therefore, the present study does not conduct offline testing of the suggested reinforcement learning model using in vivo data.

Researchers used a conventional DRL configuration to define the problem of an insulin bolus advisor. This advisor uses an agent to administer insulin and interact with the diabetes environment at distinct time intervals, ED. During timestep t, which corresponds to mealtime, the agent initially gets an observation st from the sensing devices inside the glycemic control system. Subsequently, the agent initiates an action at to administer a specific quantity of insulin bolus. Subsequently, the T1D subject's physiological condition changes to $st + 1$, and they receive the reward rt, which is determined by assessing the postprandial glucose excursion. Regarding this matter, the problem can be represented as a Markov decision process (MDP) using a tuple $\langle \mathcal{S}, \mathcal{A}, \mathcal{P}, R \rangle$ in Eq. (7.8) where $\mathcal{S}$ denotes the state space, $\mathcal{A}$ represents the action space, $\mathcal{P}$ signifies the transition functions between states, and R denotes a reward function. The agent's policy determines the allocation of actions for a specific state, as specified by π: $\mathcal{S} \to \mathcal{P}(\mathcal{A})$. The action-value function $Q\pi(st, at)$ under policy π is defined as the summation of the discounted future reward with the present state st and the selected action at. The objective of RL is to compute the best policy that maximizes the reward. Furthermore, a policy μ can be represented by associating the state with a particular action in a deterministic setting, as exemplified in that scenario: μ: $\mathcal{S} \to \mathcal{A}$. The estimated goal policy can be determined using the Bellman equation in this context:

$$Q\mu(st,at) = \mathbb{E}rt, st+1 \sim ED\left[R(st,at) + \gamma Q^{\mu}\left(st+1, \mu(st+1)\right)\right] \tag{7.8}$$

The discount factor, γ, should be chosen from the range of [0,1]. The value of $Q\mu$ can be learned through off-policy methods. Within the realm of glycemic control, the algorithm's input and output consist of the present observation of physiological states and the suggested insulin bolus, respectively. The goal is to find the optimal meal insulin bolus that improves glycemic control by solving Eq. (7.9). In a clinical setting, it is necessary to implement safety measures for insulin recommendations to prevent adverse glucose events.

The insulin bolus exerts a substantial influence on postprandial blood glucose levels, as it fluctuates based on the consumption of a meal. The task of delineating the spectrum of viable bolus insulin dosages presents a difficulty when employing value-based deep reinforcement learning techniques such as deep Q-networks [39]. Excessive intervals during training can greatly impede the process, while a restricted action set might have a detrimental effect on performance owing to the fluctuation of meals. An alternative methodology involves employing a bolus calculator to approximate the dosage and subsequently modifying it within a continuous interval, such as ±30%, surrounding this numerical number. Therefore, researchers suggest employing an actor-critic approach to enable the agent to operate within a continuous action space, using the deterministic policy gradient. The critic function $(s,\ a)$ is learned iteratively through the application of the Bellman equation, as shown in Eq. (7.9). The actor function (s) is updated based on the initial distribution J of the parameters:

$$\nabla_{\theta\mu} J \approx \mathbb{E}_{st\sim\rho}[\nabla_a Q\left(s,|a,|\theta^Q\right)\Big|_{s=st,a=\mu(st)} \nabla_{\theta\mu}\mu\left(s\middle|\theta^{\mu}\right)\Big|_{s=st}] \tag{7.9}$$

The parameters of the critic and actor are represented by θ^Q and θ^μ, respectively, while ρ denotes the state-visitation distribution. The actor determines the appropriate amount of bolus insulin to administer based on the current physiological state. Meanwhile, the critic evaluates the effectiveness of the action taken and provides guidance to the actor on any necessary adjustments. In order to acquire a comprehensive policy in a vast action-state space, deep neural networks (DNNs) are employed as nonlinear approximators to represent the actor and critic. This approach, known as deep deterministic policy gradient (DDPG) [42], involves utilizing the weights of neural networks as θ^Q and θ^μ in Eq. (7.10). Building upon the achievements of the DRL in achieving human-level control [49], researchers utilize replay memory M and fixed target networks to enhance the stability of the proposed methods. The system M stores the most recent N transitions as tuples $\langle st,\ at,\ rt,\ st+1\rangle$ in order to generate experience samples for off-policy learning. They have utilized fixed target networks to enable the segregation of neural networks for target calculation in the model training process. The target neural networks of actor Q' and critic μ' are obtained by copying weights of the current actor Q and critic μ with a fixed period $\mathscr{T}$, using soft update [42]. The loss of the critic is formulated based on the Bellman equation (7.8) and transition tuples:

$$\mathcal{L}\left(\theta^Q\right) = \mathbb{E}_{st\sim\rho}[\left(r_t + \gamma Q'\left(_{st+1},|u'\left(_{st+1}|\theta^{u'}\right),|\theta^{Q'}\right) - Q\left(s_t,|a_t,|\theta^Q\right)^2\right] \tag{7.10}$$

The insulin dose in AP systems with CGM and insulin pumps is calculated using a rather empirical approach for the conventional bolus calculator (Eq. 7.11) [14]:

$$\text{Bolus}*_t = \frac{\text{CHO}_t}{\text{ICR}} + \frac{G_t - G_T}{\text{ISF}} - \text{IOB}_t \quad (7.11)$$

The measurement of total carbohydrate intake is represented as CHO_t (in g), the ratio of insulin to carbohydrates is represented as ICR (in g/IU), the insulin sensitivity factor is represented as ISF (in mg/L/IU), the current measurement of blood glucose level from continuous glucose monitoring (CGM) is represented as G_T (in mg/dL), the desired blood glucose level is represented as G_T, and the amount of insulin present is represented as IOB [50].

7.3.4 Determination of the Optimal Insulin Bolus

The research involved the examination of several simulations in order to determine the most efficient dosage of insulin bolus for achieving optimal glycemic control in a specific participant and meal scenario. The computations of Eqs. (7.12a–7.12c) were performed by researchers for each situation, wherein several values of $f(\cdot)$ were selected from a grid designated F. A grid is a collection of numbers that are evenly spaced, represented as $\{-200 + 10k \mid k = 0, \ldots, 40\}$. Therefore, the researchers analyzed a total of 41 blood gas profiles using the given values of p and m. The profiles were quantitatively assessed by calculating the blood pm glucose risk index (BGRI). Researchers chose BGRI because it exhibits both hypoglycemia and hyperglycemic episodes with equal sensitivity, thanks to the symmetrization of the glucose scale. Therefore, it provides a concise and comprehensive representation of variations in blood glucose levels inside a single entity. Acceptable. To be more exact, when given a set of blood glucose readings (BG, $k = 1, \ldots, N$), the calculation of BGRI involves symmetrizing the glucose scale in the following way (Eq. 7.12b) [44]:

$$B = \frac{\text{CHO}}{\text{CR}} + \frac{(G_c + f(\cdot)) - G_T}{\text{CF}} - \text{IOB} \quad (7.12a)$$

$$f(\text{BG}) = 1.509\left[\log(\text{BG})^{1.084} - 5.381\right] \quad (7.12b)$$

and then computing its value as:

$$\text{BGRI} = N\sum_{k=1}^{N} 10 f(\text{BG}_k)^2 \quad (7.12c)$$

7.3.5 Insulin Sensitivity Prediction

The SI value, which is used as an indicator of the patient's current status, is determined on an hourly basis within the context of the patient's STAR (Stochastic TARgeted) treatment. The data pairs represented by {;} are generated via the stepwise time function. The prediction was derived by employing a stochastic model. In this study, a neural network-based Artificial Intelligence methodology will be used to establish the stochastic model. Therefore, the goal was to determine the function that yields the specified value using this dataset. Deep neural networks are suggested as a method of supervised machine learning to get an understanding of the correlation between input and output variables. NN-based classification models are used to predict the class of a given input. On the other hand, NN-based regression models are employed to anticipate continuous output values, which typically indicate the most probable value within a specific distribution. The primary concern pertains to the requirement of an interval, as opposed to a precise SI(t + 1) value, in the STAR protocol. Hence, a conventional regression method is inadequate for forecasting the two limits of the interval due to its absence of direct training data. The researchers created and used a classification model, together with additional postprocessing techniques, to calculate and gain insights into the conditional distribution of SI(t + 1). The codomain was divided into 128 intervals of equal size to facilitate the prediction of the distribution using a classification deep neural network. Each interval was associated with a single output class. The CDN is provided with the value as its input. The Content Delivery Network (CDN) output layer consists of 128 nodes that are linked to the stated classes. It is the responsibility of the CDN nodes to determine the probability, for each output class, that the SI domain associated with the particular class includes the expected value. Hence, the outcome can be perceived as the inequitable allocation of resources. A conventional multi-class categorization framework was used in the investigation. The activation functions employed in the buried dense layers were the tangent-hyperbolic functions. The output layer used the SoftMax function. The loss function employed in this study was the categorical cross-entropy function. The training dataset comprises SI(t) pairings associated with the one-hot encoded class number. The deep neural network for SI prediction was implemented using the TensorFlow and Keras frameworks in the Python programming language. Eighty percent of the input dataset was used during the training phase. There was a total of 20 epochs throughout the training procedure. In this case, the final result of the SI prediction is determined by applying a Gaussian distribution to the output of the deep neural network, which is considered as a histogram. The application of the STAR technique to the SI(t + 1) conditional distribution necessitates a confidence interval of 90%. Therefore, the 5th and 95th percentiles of the Gaussian distribution that was selected for analysis were used. The small interval width is a consequence of around 90% of the potential SI values falling within the range established by the two border values [51].

7.4 Conclusion and Future Scope

This chapter addressed the rapid growth of AI capacity to transform the management of insulin and glycemic control for diabetic patients. Real-time insulin dosage adjustments and the prediction of glycemic levels and potential complications were among the AI-powered strategies that were explored. These developments exhibit tremendous potential to improve patient outcomes and overall quality of life. Predicting complications such as diabetic retinopathy and nocturnal hypoglycemia provides healthcare providers and patients with proactive management strategies. With the ability to personalize insulin regimens and reduce the risk of hypoglycemia, machine learning algorithms can analyze huge datasets. Insulin bolus delivery is modified even more precisely using deep reinforcement learning algorithms that emulate the thought processes of experienced diabetologists. The potential applications of AI in diabetes management are practically limitless. By integrating data from CGM with AI systems, insulin dosing can be made more precisely and in response to individual activities and requirements in real time. Approaching, closed-loop insulin delivery systems, alternatively referred to as artificial pancreas systems, hold great potential for a future in which blood sugar levels are autonomously regulated by AI, relieving patients of the perpetual responsibility of monitoring, and adjusting their medications. However, obstacles continue to exist. It is essential to address concerns related to data privacy, guarantee fair and equal access to AI-powered technologies, and seamlessly integrate AI into preexisting healthcare systems to achieve successful implementation. AI possesses the capacity to revolutionize diabetes management through ongoing research and development, indicating a novel era of personalized, optimized glycemic control for diabetic patients across the globe.

References

1. Ellahham S. Artificial intelligence: the future for diabetes care. Am J Med. 2020;133:895–900. https://doi.org/10.1016/j.amjmed.2020.03.033.
2. Cho NH, Shaw JE, Karuranga S, Huang Y, da Rocha Fernandes JD, Ohlrogge AW, Malanda B. IDF diabetes atlas: global estimates of diabetes prevalence for 2017 and projections for 2045. Diabetes Res Clin Pract. 2018;138:271–81. https://doi.org/10.1016/j.diabres.2018.02.023.
3. Fitzmaurice C, Allen C, Barber RM, Barregard L, Bhutta ZA, Brenner H, Dicker DJ, Chimed-Orchir O, Dandona R, Dandona L, Fleming T, Forouzanfar MH, Hancock J, Hay RJ, Hunter-Merrill R, Huynh C, Hosgood HD, Johnson CO, Jonas JB, Khubchandani J, Kumar GA, Kutz M, Lan Q, Larson HJ, Liang X, Lim SS, Lopez AD, MacIntyre MF, Marczak L, Marquez N, Mokdad AH, Pinho C, Pourmalek F, Salomon JA, Sanabria JR, Sandar L, Sartorius B, Schwartz SM, Shackelford KA, Shibuya K, Stanaway J, Steiner C, Sun J, Takahashi K, Vollset SE, Vos T, Wagner JA, Wang H, Westerman R, Zeeb H, Zoeckler L, Abd-Allah F, Ahmed MB, Alabed S, Alam NK, Aldhahri SF, Alem G, Alemayohu MA, Ali R, Al-Raddadi R, Amare A, Amoako Y, Artaman A, Asayesh H, Atnafu N, Awasthi A, Saleem HB, Barac A, Bedi N, Bensenor I, Berhane A, Bernabé E, Betsu B, Binagwaho A, Boneya D, Campos-Nonato I, Castañeda-Orjuela C, Catalá-López F, Chiang P, Chibueze C, Chitheer A, Choi JY, Cowie B, Damtew S, Das Neves J, Dey S, Dharmaratne S, Dhillon P, Ding E, Driscoll T, Ekwueme D, Endries AY, Farvid M, Farzadfar F, Fernandes J, Fischer F, Ghiwot TT, Gebru A, Gopalani S,

Hailu A, Horino M, Horita N, Husseini A, Huybrechts I, Inoue M, Islami F, Jakovljevic M, James S, Javanbakht M, Jee SH, Kasaeian A, Kedir MS, Khader YS, Khang YH, Kim D, Leigh J, Linn S, Lunevicius R, El Razek HMA, Malekzadeh R, Malta DC, Marcenes W, Markos D, Melaku YA, Meles KG, Mendoza W, Mengiste DT, Meretoja TJ, Miller TR, Mohammad KA, Mohammadi A, Mohammed S, Moradi-Lakeh M, Nagel G, Nand D, Le Nguyen Q, Nolte S, Ogbo FA, Oladimeji KE, Oren E, Pa M, Park EK, Pereira DM, Plass D, Qorbani M, Radfar A, Rafay A, Rahman M, Rana SM, Søreide K, Satpathy M, Sawhney M, Sepanlou SG, Shaikh MA, She J, Shiue I, Shore HR, Shrime MG, So S, Soneji S, Stathopoulou V, Stroumpoulis K, Sufiyan MB, Sykes BL, Tabarés-Seisdedos R, Tadese F, Tedla BA, Tessema GA, Thakur JS, Tran BX, Ukwaja KN, Chudi Uzochukwu BS, Vlassov VV, Weiderpass E, Wubshet Terefe M, Yebyo HG, Yimam HH, Yonemoto N, Younis MZ, Yu C, Zaidi Z, Zaki MES, Zenebe ZM, Murray CJL, Naghavi M. Global, regional, and national cancer incidence, mortality, years of life lost, years lived with disability, and disability-adjusted life-years for 32 cancer groups, 1990 to 2015: a systematic analysis for the Global Burden of Disease Study. JAMA Oncol. 2017;3:524–48. https://doi.org/10.1001/jamaoncol.2016.5688.

4. Katsarou A, Gudbjörnsdottir S, Rawshani A, Dabelea D, Bonifacio E, Anderson BJ, Jacobsen LM, Schatz DA, Lernmark A. Type 1 diabetes mellitus. Nat Rev Dis Prim. 2017;3:1–18. https://doi.org/10.1038/nrdp.2017.16.
5. Atkinson MA, Eisenbarth GS, Michels AW. Type 1 diabetes. Lancet. 2014;383:69–82. https://doi.org/10.1016/S0140-6736(13)60591-7.
6. Dhatariya KK, Glaser NS, Codner E, Umpierrez GE. Diabetic ketoacidosis. Nat Rev Dis Prim. 2020;6:1–20. https://doi.org/10.1038/s41572-020-0165-1.
7. Chiang JL, Kirkman MS, Laffel LMB, Peters AL. Type 1 diabetes through the life span: a position statement of the American Diabetes Association. Diabetes Care. 2014;37:2034–54. https://doi.org/10.2337/dc14-1140.
8. Jacobs PG, Herrero P, Facchinetti A, Vehi J, Kovatchev B, Breton MD, Cinar A, Nikita KS, Doyle FJ, Bondia J, Battelino T, Castle JR, Zarkogianni K, Narayan R, Mosquera-Lopez C. Artificial intelligence and machine learning for improving glycemic control in diabetes: best practices, pitfalls, and opportunities. IEEE Rev Biomed Eng. 2024;17:19–41. https://doi.org/10.1109/RBME.2023.3331297.
9. Wang G, Liu X, Ying Z, Yang G, Chen Z, Liu Z, Zhang M, Yan H, Lu Y, Gao Y, Xue K, Li X, Chen Y. Optimized glycemic control of type 2 diabetes with reinforcement learning: a proof-of-concept trial. Nat Med. 2023;29:2633–42. https://doi.org/10.1038/s41591-023-02552-9.
10. Yoo JH, Kim JH. Advances in continuous glucose monitoring and integrated devices for management of diabetes with insulin-based therapy: improvement in glycemic control. Diabetes Metab J. 2023;47:27–41. https://doi.org/10.4093/dmj.2022.0271.
11. Cappon G, Vettoretti M, Marturano F, Facchinetti A, Sparacino G. A neural-network-based approach to personalize insulin bolus calculation using continuous glucose monitoring. J Diabetes Sci Technol. 2018;12:265–72. https://doi.org/10.1177/1932296818759558.
12. Chen J, Cao K, Sun Y, Xiao Y, Su X. Continuous drug infusion for diabetes therapy: a closed-loop control system design. EURASIP J Wirel Commun Netw. 2008;2008 https://doi.org/10.1155/2008/495185.
13. Khaqan A, Nauman A, Shuja S, Khurshaid T, Kim KC. An intelligent model-based effective approach for glycemic control in type-1 diabetes. Sensors. 2022;22:1–18. https://doi.org/10.3390/s22207773.
14. Pappada SM, Cameron BD. Neural network modeling approaches for patient specific glycemic forecasting. Stud Mechanobiol Tissue Eng Biomater. 2012;9:505–29. https://doi.org/10.1007/8415_2011_98.
15. Cox DJ, Gonder-Frederick L, Ritterband L, Clarke W, Kovatchev BP. Prediction of severe hypoglycemia. Diabetes Care. 2007;30:1370–3. https://doi.org/10.2337/dc06-1386.
16. Sampath S, Tkachenko P, Renard E, Pereverzev SV. Glycemic control indices and their aggregation in the prediction of nocturnal hypoglycemia from intermittent blood glucose measurements. J Diabetes Sci Technol. 2016;10:1245–50. https://doi.org/10.1177/1932296816670400.

17. Rodbard D. Interpretation of continuous glucose monitoring data: glycemic variability and quality of glycemic control. Diabetes Technol Ther. 2009;11(S1):S55–67. https://doi.org/10.1089/dia.2008.0132.
18. Rowlandson R. Prediction and management of nocturnal hypoglycaemia in diabetes. Arch Dis Child. 1987;62:1200. https://doi.org/10.1136/adc.62.11.1200-a.
19. Davies A. Prediction and management of nocturnal hypoglycaemia in diabetes. Arch Dis Child. 1987;62:1085. https://doi.org/10.1136/adc.62.10.1085.
20. Khunti K, Nikolajsen A, Thorsted BL, Andersen M, Davies MJ, Paul SK. Clinical inertia with regard to intensifying therapy in people with type 2 diabetes treated with basal insulin. Diabetes Obes Metab. 2016;18:401–9. https://doi.org/10.1111/dom.12626.
21. Khunti K, Wolden ML, Thorsted BL, Andersen M, Davies MJ. Clinical inertia in people with type 2 diabetes: a retrospective cohort study of more than 80,000 people. Diabetes Care. 2013;36:3411–7. https://doi.org/10.2337/dc13-0331.
22. Ross SA, Tildesley HD, Ashkenas J. Barriers to effective insulin treatment: the persistence of poor glycemic control in type 2 diabetes. Curr Med Res Opin. 2011;27:13–20. https://doi.org/10.1185/03007995.2011.621416.
23. Colagiuri S, Davies D. The value of early detection of type 2 diabetes. Curr Opin Endocrinol Diabetes Obes. 2009;16:95–9. https://doi.org/10.1097/MED.0b013e328329302f.
24. Griffin SJ, Borch-Johnsen K, Davies MJ, Khunti K, Rutten GE, Sandbæk A, Sharp SJ, Simmons RK, Van Den Donk M, Wareham NJ, Lauritzen T. Effect of early intensive multifactorial therapy on 5-year cardiovascular outcomes in individuals with type 2 diabetes detected by screening (ADDITION-Europe): a cluster-randomised trial. Lancet. 2011;378:156–67. https://doi.org/10.1016/S0140-6736(11)60698-3.
25. Holman RR, Paul SK, Bethel MA, Matthews DR, Neil HAW. 10-Year follow-up of intensive glucose control in type 2 diabetes. N Engl J Med. 2008;359:1577–89. https://doi.org/10.1056/nejmoa0806470.
26. Cichosz SL, Johansen MD, Hejlesen O. Toward big data analytics: review of predictive models in management of diabetes and its complications. J Diabetes Sci Technol. 2016;10:27–34. https://doi.org/10.1177/1932296815611680.
27. Kavakiotis I, Tsave O, Salifoglou A, Maglaveras N, Vlahavas I, Chouvarda I. Machine learning and data mining methods in diabetes research. Comput Struct Biotechnol J. 2017;15:104–16. https://doi.org/10.1016/j.csbj.2016.12.005.
28. Fan Y, Long E, Cai L, Cao Q, Wu X, Tong R. Machine learning approaches to predict risks of diabetic complications and poor glycemic control in nonadherent type 2 diabetes. Front Pharmacol. 2021;12:1–11. https://doi.org/10.3389/fphar.2021.665951.
29. Alhaddad AY, Aly H, Gad H, Al-Ali A, Sadasivuni KK, Cabibihan JJ, Malik RA. Sense and learn: recent advances in wearable sensing and machine learning for blood glucose monitoring and trend-detection. Front Bioeng Biotechnol. 2022;10:1–23. https://doi.org/10.3389/fbioe.2022.876672.
30. Reifman J, Rajaraman S, Gribok A, Ward WK. Predictive monitoring for improved management of glucose levels. J Diabetes Sci Technol. 2007;1:478–86. https://doi.org/10.1177/193229680700100405.
31. Sparacino G, Zanderigo F, Corazza S, Maran A, Facchinetti A, Cobelli C. Glucose concentration can be predicted ahead in time from continuous glucose monitoring sensor time-series. IEEE Trans Biomed Eng. 2007;54:931–7. https://doi.org/10.1109/TBME.2006.889774.
32. Plank J, Blaha J, Cordingley J, Wilinska ME, Chassin LJ, Morgan C, Squire S, Haluzik M, Kremen J, Svacina S, Toller W, Plasnik A, Ellmerer M, Hovorka R, Pieber TR. Multicentric, randomized, controlled trial to evaluate blood glucose control by the model predictive control algorithm versus routine glucose management protocols in intensive care unit patients. Diabetes Care. 2006;29:271–6.
33. Schlotthauer G, Gamero LG, Torres ME, Nicolini GA. Modeling, identification and nonlinear model predictive control of type I diabetic patient. Med Eng Phys. 2006;28:240–50. https://doi.org/10.1016/j.medengphy.2005.04.009.
34. Steil G, Rebrin K, Mastrototaro JJ. Metabolic modelling and the closed-loop insulin delivery problem. Diabetes Res Clin Pract. 2006;74:183–6. https://doi.org/10.1016/S0168-8227(06)70028-6.

35. Wintergerst KA, Deiss D, Buckingham B, Cantwell M, Kache S, Agarwal S, Wilson DM, Steil G. Glucose control in pediatric intensive care unit patients using an insulin-glucose algorithm. Diabetes Technol Ther. 2007;9:211–22. https://doi.org/10.1089/dia.2006.0031.
36. Steil GM, Panteleon AE, Rebrin K. Closed-loop insulin delivery—the path to physiological glucose control. Adv Drug Deliv Rev. 2004;56:125–44. https://doi.org/10.1016/j.addr.2003.08.011.
37. Foody GM, McCulloch MB, Yates WB. The effect of training set size and composition on artificial neural network classification. Int J Remote Sens. 1995;16:1707–23. https://doi.org/10.1080/01431169508954507.
38. Pappada SM, Cameron BD, Rosman PM. Development of a Neural Network for Prediction of Glucose Concentration in Type 1 Diabetes Patients. Journal of Diabetes Science and Technology. 2008;2(5):792–801. https://doi.org/10.1177/193229680800200507.
39. Mnih V, Kavukcuoglu K, Silver D, Rusu AA, Veness J, Bellemare MG, Graves A, Riedmiller M, Fidjeland AK, Ostrovski G, Petersen S, Beattie C, Sadik A, Antonoglou I, King H, Kumaran D, Wierstra D, Legg S, Hassabis D. Human-level control through deep reinforcement learning. Nature. 2015;518:529–33. https://doi.org/10.1038/nature14236.
40. Qian N. On the momentum term in gradient descent learning algorithms. Neural Netw. 1999;12:145–51. https://doi.org/10.1016/S0893-6080(98)00116-6.
41. Chen Y, Chen Z, Zhao L, Li S, Ying Z, Yu P, Yan H, Chen H, Yang C, Zhang J, Meng Q, Liu Y, Cao L, Shen Y, Hu C, Huang H, Li X, Bian H, Li X. Real-time artificial intelligence assisted insulin dosage titration system for glucose control in type 2 diabetic patients: a proof of concept study. Curr Med. 2023;2 https://doi.org/10.1007/s44194-023-00020-7.
42. Nguyen M, Jankovic I, Kalesinskas L, Baiocchi M, Chen JH. Machine learning for initial insulin estimation in hospitalized patients. J Am Med Inform Assoc. 2021;28:2212–9. https://doi.org/10.1093/jamia/ocab099.
43. Boughton CK, Hovorka R. Advances in artificial pancreas systems. Sci Transl Med. 2019;11:3–6. https://doi.org/10.1126/scitranslmed.aaw4949.
44. Cappon G, Vettoretti M, Marturano F, Facchinetti A, Sparacino G. Optimal insulin bolus dosing in type 1 diabetes management: neural network approach exploiting CGM sensor information. In: Proceedings of the annual international conference of the IEEE Engineering in Medicine and Biology Society (EMBS), Jul 2018. p. 340–3. https://doi.org/10.1109/EMBC.2018.8512250.
45. Tyler NS, Mosquera-Lopez CM, Wilson LM, Dodier RH, Branigan DL, Gabo VB, Guillot FH, Hilts WW, El Youssef J, Castle JR, Jacobs PG. An artificial intelligence decision support system for the management of type 1 diabetes. Nat Metab. 2020;2:612–9. https://doi.org/10.1038/s42255-020-0212-y.
46. Lee M, Gatton TM, Lee KK. A monitoring and advisory system for diabetes patient management using a rule-based method and KNN. Sensors. 2010;10:3934–53. https://doi.org/10.3390/s100403934.
47. Sun Q, Jankovic MV, Budzinski J, Moore B, Diem P, Stettler C, Mougiakakou SG. A dual mode adaptive basal-bolus advisor based on reinforcement learning. IEEE J Biomed Health Inform. 2019;23:2633–41. https://doi.org/10.1109/JBHI.2018.2887067.
48. Agianniotis A, Anthimopoulos M, Daskalaki E, Drapela A, Stettler C, Diem P, Mougiakakou S. GoCARB in the context of an artificial pancreas. J Diabetes Sci Technol. 2015;9:549–55. https://doi.org/10.1177/1932296815583333.
49. Li K, Liu C, Zhu T, Herrero P, Georgiou P. GluNet: a deep learning framework for accurate glucose forecasting. IEEE J Biomed Health Inform. 2020;24:414–23. https://doi.org/10.1109/JBHI.2019.2931842.
50. Zhu T, Li K, Kuang L, Herrero P, Georgiou P. An insulin bolus advisor for type 1 diabetes using deep reinforcement learning. Sensors (Switzerland). 2020;20:1–15. https://doi.org/10.3390/s20185058.
51. Benyó B, Paláncz B, Szlávecz Á, Szabó B, Anane Y, Kovács K, Chase JG. Artificial intelligence based insulin sensitivity prediction for personalized glycaemic control in intensive care. IFAC-PapersOnLine. 2020;53:16335–40. https://doi.org/10.1016/j.ifacol.2020.12.659.

Hormone Balancing Through Nutrition: Nutritional Strategies and AI Tools to Balance Hormones Associated with PCOS

8

K. S. Hemanth, Noorain Fathima, and G. D. Sridhar

8.1 Introduction

8.1.1 Global Reach of PCOS

Polycystic ovary syndrome (PCOS), identified by Stein and Leventhal in 1935, is a common hormonal dysfunction among women of reproductive age, marked by hormonal disturbances, irregularities in menses, and the presence of small ovarian follicular vesicles. The diverse clinical presentation of PCOS includes menstrual irregularities, hirsutism, acne, infertility, and metabolic imbalances, including impaired insulin sensitivity, obesity, and diabetes mellitus type 2. It also includes amenorrhea, oligomenorrhea, obesity, male pattern hair loss, and reproductive disorders. These symptoms affect the overall quality of women's life, mental health, and reproductive health and vary across different populations, with some women experiencing only mild symptoms while others severe symptoms [1, 2].

The occurrence of PCOS may differ based on the diagnostic criteria that are utilized, but it is estimated to affect 3.4% of women globally and up to 18% in some community-based studies. From a healthcare system perspective, PCOS is associated with high healthcare costs due to the need for long-term management of metabolic disturbances and reproductive health issues. The disorder is also associated with a higher risk of complications during pregnancy, such as gestational diabetes, hypertension, and preterm birth [3, 4].

K. S. Hemanth (✉)
Department of Computer Science, Christ University, Bangalore, Karnataka, India
e-mail: hemanth.ks@christuniversity.in

N. Fathima · G. D. Sridhar
School of Computer Science and Application, REVA University, Bangalore, Karnataka, India

R. Kumar et al. (eds.), *AI-Based Nutritional Intervention in Polycystic Ovary Syndrome (PCOS)*, https://doi.org/10.1007/978-981-96-2120-0_8

8.1.2 Limitations of Current Treatments

The management of polycystic ovary syndrome (PCOS) traditionally involves both pharmacological and non-pharmacological methods aimed at addressing the symptoms associated with the condition.

8.1.2.1 Pharmacological Approaches

Pharmacological interventions commonly include the use of oral contraceptives, metformin, and anti-androgens, which help regulate menstrual abnormalities and manage hirsutism and acne. Oral contraceptive pills (OCPs) work by inhibiting LH secretion, thereby reducing the production of androgens. Insulin sensitizers, such as metformin and thiazolidinediones, have proven to increase insulin sensitivity as well as activate ovarian release in PCOS.

Anti-androgens, such as spironolactone, flutamide, and finasteride, are employed to reduce excessive hair growth and other androgen-induced complications in PCOS by blocking the action of testosterone.

While these medications can provide symptomatic relief, they do not address the underlying causes of PCOS, such as insulin resistance and hormonal imbalances. Moreover, long-term use of these medications results in side effects and difficulties, such as weight gain, mood changes, and liver damage [2, 5].

8.1.2.2 Non-pharmacological Approaches

Non-pharmacological approaches include lifestyle modifications, dietary changes, and exercise. These approaches have been shown to be effective in managing PCOS.

Lifestyle modifications, such as consistent physical exercise and a healthy body weight, are crucial for PCOS management, along with adopting a low-glycemic index (LGI) diet and achieving weight loss, which have been shown to improve insulin resistance, cholesterol levels, waist circumference, and testosterone levels in PCOS patients.

Supplementation with vitamins and minerals, such as bioflavonoids, carnitine, alpha-lipoic acid, chromium picolinate, calcium, magnesium, selenium, and zinc, has shown an improvement in insulin sensitivity and hormonal balance in PCOS.

Despite of providing relief from symptoms, the conventional methods overlook the primary causes of the condition. This has led to the development of a comprehensive and personalized approach that combines the existing approaches with artificial intelligence for effective PCOS management [2, 5].

8.1.3 The Rise of AI in Healthcare

Healthcare AI is transforming different medical fields with its potential for personalized medicine and precision therapeutics like analyzing diagnostic images or corresponding symptoms and biological indicators from electronic health records (EHRs) to identify and diagnose the condition. Applications of AI in healthcare include genetics-based solutions, drug discovery and development, medical visualization, and medical robotics by enhancing the work of healthcare professionals. The market for AI in healthcare is projected to grow rapidly, reaching USD 150 billion by 2026.

Technological advancements, like deep learning, have facilitated the rapid growth of AI-powered healthcare tools and technology. For instance, convolutional neural networks (CNNs) are used in image recognition to identify features of medical images and classify them based on those features.

Genetics-based solutions involve identifying patterns in genetic datasets and linking them with EMRs to develop individualized genetic medicines. AI can streamline drug discovery and development by assessing chemical properties of drugs and activity, formulating new drug molecules, analyzing drug-receptor interactions, and predicting drug reactions. For example, Deep Genomics, a HealthTech company, detects patterns and trends in the vast genetic dataset and electronic medical records (EMRs) to correlate them to determine treatment objectives, either existing or new treatment objectives, aiming to create personalized genetic treatments. AI is implemented throughout all stages of their process in discovering and developing drug, which includes identifying targets, refining leads, assessing toxicity, and designing groundbreaking trials.

Immersive technologies can be embedded in healthcare systems, from medical education to patient care. These technologies can enhance learning experiences for medical students and specialists, provide immersive therapy for patients, and assist in complex surgical procedures. Wearable health devices (WHDs) and remote monitoring can help detect early signs of disease and facilitate communication between patients and healthcare workers without disrupting daily routines [6].

8.1.4 AI for Hormonal Balance

AI has been widely used in the field of medicine to enhance patient health results. Machine learning and deep learning algorithms can process medical data efficiently, such as biomarkers and clinical images, and have been used for computerized diagnosis, patient triage, severity diagnosis, drug discovery, treatments, prognosis, and decision-making assistance.

AI-powered tools for PCOS management focus on hormonal balancing by analyzing patient data and providing personalized dietary recommendations. Machine learning and deep learning algorithms are utilized to provide personalized dietary recommendations to optimize hormonal balance in PCOS patients. The potential limitations of using AI-powered tools in PCOS management include issues related to data privacy and security.

Organization of Chapter

The rest of the chapter is organized as follows: Section 8.2 illustrates AI-powered personalized nutrition for PCOS. Section 8.3 focusses on critical considerations for AI in healthcare. Section 8.4 highlights the future of PCOS care with care with AI. And finally, Sect. 8.5 concludes the chapter.

8.2 AI-Powered Personalized Nutrition for PCOS

8.2.1 The Data Landscape

PCOS is a complex disorder that involves various types of data: genetic data, biomarkers, dietary habits, and lifestyle factors. PCOS is a polygenic and multifactorial disease, meaning it involves a variety of genes that affect steroidogenesis, gonadotrophic activity and regulation, insulin activity and discharge, body mass index, and persistent inflammation. Understanding these genetic factors can help in better understanding the pathogenesis of PCOS and developing targeted therapies. Hormonal (FSH, LH, FSH/LH, hCG, TSH), metabolic (weight, BMI, RBS), and inflammatory biomarkers play a significant role in PCOS diagnosis and management. In PCOS, there is often an imbalance in the levels of these hormones, with higher levels of LH and lower levels of FSH. This imbalance can contribute to the irregular menstrual cycles and infertility that are common in PCOS. Women diagnosed with PCOS have a higher tendency to be overweight or obese, which can contribute to insulin resistance, a key feature of PCOS. Lifestyle factors, including diet, are crucial in PCOS management. Women with PCOS are often advised to follow a healthy diet to manage their weight and insulin levels. Other lifestyle factors, such as physical activity, regular exercise, and stress management, are also important in PCOS management [7, 8].

8.2.1.1 Data Quality and Standardization

In the context of PCOS, data quality and standardization are important for ensuring the reliability and accuracy of the AI system. AI models learn patterns from the training data. If the data includes noise or outliers, the AI model may learn inaccurate patterns, resulting in less accurate predictions. For instance, the dataset may include some women who have been incorrectly diagnosed with PCOS. The AI model may learn patterns from this data that are not representative of true PCOS cases, leading to poor predictions and incorrect diagnoses in the future.

AI models perform well when the features are on a comparable scale. If the features are not scaled, the model may give more importance to some features that have a larger range of values, leading to biased predictions. In addition, AI models may not perform well if the data they are trained on is not consistent in its representation. For example, if the ultrasound images are not preprocessed consistently, the model may not be able to learn the patterns effectively.

AI models need to generalize well to new, unseen data. If the data quality and standardization are not considered during the model training phase, the model might not generalize well to unseen data, leading to poor predictions that may not be easily interpretable. This may make it difficult to understand the reasons behind the predictions, for example, if the model utilizes data from women with PCOS who have a specific set of symptoms and then applied to a new dataset of women with PCOS who have different symptoms, The model may not be able to generalize to the new dataset, leading to poor predictions.

Accurate predictions and recommendations based on AI models require high-quality and standardized data. In the case of PCOS, accurate data will enable health-care professionals to make informed treatment decisions, potentially improving patient outcomes [9].

8.2.1.2 Recommendations to Address the Data Quality and Standardization Issues

To ensure that the dataset includes a variety of patients with different characteristics, ages, and weight ranges, it is recommended to collect data from multiple centers or hospitals rather than relying on data from a single source. This can aid in ensuring that the dataset reflects the larger population of women identified with PCOS and minimizes the bias.

For instance, the dataset could include women with PCOS from a variety of age ranges, including adolescents, young adults, and postmenopausal women. It could also include women with PCOS who have a range of weight and BMI values, from underweight to obese.

To further enhance the data quality and standardize it, preprocessing techniques such as resizing ultrasound images to a standard size, normalizing the pixel values to a standard range, and normalizing numerical features such as hormonal and metabolic biomarkers to a standard scale can be applied.

Cross validation is another technique that can be used to ensure that the dataset is representative and does not contain biases. This involves randomly partitioning the dataset into many folds (subsets), training and testing the AI algorithm on each fold. This can help ensure that the model can perform well on a variety of data subsets, rather than just a single subset.

By implementing these techniques, the data quality and standardization can be improved, leading to more accurate and reliable AI models for detecting and diagnosing the disorder [9].

8.2.2 AI Algorithms and Models

Linear discriminant analysis (LDA) and principal component analysis (PCA) are techniques that can be used in hormone balancing for PCOS to reduce the dimensionality of complex hormone data while preserving the essential information. LDA is a supervised technique that distinguishes between different groups, such as healthy individuals and those with PCOS. On the other hand, PCA is an unsupervised method that retains the originality of the dataset by finding a new set of variables called principal components, which are linear combinations of the original variables.

SGD is an optimization technique that can improve the performance of regression models used to predict hormone levels based on various factors. Linear, polynomial, and Lasso regression techniques can be applied to identify the relationships between independent variables (such as lifestyle factors, age, or genetic markers) and the dependent variable (hormone levels). Naive Bayes, decision trees, and SVM can be used for classification tasks, distinguishing between healthy individuals and those with PCOS based on hormone data and other relevant factors. Clustering techniques like DBSCAN, GMM, and agglomerative clustering can reveal hidden patterns and subgroups in hormone data, aiding in the identification of different PCOS phenotypes.

A priori algorithm and stacking can be used to discover frequent itemsets and association rules in patient data, helping to identify connections between various factors and PCOS risk. Monte Carlo, Q-learning, ANN, CNN, and LSTM-RNN can be employed to analyze complex, large-scale hormone data and predict hormone levels and PCOS risk based on a multitude of factors.

8.2.3 Generating your Hormonal Profile

AI, particularly machine learning (ML) techniques, can analyze individual data to create a comprehensive metabolic and hormonal profile for PCOS (polycystic ovary syndrome) patients, aiding in personalized treatment plans. The process includes collecting and preprocessing data, feature selection, model building and optimization, model evaluation, and generating a personalized profile.

Data collection and preprocessing: Patient data like medical history, blood tests (hormone levels, glucose, etc.), anthropometric measurements (weight, BMI, waist circumference), and lifestyle habits (diet, exercise) are collected. Missing values are imputed, and outliers are handled to ensure data quality. Categorical data might be encoded numerically (if required).

Feature selection: ML algorithms cannot process all data effectively. Feature selection methods like mutual information or recursive feature elimination are used to identify the most significant features (e.g., specific hormone levels, BMI) that best predict the presence or severity of PCOS.

Model training and optimization: Machine learning algorithms are trained on cleaned and formatted data. These models can be used to identify patterns that distinguish between healthy and unhealthy patients based on various health metrics. Hyperparameter optimization techniques, such as SGD, are used to optimize the model's internal settings for better performance. Hyperparameters are the parameters that are not internally learned from the data but instead are configured before the learning process begins, such as the maximum depth of a decision tree.

Model evaluation: Evaluation metrics like accuracy, precision, recall, F1-score, and ROC AUC access the model's capability to correctly classify individuals with and without PCOS. To explain how each feature contributes to the model's prediction, techniques like SHAP values or LIME are applied, thereby increasing trust and transparency.

Generating a personalized profile: The trained and evaluated model predicts the likelihood of PCOS based on an individual's data, creating a unique picture of the individual's hormonal and metabolic state. This personalized profile, built upon AI analysis, empowers healthcare professionals to address the root causes of PCOS rather than just managing symptoms and predicting the potential complications associated with PCOS, allowing for proactive interventions and preventative measures [7, 8, 10].

8.2.4 AI-Powered Dietary Recommendations

8.2.4.1 Adaptive Meal Plans

AI algorithms can generate adaptive meal plans that adjust in real time based on various factors, including blood sugar fluctuations, hormone levels, and activity data, to benefit individuals with PCOS (polycystic ovary syndrome). By optimizing insulin sensitivity, androgen control, and overall metabolic health, these systems can contribute to improved PCOS management and overall well-being. For instance, if the system spots an increase in blood sugar levels, it may suggest a low-glycemic index meal to help stabilize blood sugar. Similarly, if the system detects elevated testosterone levels, it may suggest a meal plan that is rich in fiber and omega-3 fatty acids, which have been shown to help reduce testosterone levels in PCOS patients. The system can also incorporate activity data to further optimize meal plans. For example, if the patient has been sedentary for an extended period, the system may suggest a meal plan that is lower in calories to help prevent weight gain.

8.2.4.2 Optimizing Insulin Sensitivity

Insulin sensitivity is crucial for individuals with PCOS, as 35–80% of them have insulin resistance. AI algorithms can monitor an individual's blood sugar levels after meals. AI systems can identify which foods trigger spikes and adjust meal plans and timing accordingly to maintain stable blood sugar levels and minimize insulin resistance. AI algorithms can also customize the meal plan's macronutrient composition (proteins, fats, and carbohydrates) based on an individual's specific needs and insulin response. Suppose the patient has a high insulin response to carbohydrates. The system may suggest a meal plan that is lower in carbohydrates and higher in protein and fat. Conversely, if the patient has a low insulin response to carbohydrates, the system may suggest a meal plan that is higher in carbohydrates and lower in protein and fat.

8.2.4.3 Androgen Control

Elevated androgen levels in women with PCOS can lead to various symptoms. AI-powered meal plans can help control androgen levels by suggesting that foods like spearmint, flaxseeds, and soy are anti-androgenic and by finding the best macronutrient composition to help control androgen levels, like eating more fiber and less refined carbohydrates.

AI-driven adaptive meal plans can also contribute to overall metabolic health in PCOS by analyzing an individual's energy expenditure and caloric intake as shown in Fig. 8.1. AI systems can ensure that meal plans include a variety of nutrient-dense foods, providing all the necessary macronutrients, vitamins, and minerals for optimal metabolic function. AI algorithms can identify anti-inflammatory foods and

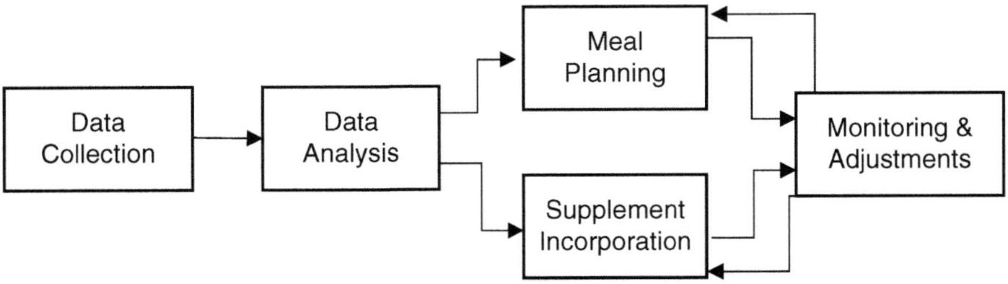

Fig. 8.1 Flowchart for the steps involved in AI-powered PCOS management

incorporate them into meal plans to help reduce overall inflammation in individuals with PCOS. By continuously analyzing real-time data and adjusting meal plans accordingly, AI algorithms can significantly contribute to optimizing insulin sensitivity, androgen control, and overall metabolic health in individuals with PCOS [11–14].

8.2.5 Real-World Success Stories

8.2.5.1 Personalized Nutrient Optimization

AI-generated dynamic meal plans: AI algorithms can generate dynamic meal plans that adjust in real time based on blood sugar fluctuations, hormone levels, and activity data, optimizing insulin sensitivity, androgen control, and overall metabolic health in PCOS. These meal plans can be tailored to individual dietary preferences, allergies, and intolerances.

Increased oxidation of fasting fat: A low-starch and dairy diet rich in natural animal protein, low-starch eatables, and high-calorie cheese has been shown to increase the breakdown of stored fat following a nutrition plan in obese women having PCOS, leading to a positive change in waist-to-hip ratio, adipose tissue, body weight, and fasting blood sugar, HbA1c, and free testosterone.

Weight loss and improvement of insulin resistance: A low-starch and dairy diet consisting of natural animal protein, fish and shellfish, eggs, low-starch vegetables, low-glycemic fruits, avocados, olives, nuts, seeds, fats, red wine, and fresh lipid-rich cheese has been shown to lead to a noticeable decrease in all body measurements, enhancing insulin sensitivity, and reduced levels of both overall and active testosterone in obese women with PCOS.

Synthesis of inflammatory mediators: A 3-month reduction diet, containing five meals a day with lowered glycemic index carbohydrates, lean protein, fish, nuts and seeds, legumes, and fruits and vegetables with low GI, has been shown to facilitate the synthesis of inflammatory mediators in women with PCOS.

Adherence to the Mediterranean diet: Women diagnosed with PCOS have been shown to consume refined olive oil, legumes, fish, nuts, simple carbohydrates, full fat, saturated triglycerides, polyunsaturated fatty acids, and n-6. Adherence to the Mediterranean diet has been directly correlated with women diagnosed with PCOS and exhibiting a distinct physique marked by limited polyhydroxyalkanoates (PHAs) and no fat.

Low-calorie hypocaloric diet: A low-calorie hypocaloric diet, rich in lean meat, whole grains, low-fat dairy, non-starchy vegetables, and vegetable oils, has been shown to lead to similar improvements in physical and nutritional parameters of obese women. Among women having PCOS, menstrual periods, biochemical and medical characteristics showed improvement after the 6-month period.

aMED and DASH diets: The aMED and DASH diets have been shown to improve the appearance of the ovaries; improve insulin sensitivity, blood sugar imbalance, high androgen levels, and obesity; cause satiety and weight loss; reduce intake of red meat and increase protein consumption from fish and dairy; and reduce beverage and sodium intake, increasing glucose regulation, reducing insulin resistance, and improving abdominal adiposity.

Ketonic Mediterranean diet: A ketonic Mediterranean diet with plant extracts has been shown to significantly reduce insulin, cholesterol, triglycerides, androgens, LH, and the LH/FSH fraction, leading to the remission of hormonal abnormalities of PCOS in obese women with PCOS [12].

8.2.5.2 Predictive Insights and Proactive Adjustments

AI models have the prospect to anticipate hormonal imbalances among women having PCOS by analyzing individual trends in hormone levels and other relevant health data. These models can learn from previous patterns in the data and make predictions about future hormonal states.

By incorporating environmental factors, such as lifestyle habits and exposure to certain chemicals, the predictions of the AI models can become even more accurate. This is because these factors play a major role in the development of hormonal imbalances in women with PCOS.

The ability to anticipate hormonal imbalances in women with PCOS can empower both patients and healthcare professionals to make proactive dietary adjustments to prevent flare-ups and maintain hormonal equilibrium. For example, if an AI model predicts that a patient's testosterone levels are likely to increase soon, a healthcare professional could recommend a low-carbohydrate diet, which has been shown to decrease testosterone levels in women with PCOS.

Patients can use this information to make personalized dietary and lifestyle habits. For example, patients could choose to eat more whole foods, such as fruits and vegetables, and engage in consistent exercise, which have been shown to improve hormonal balance among women diagnosed with PCOS [7, 15–17].

8.2.5.3 Case Studies and Real-World Applications

PCOS is an endocrine dysfunction among reproductive-aged females. One of the ways to manage PCOS is through diet and nutrition. However, knowing which foods to eat or avoid can be complicated and time-consuming. This is where AI-powered personalized nutrition comes in.

Case Study 1 (Anonymized)

Background: Maria (anonymous), a 30-year-old woman with PCOS who has been struggling with irregular periods, weight gain, and acne. She is interested in improving her health and reducing her symptoms through diet and lifestyle changes.

Data collection: Maria's healthcare provider collects data on her hormone levels, dietary habits, sleep patterns, physical activity, and stress levels. This information is then used to create a personalized nutrition plan for Maria.

AI-powered analysis: An AI-powered algorithm analyzes Maria's data and identifies specific dietary patterns and nutrients that may be contributing to her PCOS symptoms. The algorithm also considers Maria's individual preferences, lifestyle, and cultural background to create a tailored nutrition plan.

Personalized nutrition plan: Based on the AI-powered analysis, Maria's healthcare provider recommends a diet low in refined carbohydrates and high in fiber, with a focus on whole foods, lean proteins, and healthy fats. The plan also includes specific recommendations for portion sizes, meal timing, and nutrient ratios.

Follow-up and monitoring: Maria's healthcare provider monitors her progress through regular check-ins, hormone-level assessments, and symptom tracking. The AI-powered algorithm continues to analyze Maria's data and adjust her nutrition plan as needed.

Result: After 6 months of following her personalized nutrition plan, Maria experiences significant improvements in her PCOS symptoms. Her menstrual cycles become more regular, her weight decreases, and her acne clears up. Maria's healthcare provider attributes these improvements to the AI-powered personalized nutrition plan, which allowed Maria to make targeted and data-driven changes to her diet and lifestyle.

Case Study 2

Background: Determine the nutrients in women with polycystic ovary syndrome (PCOS), and compare the findings with the existing dietary guidelines for the Polish population.

Methods: The study involved 54 women in their reproductive age having PCOS based on the Rotterdam criteria. The women were assessed using physical measurements, body mass ratio (BMR), and waist-hip circumference ratio (WHR) calculations. The research employed a quantitative evaluation of the participants' dietary habits, utilizing a 3-day food diary and records of food intake from the previous 24 h. This data was entered into DIETA 5.0, a dietary software program, which computed the mean consumption of energy, nutrients, vitamins, minerals, cholesterol, and dietary fiber. These findings were then compared with the dietary recommendations set forth by Polish authorities.

Results: The results showed that the examined group had an average waist circumference of 98.71 ± 13.6 cm and an average WHR of 0.92 ± 0.08. The average BMI was also elevated at 28.91 ± 5.54 kg/m^2. The risk of insufficient protein intake was high in 36.7% of the examined women. The highest risk of deficiency in minerals was related to calcium (634 mg), potassium (3493 mg), and magnesium (250.1 mg). The percentage of women at risk of insufficient vitamin intake was as follows: 70.4% for folic acid, 36.7% for vitamin C, and 26.7% for vitamin B12. The average consumption of vitamin D was at the level of 3.4 μg. The proportion of individuals with an excessive cholesterol intake was at 40.74%. Up to 83.3% of patients had dietary fiber intake below the recommended level (<25 g).

Conclusion: In the dietary regimen of women having PCOS, an increased consumption of folate, vitamin C, vitamin D, B12 supplement, dietary roughage, and calcium should be emphasized. Reducing the intake of fats, saturated lipids, and cholesterol is recommended to lower the risk of diabetes and cardiovascular diseases. Certain patients may benefit from dietary supplementation with potassium, magnesium, and zinc. Emphasizing a well-balanced diet is essential in the management of PCOS according to the Rotterdam criteria [18].

8.3 Critical Considerations for AI in Healthcare

8.3.1 Limitations and Uncertainties

Artificial intelligence (AI) has made great achievements in recent years, with many decision-making tasks now relying on AI technology. However, these systems are not without their limitations and uncertainties. For example, even with advanced camera and sensing technologies, autonomous vehicles can struggle to accurately identify unfamiliar objects or animals and adapt to challenging environmental conditions like heavy rain, flooding, or mud puddles. This can make it difficult to ensure that AI-enabled decision-making applications can keep up with a changing world and maintain their performance over time.

Another challenge is the complexity of AI models, which can make it challenging to understand the explanation behind the decisions. This lack of transparency can result in distrust and limit the adoption of AI technologies in certain domains. Additionally, the training data can contain biases that may negatively impact the fairness and accuracy of AI-enabled decision-making applications. These biases can come from a variety of sources, such as historical data that may not accurately represent current or future scenarios or from the way data is collected, processed, or analyzed.

AI-enabled decision-making applications can also face ethical dilemmas that are difficult to address. For example, autonomous vehicles may need to prioritize passenger safety over pedestrian safety in certain situations, which raises moral and ethical concerns. To ensure the long-term success of AI-enabled decision-making applications, it is important to address these limitations and uncertainties by improving the transparency, fairness, and robustness of AI systems, as well as ensuring that they can adapt to a wide range of situations and contexts. This will establish trust in AI technologies and their ethical and responsible use [19–22].

8.3.2 Human Expertise and Collaboration

Even though the idea of AI replacing doctors is compelling, it is not developed to substitute doctors. Rather, AI can redefine roles and enhance effectiveness, as evidenced by LLM-driven digital assistants and conversation summarizers. AI has integrated into healthcare services without displacing physicians. AI-assisted systems, such as those with ultrasound or MRI machines, contribute to the process of diagnosis, while the advancement of voice recognition technology in dictation devices improves the efficiency of radiology note-taking.

Latest advancements in AI, such as large language models (LLMs) and generative AI, have shown highly intricate, evolving at a rapid speed, and possessing extensive capabilities, leading us to question their value and application. For instance, a healthcare LLM can be trained on a dataset of PCOS-related medical records, clinical trials, and treatment outcomes to generate a personalized medical plan for a patient according to their medical history, symptoms, and other relevant factors. This can enable healthcare professionals to make better decisions and enhance patient outcomes. These developments can lead to more efficient and organized healthcare system by repurposing (not replacing) the roles of medical professionals. This collaboration between AI and doctors can lead to enhanced diagnostic accuracy, better care coordination, and enhanced patient benefits.

In the healthcare sector, human-in-the-loop (HITL) systems could be used where trained medical professionals collaborate with AI. They manage, validate, and offer guidance throughout the procedure, interpret AI-generated outputs, and offer suggestions to enhance the AI's capability and effectiveness. Recent research indicates that AI, when merged with expert human assessment, can improve the accuracy of diagnoses and clinical decisions, highlighting the cooperative relationship between AI and medical professionals. This partnership could address differences, especially in resource-limited settings like rural areas or developing countries, by enhancing assessment, clinical communication, and education and mitigating language constraints.

To make sure that AI implementations are successful, it's vital to have thorough evaluation approaches and assessment systems that focus on validating, verifying, evaluating the usefulness, and promoting the adoption of AI. This involves revising organizational policies and protocols to make it easier to adopt AI while also addressing moral and lawful considerations such as assuring compliance, confidentiality, and security [20].

8.3.3 Data Privacy and Security

Advances in artificial intelligence (AI) are revolutionizing healthcare, with AI technologies being increasingly integrated into healthcare systems for various applications, such as assessing diagnostic images, radiation cancer treatment and therapy, organ distribution, and robot-assisted surgery. The rapid progress in this field, however, raises ethical concerns surrounding data collection, storage, and ownership, particularly in the context of commercial healthcare AI.

Ethical concerns: AI has some unique features, such as being susceptible to specific kinds of mistakes and biases and having the "black box" problem. This signifies that the methods and decision-making employed by learning algorithms to arrive at conclusions can be difficult for people to understand. This same lack of transparency also applies to the usage of health and personal information, which highlights the importance of implementing appropriate safeguards to protect privacy and ensure individuals maintain control over their own information. Biased data incorporated into AI algorithms can lead to discriminatory healthcare decisions, perpetuating discrepancies in healthcare outcomes among diverse demographic segments. Healthcare practitioners and patients must understand AI systems' decision-making processes. Encouraging transparency and holding users responsible for their decisions are important for establishing trust in AI systems.

Regulatory measures: Regulations should mandate that personal health information remains in the realm from which it is collected, with limited exceptions, to ensure robust privacy protection. Necessary precautions should be established to maintain privacy, particularly in public-private collaborations, given the challenge posed by AI algorithms requiring access to extensive patient data and the potential risks of privacy breaches from complex algorithmic systems. With concerns about the potential misuse of patient health information by corporations, there is a growing demand for increased regulatory control of big data health research and technology. Public confidence in commercial healthcare AI is limited, with just 11% of American adults willing to disclose health data to tech firms. Hospitals should refrain from sharing the patient health information that isn't fully anonymized with companies, and detailed contracts should be prepared to clarify the rights and responsibilities of all parties involved, considering the legal risks that private AI developers and operators may face when handling large volumes of patient data.

8.3.4 Regulatory Landscape and the Future

Artificial intelligence (AI) holds the promise of transforming healthcare by enhancing diagnosis, treatment, and patient results. However, implementing AI-powered interventions in clinical practice faces several challenges due to the complex regulatory landscape and ethical considerations [23, 24].

8.3.4.1 Current Regulatory Landscape

The regulatory landscape surrounding AI in healthcare is complex and constantly changing. In the USA, the Food and Drug Administration (FDA) manages the regulation of AI-driven medical devices. The FDA has released a discussion paper on AI and machine learning (ML) in medical devices, outlining the agency's approach to regulating these technologies. The European Union has also released guidelines on AI, including a proposal for a regulatory framework for AI.

For example, an AI model that is used to forecast the risk of developing PCOS derived from patient symptoms and medical history would likely be classified as a low-risk device. This means that it would be subject to less stringent regulation compared to a high-risk device, such as an AI model used for automated insulin delivery in patients with diabetes.

However, even low-risk devices would still need to meet certain regulatory requirements, such as obtaining clearance or approval from the FDA, before being marketed in the USA. The FDA has proposed a pre-certification program for AI-powered medical devices, which would allow developers to demonstrate their ability to develop and maintain safe and effective devices. This program is designed to reduce the regulatory burden for low-risk devices while still ensuring patient safety [6, 25].

8.3.4.2 Challenges in Implementing AI-Powered Interventions

In spite of the potential advantages of AI in healthcare, numerous issues must be addressed to ensure safe and effective implementation. AI technologies have become increasingly vital in the world of healthcare, yet they come with their own unique set of issues. A primary issue is the protection and security of patient data, as AI models need extensive data to function. Healthcare institutions need to give importance to safeguarding data privacy and security to guarantee the confidentiality of patient information. Another challenge is the perpetuation of biases in healthcare by AI algorithms, which can occur if they are trained using biased data. It is crucial to prioritize fairness and eliminate biases in AI algorithms to promote equitable healthcare.

Transparency and explainability are also critical factors to consider when implementing AI technologies in healthcare. AI algorithms can be complex and challenging to understand, making it imperative to assure they are transparent and explainable to build trust with healthcare providers and patients. Lastly, regulatory compliance is a crucial aspect to consider, as AI-powered medical devices must adhere to regulatory requirements, including those related to safety, efficacy, and data privacy. Ensuring compliance can be challenging due to the constantly evolving nature of AI technology. By addressing these challenges, healthcare organizations can effectively utilize AI to enhance patient care while also preserving privacy, fairness, and regulatory compliance [25].

8.4 The Future of PCOS Care with AI

The rapid advancement of AI and data science technologies, such as deep learning, has opened new possibilities for healthcare applications. Deep learning has demonstrated potential results in various medical tasks, including image analysis, natural language processing, and drug discovery. In precision medicine, AI can facilitate and enhance personalized care by customizing healthcare interventions for individuals or groups according to their health condition, diagnostic information, or therapeutic effect. Important areas for AI in personalized medicine include intricate algorithms, connected health applications, and omics examinations.

In pharmacological discovery and development, AI can streamline the process by efficiently classifying potential drug compounds and predicting their properties and activity. AI models can also aid in the design of new drug molecules, drug-target interactions, and drug response prediction.

In the interpretation of medical images and videos, AI can provide diagnostic and surgical support. Deep learning methods, such as convolutional neural networks, have shown promising results in medical image recognition tasks.

Patients can also benefit from AI through personalized recommendations and remote monitoring. Wearable health devices and telehealth applications can generate large volumes of data that can be used to enhance patient outcomes and inform clinical decision-making. By utilizing the power of AI, healthcare organizations can provide more personalized and effective care to patients while also improving efficiency and accuracy [6].

8.4.1 Personalized, Proactive, and Data-Driven

AI-powered personalized nutrition plays an important role in guiding individualized treatment plans, anticipating potential issues, and empowering patients actively involve in supervising their health. By assessing a patient's medical history, genetic composition, and behavioral lifestyle, AI can create customized nutrition plans to help manage weight, balance hormones, and improve insulin sensitivity.

Moreover, AI can predict issues such as insulin resistance before they become problematic, allowing for proactive treatment and prevention of complications like diabetes and cardiovascular disease. Additionally, AI-powered tools can empower patients by providing real-time data and insights, increasing their awareness of the impact of lifestyle choices on their PCOS symptoms, and motivating them to make positive changes.

Some examples of AI-powered nutrition apps that can offer nutritional advice and guidance include MyFitnessPal, Lose It!, SnapCalorie, and RxFood. These apps use AI technology like image recognition and conversational platforms to offer accessible diet information and advice for individuals who may not have access to a dietitian. By integrating AI through photo recognition and conversational interfaces, these apps can offer personalized nutrition recommendations and feedback based on users' dietary habits, aims, and nutrition-related questions.

AI assesses a patient's medical record, lifestyle, and dietary preferences to provide tailored nutrition recommendations. This individualized approach can help address specific nutritional needs and improve overall health outcomes. By proactively addressing potential issues identified through large datasets and patterns, AI can help avoid the development of more severe health problems related to PCOS. Patients can improve adherence to treatment plans and make informed decisions about their health with the help of AI-powered nutrition guides. Integrated into electronic health records, AI can provide healthcare providers with access to the latest information to ensure effective patient care. As a cost-effective solution, AI-driven nutrition guides can help reduce the burden of PCOS on patients and the healthcare system by improving adherence to treatment plans and preventing the development of more severe health problems [26].

8.4.2 Integration with Existing Interventions

AI-powered dietary recommendations can be seamlessly integrated with other therapeutic strategies for PCOS, including lifestyle modifications, exercise programs, and complementary therapies. The following discussion explores the potential for such integration:

Lifestyle modifications: Lifestyle modifications, such as dietary modifications, increased exercise, and behavioral treatments, are important in PCOS management. AI-powered dietary recommendations can complement these modifications by providing personalized and evidence-based guidance to women with PCOS.

Exercise programs: Exercise is a crucial component of PCOS management, as it helps improve insulin sensitivity, weight management, and overall health. AI-powered recommendations can be integrated with exercise programs to optimize the benefits of both interventions. For instance, AI can help create personalized exercise plans based on users' individual needs, preferences, and progress. This can include suggestions for various types of exercises, intensity levels, and durations, as well as real-time feedback during workouts to ensure proper form and intensity.

Complementary therapies: Complementary therapies, such as acupuncture, yoga, and mindfulness meditation, can help alleviate PCOS symptoms and improve overall well-being. AI-powered recommendations can be integrated with these therapies to enhance their effectiveness. For example, AI can help identify the most appropriate complementary therapies based on users' specific PCOS symptoms, health history, and lifestyle factors. Additionally, AI can provide personalized guidance on how to incorporate these therapies into daily routines and monitor users' progress to ensure they are receiving the maximum benefits.

Behavioral interventions: Behavioral interventions, such as cognitive behavioral therapy (CBT) and mindfulness meditation, can also be integrated with AI-powered dietary recommendations to enhance involvement and adoption to healthy lifestyle changes. CBT has been shown to improve the standard of living and reduce psychological exhaustion in women with PCOS, while mindfulness meditation can reduce perceived stress, depressive symptoms, and fasting blood glucose [27, 28].

8.4.3 Building a Collaborative Ecosystem

Collaborative ecosystems are essential for creating a robust and accessible ecosystem for personalized AI-powered healthcare. By bringing together healthcare professionals, researchers, data scientists, and technology developers, we can collectively create value propositions that are greater than what can be achieved individually. This collaboration can help address the unique challenges of PCOS and improve patient outcomes.

There are three main components to establishing a collaborative data environment for personalized AI-powered healthcare in PCOS: the business ecosystem, the data ecosystem, and the collaborative data ecosystem.

Business ecosystems: A commercial arrangement among two or more companies to collectively create value propositions for personalized AI-powered healthcare in PCOS. Participants in this ecosystem, whether orchestrators or participants, have their brands present in the value propositions.

Data ecosystems: A partnership between multiple organizations to share and manage data related to PCOS, with the goal of creating value and innovation. A fundamental challenge in these data ecosystems is the existence of data silos, where data is locked in different departments, business units, or technologies under different data sovereignty and ownership.

Collaborative data ecosystems: A collaborative data ecosystem for personalized AI-powered healthcare in PCOS would require a new approach to collaboration that goes beyond the scope of internal projects. This collaboration would enable co-creation and innovation, analysis, and drawing insights from data to derive value from it.

When establishing a collaborative data environment for personalized AI-powered healthcare in PCOS, it is necessary to consider the effect of the ecosystem on the rest of the industry innovatively, the interoperability and scalability of the ecosystem, and its ability to actively address privacy, security, sovereignty and protect the IP of all parties [29–31].

8.5 Conclusion

Polycystic ovary syndrome (PCOS) is a prevalent disorder affecting reproductive-age women across the globe, distinguished by hormonal imbalances, irregular menstrual cycles, and small cysts in the ovaries. Its diverse clinical presentation and significant burden on individual and healthcare system levels necessitate effective management strategies. Conventional management approaches, both pharmacological and non-pharmacological, have limitations in addressing the root causes and achieving personalized care. The advancement of AI in healthcare offers potential solutions for personalized medicine and precision therapeutics, including the optimization of hormonal balance through dietary interventions in

PCOS management. AI-powered tools can analyze individual data, generate comprehensive metabolic and hormonal profiles, and provide personalized dietary recommendations, addressing the unique needs of PCOS patients. Building a collaborative ecosystem among healthcare professionals, researchers, data scientists, and technology developers is essential for creating a robust and accessible AI-powered healthcare ecosystem in PCOS.

References

1. Shrestha A, Dixit A, Zaidi A. Assessment of lifestyle and diet modification of patients suffering from polycystic ovarian disease (PCOS) in North India. J Food Nutr Sci. 2019;7(4):60. https://doi.org/10.11648/j.jfns.20190704.12.
2. Begum M, Areen S. Optimizing polycystic ovarian disorder (PCOS) treatment with personalized lifestyle and nutrition strategies. J Clin Med Res. 2023:1–8. https://doi.org/10.46889/jcmr.2023.4306.
3. Szczuko M, et al. Nutrition strategy and lifestyle in polycystic ovary syndrome—narrative review. Nutrients. 2021;13(7):2452. https://doi.org/10.3390/nu13072452.
4. Faghfoori Z, Fazelian S, Shadnoush M, Goodarzi R. Nutritional management in women with polycystic ovary syndrome: a review study. Diabetes Metab Syndr Clin Res Rev. 2017;11:S429–32. https://doi.org/10.1016/j.dsx.2017.03.030.
5. Rashid R, et al. Polycystic ovarian syndrome-current pharmacotherapy and clinical implications. Taiwan J Obstet Gynecol. 2022;61(1):40–50. https://doi.org/10.1016/j.tjog.2021.11.009.
6. Bohr A, Memarzadeh K. The rise of artificial intelligence in healthcare applications. Artif Intell Healthc. 2020:25–60. https://doi.org/10.1016/b978-0-12-818438-7.00002-2.
7. Elmannai H, El-Rashidy N, Mashal I, Alohali MA, Farag S, El-Sappagh S, Saleh H. Polycystic ovary syndrome detection machine learning model based on optimized feature selection and explainable artificial intelligence. Diagnostics. 2023;13(8):1506. https://doi.org/10.3390/diagnostics13081506.
8. Aggarwal S, Pandey K. Early identification of PCOS with commonly known diseases: obesity, diabetes, high blood pressure and heart disease using machine learning techniques. Expert Syst Appl. 2023;217:119532. https://doi.org/10.1016/j.eswa.2023.119532.
9. Alamoudi A, Khan IU, Aslam N, Alqahtani N, Alsaif HS, Al Dandan O, et al. A deep learning fusion approach to diagnosis the polycystic ovary syndrome (PCOS). Appl Comput Intell Soft Comput. 2023(1):9686697. https://doi.org/10.1155/2023/9686697.
10. Sarker IH. Machine learning: algorithms, real-world applications and research directions. SN Comput Sci. 2021;2(3):160. https://doi.org/10.1007/s42979-021-00592-x.
11. Azzaro MG. PCOS meal plan: what to eat to help with symptoms and support overall health. EatingWell, 14 Jan 2024. https://www.eatingwell.com/article/7920027/pcos-meal-plan/.
12. Xenou M, Gourounti K. Dietary patterns and polycystic ovary syndrome: a systematic review. Maedica. 2021;16(3):516. https://doi.org/10.26574/maedica.2020.16.3.516.
13. Lofton T, KFF Health News. How ChatGPT can help you meal plan, even with dietary restrictions. Washington Post, 2 May 2023. https://www.washingtonpost.com/wellness/2023/05/02/chatgpt-ai-meal-planning-diet/.
14. Calcaterra V, Verduci E, Cena H, Magenes VC, Todisco CF, Tenuta E, et al. Polycystic ovary syndrome in insulin-resistant adolescents with obesity: the role of nutrition therapy and food supplements as a strategy to protect fertility. Nutrients. 2021;13(6):1848. https://doi.org/10.3390/nu13061848.
15. AI, machine learning can help diagnose polycystic ovary syndrome. National Institute of Environmental Health Sciences. https://factor.niehs.nih.gov/2023/11/papers/AI-diagnose-polycystic-ovary-syndrome.

16. AI and machine learning can successfully diagnose polycystic ovary syndrome. ScienceDaily, 23 Sept 2023. https://www.sciencedaily.com/releases/2023/09/230918153140.htm.
17. Barrera FJ, Brown ED, Rojo A, Obeso J, Plata H, Lincango EP, et al. Application of machine learning and artificial intelligence in the diagnosis and classification of polycystic ovarian syndrome: a systematic review. Front Endocrinol. 2023;14:1106625. https://doi.org/10.3389/fendo.2023.1106625.
18. Szczuko M, Skowronek M, Zapałowska-Chwyć M, Starczewski A. Quantitative assessment of nutrition in patients with polycystic ovary syndrome (PCOS). Rocz Panstw Zakl Hig. 2016;67(4):419–26. https://pubmed.ncbi.nlm.nih.gov/27925712.
19. Ueda D, Kakinuma T, Fujita S, Kamagata K, Fushimi Y, Ito R, et al. Fairness of artificial intelligence in healthcare: review and recommendations. Jpn J Radiol. 2023;42(1):3–15. https://doi.org/10.1007/s11604-023-01474-3.
20. Sezgın E. Artificial intelligence in healthcare: complementing, not replacing, doctors and healthcare providers. Digital Health. 2023;9 https://doi.org/10.1177/20552076231186520.
21. Wu J, Shang SSC. Managing uncertainty in AI-enabled decision making and achieving sustainability. Sustainability. 2020;12(21):8758. https://doi.org/10.3390/su12218758.
22. Davenport TH, Kalakota R. The potential for artificial intelligence in healthcare. Future Healthc J. 2019;6(2):94–8. https://doi.org/10.7861/futurehosp.6-2-94.
23. Murdoch B. Privacy and artificial intelligence: challenges for protecting health information in a new era. BMC Med Ethics. 2021;22(1):122. https://doi.org/10.1186/s12910-021-00687-3.
24. Renfro M. The ethics of AI in healthcare. HITRUST Alliance, 21 Nov 2023. https://hitrustalliance.net/the-ethics-of-ai-in-healthcare/.
25. Alowais SA, Alghamdi SS, Alsuhebany N, Alqahtani T, Alshaya AI, Almohareb SN, et al. Revolutionizing healthcare: the role of artificial intelligence in clinical practice. BMC Med Educ. 2023;23(1):689. https://doi.org/10.1186/s12909-023-04698-z.
26. Krishanga. Turning data into diagnosis: AI and ML to transform PCOS detection. Medindia, 23 Sept 2023. https://www.medindia.net/news/healthwatch/turning-data-into-diagnosis-ai-and-ml-to-transform-pcos-detection-213570-1.htm.
27. Lee H, Lee SH. Effectiveness of an integrated mobile application for lifestyle modifications in overweight women with polycystic ovarian syndrome: a randomized controlled trial. Life. 2023;13(7):1533. https://doi.org/10.3390/life13071533.
28. Cowan S, Lim S, Alycia C, Pirotta S, Thomson R, Gibson-Helm M, et al. Lifestyle management in polycystic ovary syndrome—beyond diet and physical activity. BMC Endocr Disord. 2023;23(1):14. https://doi.org/10.1186/s12902-022-01208-y.
29. Stafie CS, Sufaru IG, Ghiciuc CM, Stafie II, Sufaru EC, Solomon SM, Hancianu M. Exploring the intersection of artificial intelligence and clinical healthcare: a multidisciplinary review. Diagnostics. 2023;13(12):1995. https://doi.org/10.3390/diagnostics13121995.
30. Healthcare ecosystem drives collaboration and accelerates digital. Healthcare IT News, 16 Aug 2021. https://www.healthcareitnews.com/news/emea/healthcare-ecosystem-drives-collaboration-and-accelerates-digital-transformation.
31. Hwesterman. Building a collaborative ecosystem for AI in healthcare in low- and middle-income economies. Atlantic Council, 7 Sept 2020. https://www.atlanticcouncil.org/content-series/smart-partnerships/building-a-collaborative-ecosystem-for-ai-in-healthcare-in-low-and-middle-income-economies/.

Micronutrient Optimization: An In-Depth Look at Vitamins and Minerals Critical for PCOS Management and AI's Role in Ensuring Adequate Intake

9

Shaik Khaja Mohiddin, Shaik Sharmila, and Anand Nayyar

9.1 Introduction

It is a common endocrine disease affecting 6–12% of women worldwide in the reproductive age. PCOS can manifest in a variety of symptoms, including irregular menstruation periods, polycystic ovaries, and high testosterone levels. This disease's pathophysiology is likely due to a complex interplay of genetic, hormonal, and environmental issues, affecting its presentation. In addition to the reproductive complications mentioned ahead, PCOS is associated with several comorbidities, including obesity, type 2 diabetes, insulin resistance, and cardiovascular morbidity. Consequently, the holistic approach to the management and treatment of PCOS has been of utmost importance. This disease is prevalent, has a severe negative impact on women's health and quality of life, and is also associated with general morbidity. Hence, research and education concerning PCOS must always be a priority. Patients must understand how and why PCOS manifests and affects women's health, as should all professionals involved in educating about the importance of lifestyle choices in PCOS therapy.

Affecting 5–10% of women of childbearing age with estimates that 10% of US women have taken the medication "off-label," polycystic ovary syndrome is the

S. K. Mohiddin (✉)
Department of CSE, Koneru Lakshmaiah Education Foundation,
Vaddeswaram, Andhra Pradesh, India
e-mail: mail2mohiddin@kluniversity.in

S. Sharmila
Department of IT, Vignan Nirula Institute of Technology and Science for Women,
Guntur, Andhra Pradesh, India

A. Nayyar
School of Computer Science, Duy Tan University, Da Nang, Vietnam
e-mail: anandnayyar@duytan.edu.vn

R. Kumar et al. (eds.), *AI-Based Nutritional Intervention in Polycystic Ovary Syndrome (PCOS)*, https://doi.org/10.1007/978-981-96-2120-0_9

most common endocrinopathy. Various diagnostic criteria have been formulated, the majority of which are based on the triad polycystic ovarian morphology, oligo-ovulation, and hyperandrogenism or hyperandrogenemia. Most instances have insulin resistance, and compensatory hyperinsulinemia promotes hyperandrogenism by overstimulation of ovarian androgen secretion and selective inhibition of the synthesis of the circulating sex hormone-binding globulins in the liver. Insulin resistance in PCOS has been considered to be primarily linked to adipose malfunction. PCOS is the product of the joint contributions of environmental and genetic factors. Many morbidities are related to this disorder, including mood and eating disorders, type 2 diabetes mellitus, obstetrical difficulties, infertility, and coronary heart disease. Despite the disease burden, it may be more prevalent in modern society due to the several evolutionary rewards of the syndrome, such as smaller family sizes, a reduction in mortality associated with birth, increased muscle mass, and more extensive energy storage. PCOS cannot be treated successfully without identifying its essential features and adequately ruling out other causes of hyperandrogenism/oligo-ovulatory disorders. The principal treatment goals are to combat the hyperandrogenic signs, promote ovulation, and prevent cardiometabolic system-related effects.

PCOS manifests itself clinically in a variety of ways. Menstrual irregularities, clinical signs of hyperandrogenism, and infertility are common reasons why women with PCOS seek medical attention. Oligomenorrhea, amenorrhea, and protracted irregular monthly flow are among the menstrual abnormalities frequently linked to PCOS. Two nonetheless, regular menstruation is experienced by 30% of women with PCOS. About 30–40% of women with amenorrhea and 85–90% of women with oligomenorrhea will develop PCOS. More than 80% of women who have androgen excess symptoms also have PCOS. In as many as 70% of women with PCOS, hirsutism is a prevalent clinical manifestation of hyperandrogenism. An adapted Ferriman-Gallwey scoring system is used to assess hirsutism. Seven sites, namely, the upper lip, chin/face, chest, back, abdomen, arms, and thighs, are assessed for hair development using this instrument. When terminal hair development is absent, a score of 0 is assigned, and when substantial growth is present, a score of 4. A total score of 8 or higher indicates hirsutism. Through ultrasonography, polycystic ovaries are seen in over 90% of women with hirsutism who are typically menstruating. Not only that, but 50% of women with less severe undesired hair growth has PCOS. Hyperandrogenism can also be indicated by acne; however, it is less common in PCOS and less specific than hirsutism. Between 15% and 30% of adult PCOS-afflicted women have acne at first. The variation in 5α-reductase expression between the hair follicle and the sebaceous gland, and the consequent increase in dihydrotestosterone in the hair follicle, may be the cause of the disparity in the prevalence of hirsutism and acne. Of the women who presented with severe acne, more than 40% had PCOS as their diagnosis. According to some specialists, women who arrive with acne should be questioned about their menstrual history and checked for additional hyperandrogenism symptoms. Of women with PCOS, 40% experience infertility. Anovulatory infertility is most frequently caused by PCOS. Ninety to ninety-five percent of anovulatory women who visit infertility clinics have PCOS. Primordial and secondary follicle counts are noticeably higher in PCOS-affected women, although primordial follicle counts are normal. But once follicles get to a diameter of 4–8 mm, expansion of the follicles is stopped due to disruptions in components essential in normal follicular development. Ovulation does not occur because of the absence of a dominant follicle. Furthermore, spontaneous abortion rates are higher in PCOS, ranging from 42% to 73%.

One of the most usual endocrine illnesses among women is polycystic ovary syndrome. This condition is characterized by a combination of irregular ovulation or anovulation, high androgen levels, and polycystic ovaries. Ovulatory dysfunction is the major responsible factor and presents as anovulatory menses, irregular ovulatory menses, and ovulatory dysfunction without obvious menses. Hyperandrogenism can be manifested either by individual symptoms of clinical hyperandrogenism and biochemical proof of hyperandrogenemia or by biochemical evidence only. The last condition is termed "core cut syndrome."

PCO can be diagnosed solely based on the ultrasound image it creates. Polycystic ovarian morphology is determined by ovarian ultrasound. The PCO term defines the existence of more than the usual number of preantral follicles in one or both ovaries. Finally, PCOS has a wide range of clinical manifestations and can be broken down into many phenotypes based on the presence or absence of three specific criteria. Polycystic ovary syndrome is a diagnosis of elimination and is primarily identified by an excess of androgens, ovulatory function toxicity, accompanied by polycystic ovaries. PCOS is associated with numerous metabolic abnormalities such as obesity, insulin insensitivity, poor glucose metabolism, and the possibility of type 2 DM. Dyslipidemia is also abundant, a sickness characterized by elevated low-density lipoprotein and triglyceride levels and low high-density lipoprotein levels. In addition to the women's PCOS group [1], there is a large portion of cardiovascular and metabolic diseases. Thus, recent studies have discovered that women with PCOS are far more likely to produce CVD in the future and that PCOS has recently been linked to psychological health, with a higher probability of experiencing depression and anxiety symptoms and poor self-confidence.

Familial clustering and the results of twin studies showed that PCOS might have a genetic basis. For example, if the person has the mother or sister with PCOS, this individual has 50% of the possibility to have PCOS. The correlation of PCOS was twice as high between monozygotic twin sisters compared to the dizygotic twins. Several genetic models suggested that approximately 70% of the variance might be attributed to the hereditary causes. Furthermore, robust evidence indicated that metabolic syndrome, hypertension, and dyslipidemia clustered in the immediate family members, both mothers, fathers, sisters, and brothers of PCOS probands. This could suggest that the genetic architecture of PCOS is polygenic one, presenting a complex genetic inheritance pattern. Even though PCOS is a phenotypically and clinically relevant, highly heritable disorder, its exact molecular cause remains poorly understood. Two common approaches are utilized to delineate genes or genetic variants underlying complex genetic disorders, such as PCOS: candidate gene approach and genome-wide association study (GWAS).

Candidate gene studies are credited when it comes to confirming and explaining the functional effects of gene loci identified by a GWAS to comprehend their clinical relevance. Several candidate gene investigations have been performed in PCOS, and they have identified a substantial number of SNPs that could contribute to the genetic basis of PCOS. These studies represent a fruitful approach to identifying genetic variations that are either causative of a disorder or members of a set of genes that cause the disorder. Nonetheless, candidate gene studies frequently confront a few common limitations. They include a small sample size, which might limit statistical power, as well as the existence of confounding variables that may result in contradictory results. These variables include ancestry, diagnostic criteria, body mass index, source, and participant ethnicity. The possible reasons for contradictory results may be attributed to the most studies' limitations. Most previous research was limited in that only one or two genotyped SNPs in the gene of interest had been examined, rather than covering the whole gene. On the other hand, GWAS studies, which are hypothesis-free, are sometimes mistakenly assumed to have identified the specific causative genes. Instead, they simply provide information on a particular genomic region that demonstrates significant association with the trait under study. The identified gene loci may have a direct impact on the gene function if they are located within or near a gene. Alternatively, they may regulate the activity of a gene located either up or down in the genome.

Organization of Chapter

The rest of the chapter is organized as follows: Section 9.2 illustrates the concept of PCOS. Section 9.3 focuses on role of micronutrients in PCOS. Section 9.4 highlights PCOS symptoms and effects. Section 9.5 enlightens challenges in nutritional management of PCOS. Section 9.6 discusses personalizing PCOS care with AI followed by concept embarking on integrating AI with micronutrient optimization in Sect. 9.7. Section 9.8 focuses on implications for healthcare providers. And, finally, Sect. 9.9 concludes the chapter.

9.2 Understanding PCOS

Polycystic ovary syndrome is a condition that occurs when a person has signs related to high androgen levels [2]. Androgens are typically thought of male sex hormones. Nevertheless, when generated in smaller amounts, they do a fundamental role in guaranteeing the female reproductive system's efficiency. Most patients with PCOS are women in their reproductive years exhibiting symptoms such as weight gain, a lack of regular menses, increased body hair, hair loss or balding around the top of the head, acne or shiny skin, and sometimes inability to conceive. An insufficiency of certain hormones might impair ovarian follicle development, resulting in irregular ovulation [3]. The incidence of polycystic ovary syndrome among Indian women ranges from 8.2% to 22.5%, varying based on geography, life circumstances, diet, and perhaps other factors [4]. This endocrinopathy significantly influences the patients' lifestyle and can result in clinical depression, anxiety, eating disorders, and obstructive apnea during sleep. Furthermore, metabolic syndromes are prone to cardiovascular diseases, female endometrial cancer, and type 2 diabetes

[5, 6]. The specific etiology of PCOS has not yet been discovered. Certain investigations demonstrate that cells acquire resistance to insulin in the blood, causing blood sugar to rise. It is also important to note that a neck and armpits skin brownish glove, or insulin resistance, is not related to clinical diabetes but that limited exercise and poor diet are major reasons for developing PCOS in women [7].

In clinical scenarios, ultrasound is the most applied imaging technology for diagnosing ovarian disorders. It exhibits numerous benefits compared to other medical imaging technologies like computed tomography and MRI. The justification for using ultrasonography in this examination is that it is a cheaper and more accessible method that provides immediate actual results while being safer. This imaging technology also offers a significant possibility to develop a deep learning model for automatic analysis. It enables improved objectivity and diagnostic precision in this investigation. Deep learning is a powerful solution employed in image analysis and computer vision. The use of clinical data and ultrasound pictures enables the classification of PCOS stages in this study as it helps detect the disease. Polycystic ovary syndrome the varied criteria and symptoms make it necessary to test blood, ultrasound study and accurately record the dates of the menstrual cycle. Hence, the variety of symptoms of the disease and the lack of the only indicator or the only diagnostic method according to doctors lead to the need to ask for several test results and unnecessary radiological research. Therefore, the diagnosis approach of the PCOS is "by removing" the unnecessary symptoms and based on the scarce areas of the path mechanism of PCOS. On the other hand, it is necessary to diagnose the disease quickly and effectively, as this disease immediately leads to ovarian disfunction. This results in an immediate risk of infertility and the subsequent risk of gynecological diseases and emotional discomfort to patient due to the loss of human and financial resources. As such, relevant imagery is used to evaluate ovary morphology using ultrasound picture and image processing. Currently, the polycystic ovary morphology is diagnosed on ultrasound images by manual analysis. The current method of diagnosing this image-based investigation relies on the specialist, who has a lot of experience and knows the answers due to the photo of the same instance. Sometimes, the differential diagnosis can be subjective between two professionals. Furthermore, the good diagnostic correctness of ultrasound is found in expert professionals than nonexperts' physicians. Nonetheless, there are inadequate numbers of professional examiners, especially in poor regions, to perform these analyses. In addition, the professional radiologist manually counts follicle quantities depending on their size in the ovary image. This is a difficult and complex operation for the radiologist due to the variant size of the follicles and their linkage with vessels and tissues. Furthermore, this results in artifacts and echo noise in the image. The uncertainty of the diagnosis leads to long-term fertility and hormonal consequences of women. Additionally, this computational picture diagnostic system is a prospective option for errors in the diagnosis, leading to discomfort to the patient. Hence, the computer-aided system for the decision of the gynecologist is to be recommended.

Polycystic ovary syndrome affects nearly 10% of women of childbearing age. It is a multifaceted endocrine disease characterized by polycystic ovaries, menstrual irregularity, and elevated testosterone levels. Nutrition is an important way to impact hormonal imbalances and improve the quality of life, thereby being vital for improving diet inadequacies. Specifically, micronutrient deficiencies can be addressed through diet modifications. Due to the absence of known etiologies, present medicine lacks other non-pharmacological assistance opportunities in contemplation of patient outcomes [8]. Polycystic ovary syndrome is a hormonal problem that affects several women of childbearing age. Although the root reason is still unknown, genetics, insulin resistance, and persistent inflammation play a vital role [9]. Diabetes, cardiovascular disease, and metabolic syndrome are among the health conditions that PCOS exacerbates. For these risks to be reduced and life quality to be enhanced, early diagnosis and efficient management are essential [10].

Micronutrients are essential for good health because they boost immune system and metabolism, two processes that are particularly important for people with PCOS [11]. Because PCOS affects the hormone and metabolic systems, women may need certain micronutrients. For instance, magnesium may help insulin sensitivity and metabolic profiles [12], inositol can enhance ovarian function and insulin sensitivity [13], vitamin D is connected to menstrual regularity, and insulin resistance and omega-3 fatty acids can lower cardiovascular risks [14]. It is recommended that individuals get these nutrients in a proper diet; however, to successfully address specific health needs, supplementing should be explored under medical advice.

IR, oxidative stress [15], a sedentary lifestyle, and eating behavior can undoubtedly exacerbate insulin resistance and blood insulin levels, causing obesity and severe PCOS symptoms [16]. The role of several micronutrients in IR and IR alleviation has been discussed in previous studies [17]. Selenium is an essential mineral with antioxidant properties, as it prevents free radicals, playing a crucial role in the pathways that activate reactive oxygen species (ROS) signals [18]. Selenium and other antioxidants are inversely related to women's serum CRP as they have anti-inflammatory properties. A high intake of Se can decrease oxidative stress and inflammation-induced diseases by altering lipid metabolism [19]. Patients with PCOS registered low serum Se levels. It has been observed that prescribing selenium supplements improves parameters associated with insulin metabolism, as well as TG and VLDL levels [20]. Consumption of the marker of inflammation, salicylic acid, has been negatively correlated with MetS as well as dietary selenium intake across studies [21]. In Zagrodzki et al.'s [22] work, however, no differences were found in Se serum levels between PCOS patients and healthy people. Moreover, Mohammed Hosseinzadeh et al. [23] showed no positive effect of Se supplementation in PCOS patients and even suggested that Se might deteriorate the IR condition in these patients. It is interesting to note that Obeid et al. [24] on the other hand, reported a direct correlation between Se in the blood and MetS components sic.

Another crucial group of micronutrients that could reduce OS impact is carotenoids. According to Sy et al. [25], carotenoids could enhance IR. Another micronutrient that could increase the effect of insulin is chromium. Thus, it is vital for the metabolism of fats and carbohydrates. Cr supplements are thought to improve type 2 diabetic patients' MetS parameters and insulin susceptibility. All the effects of Cr supplementation might include the OS status of PCOS patients, decreased CVD risk, and glycemic index. Zinc is a cofactor of antioxidant enzymes and among the essential components of the enzyme superoxide dismutase. Thus, the crucial component has been identified to contribute significantly to the reduction of markers of inflammation and IR. The genes associated with vitamin D regulation influence BP homeostasis, lipid and glucose metabolism, and vitamin D level regulation. Vitamin D might halt OS and inflammation by preventing DNA destruction at the cellular level. Therefore, vitamin D in PCOS women has been found to link with obesity, insulin resistance, and hypertension. Vitamin D treatment for PCOS women also improves the IR in MeS and metabolic profiles and reduces total testosterone and subcutaneous fat. Vitamin D, on the other hand, and inflammation-linked factors have an inverse connection with BP vitamin D and signs of MeS disorders, like impaired glucose metabolism, BP regularity issues, and stomach obesity.

Polycystic ovary syndrome afflicts about 10% of women of reproductive age and is a multifaceted endocrine disease characterized by the presence of polycystic ovaries, irregular menstruation, and elevated testosterone level. One of its most complex aspects is that it is impossible to manage it effectively due to a multicausal etiology comprising genetic, hormonal, and environmental characteristics. However, nutrition plays a key role in this process as the consumption of micronutrients reduces the intensity of its symptoms and contributes to the high quality of patients' lives. A change in metabolic imbalance and hormonal function can help overcome this from a non-pharmacological support perspective. The risk factors related with PCOS are not well known, but genetics, insulin resistance, and inflammation are known to play a role. The health conditions that PCOS exacerbates are diabetes, cardiovascular diseases, and metabolic syndrome. For these risks to be mitigated and quality of life improved, it is important to be accurately diagnosed and effectively managed. The role of micronutrients is vital for human health; they enhance the immune system and metabolism, the two most important processes for these patients. Thus, women with PCOS experience an imbalance in the hormone and metabolic systems and may particularly need certain microelements. For example, magnesium can help with insulin sensitivity and metabolic profiles; inositol, ovarian function improvement and insulin sensitivity; vitamin D, menstrual regularity and insulin resistance; and omega-3 fatty acid, blood pressure reduction. It is considered that all of them can be consumed at an adequate level with the food we eat; however, supplements can be useful in solving certain health problems and can be considered if diagnosed by a physician.

9.3 Role of Micronutrients in PCOS

Micronutrients also play a significant role in maintaining hormonal balance, something that is of particular significance to people with PCOS. For example, zinc is known to assist in the creation and regulation of additional reproductive hormone, as well as regulation of testosterone levels. Selenium, in turn, plays a role in the manufacturing of thyroid hormone, which is also vital for hormonal regulation more generally. All of these nutrients, and numerous others, have an impact on hormone synthesis, secretion, and action as a result, influencing diverse PCOS symptoms.

Thus, proper levels of these essential micronutrients might be another component to traditional care if they are to have the possibility to be addressed as a strategic approach to PCOS hormonal imbalances. Micronutrients play an important role in maintaining hormonal balance, and consumption of supplements of such vitamins and minerals such as inositol, magnesium, and vitamin D has been proven to influence insulin sensitivity and androgen levels. By assisting in rebalancing the hormone status, the adequate intake of minerals can assist in alleviating some of the main PCOS symptoms.

However, given the continued nature of the PCOS, effective techniques must be established to mitigate and instrument practical control mechanisms, in both short and long terms. Presently, it is generally acknowledged that lifestyle actions, including a healthy diet and physical exercise, constitute the foundation for PCOS treatment. In the short term, these interventions are well-suited to weight management and the potential risk of cardiovascular disease reduction. However, although the 2023 International PCOS Guidelines supported lifestyle as the foundation of PCOS treatment, diet evidence in PCOS is generally inadequate to advocate a particular diet, and there is a scarcity of robust data that support the design on any special diet for women with PCOS other than creating recommendations based on the National Population-Based Dietary Guidelines. Although lifestyle interventions are the primary treatment for PCOS, pharmaceutical drugs are also primarily administered. Pharmacological treatments are used to enhance the metabolic and reproductive aspects of lifestyle interventions. However, due to the presence of a variety of overlapping symptoms experienced by most patients, it may be impossible to implement a standardized framework to address each of the conditions experienced by every individual.

As a result, some women may seek alternative or adjunct treatment methods. Nutraceuticals or specific micronutrients have emerged as an adjunct therapeutic alternative to lifestyle and/or pharmacological interventions for chronic diseases. Nutraceuticals have been previously described as the derivatives of nutrients or extracts of foods or plants or animals that can have a pharmacological effect. Furthermore, there is strong evidence that women with PCOS use complementary medicines actively to manage PCOS symptomatology. In the previous study, it was reported that more than 70% of the 493 Australian women with PCOS used complementary medicine during the last year. The most frequently used complementary medicine was micronutrient supplementation, which included vitamins, minerals, fish oil capsules, and herbal remedies. Moreover, more than a third of the women believed the beneficial effect of complementary medicine on the symptoms of polycystic ovary syndrome and only a small part of the women indicated the negative effects of CMs, and this usually happens after the nutritional and herbal supplements intake. The use of nutraceutical and micronutritive supplementation for the treatment of PCOS has not yet given accurate results based on prior systematic reviews; in addition, potential limitations were found, such as differences in study designs, sample sizes, what patients were enrolled in the studies, and insufficient control mechanisms. There are dietary and physical activity multimodal interventions as a means of PCOS treatments. Still, no direct evidence or recommendations exist on the nutrients applied in these interventions [26]. According to the popularity use of nutritional supplements, they can be used for the management of PCOS. However, a thorough study is needed to measure the overall efficacy and safety based on the current comprehensive and diverse data. Therefore, a systematic scoping review is required before such a full range of synthesis is held, as this facilitated synthesis provides the basis for organizing and summarizing relevant literature up to the present general conditions [27].

9.3.1 Nutrient Interactions and Metabolic Processes

Obesity and insulin resistance are two metabolic disorders that are frequently seen in PCOS patients. Micronutrients are important for metabolic pathways. For instance, lipid profiles can be improved by omega-3 fatty acids, while insulin sensitivity can be increased by chromium. Designing dietary solutions to address metabolic dysfunctions in PCOS is made easier with an understanding of these nutritional relationships. Nutrient interactions are critical in PCOS individuals' control over the way their bodies metabolize carbohydrates, lipids, and proteins [28]. One example is that magnesium and vitamin B are required for enzymatic processes to drive glucose metabolism and cellular energy generation. This directly influences insulin sensitivity. Furthermore, the trace mineral chromium enhances insulin function; therefore, glucose is more easily soaked up and utilized. In addition to the fact that oxidation is generally heightened in metabolic illnesses like PCOS, antioxidants such as vitamins C and E may reduce it owing to their interaction [29]. This well-balanced view of the metabolic aspects of PCOS serves as a basis for the importance of a well-balanced nutrition that contains the essential micronutrients necessary to maintain metabolic health and reduce the likelihood of problems.

9.3.2 Key Nutrients and Reproductive Health

There might also be a link between dietary status and the problems associated with PCOS-related infertility. Omega-3 fatty acids, vitamin B12, and folic acid are essential for genitalia's head health since the three of them seem to enhance not only ovulation but also the primordial phase of embryogenesis. Thus, modulating the dietary consumption of these agents may be beneficial for women with PCOS in terms of improved reproductive health.

9.4 PCOS Symptoms and Effects

Polycystic ovary syndrome, for example, is a frequent hormonal disorder among patients of reproductive age. PCOS clinical presentation can be very varied and ranges vastly from one person to another. The most common clinical signs include lengthened and infrequent menstrual periods, as well as copiousness in diameter androgens, severe cystic acne, hirsutism, and a male pattern of hair fall. A significant portion of the populace is described by the existence of polycystic ovaries, large cystic enlargement of the ovary containing many small sacs loaded to the brim with fluid, a process that interferes with normal ovulation. In addition to the reproductive sphere, PCOS has a particularly detrimental effect on general health. Figure 9.1 and Tables 9.1 and 9.2 highlight various effects and symptoms of PCOS.

PCOS sufferers frequently suffer from insulin resistance, a phenomenon that sensitizes patients to the development of type 2 diabetes and increases the likelihood of developing gestational diabetes or other metabolic disorders. Psychological disorders in ideological patients are also observed. Eating disorders are common among such persons, in addition to a higher incidence of mood disorders such as anxiety and depression. In many cases, obesity in these patients is observed, which

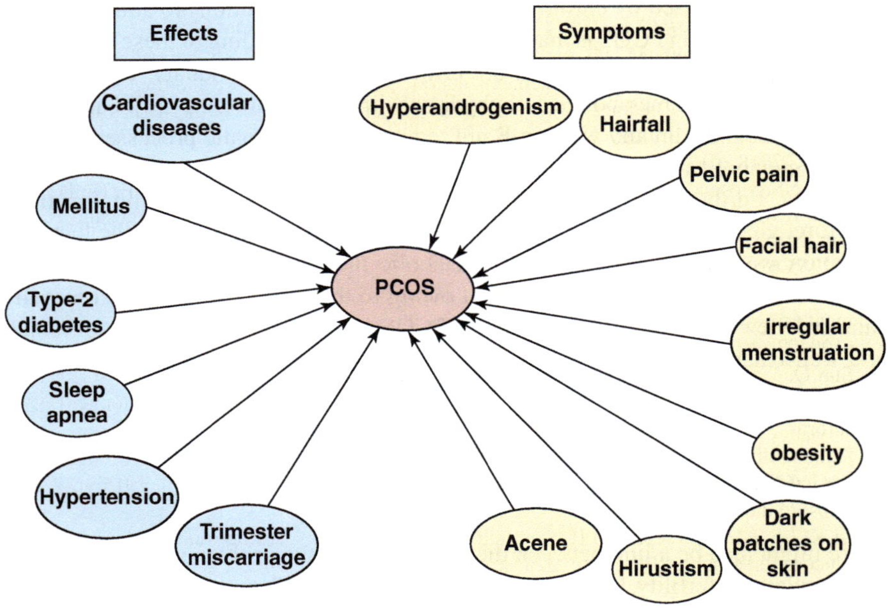

Fig. 9.1 Effects and symptoms of PCOS

Table 9.1 Showing various effects of PCOS

Effects
Cardiovascular: Causes heart diseases; women with PCOS are more likely to have heart disease due to high blood pressure, high cholesterol, and obesity
Trimester miscarriage: Pregnant women with PCOS are likely to have miscarriages due to high levels of hormones and possibly embryos' development level
SD mellitus type 2: Is at high risk for developing type 2 diabetes due to insulin resistance
Sleep apnea: More common in women with PCOS, women and women who are obese
Hypertension: Can develop high blood pressure level

Table 9.2 Showing various symptoms of PCOS

Symptoms
Hyperandrogenism: Too many male hormones, which often lead to symptoms like acne, hirsutism, and sometimes severe levels of hair loss
Hair fall: Common in PCOS as hormonal imbalances disrupt the hair growth cycle of the hair and leads to an increase in hair shedding
Pelvic pain: Pelvic pain is often linked to irregular monthly cycles or ovarian cysts, which is a hallmark of PCOS
Facial hair: An excess of hair growth on the face, a condition called hirsutism caused by high levels of male hormones
Irregular monthly cycles: The most common symptom of PCOS
Acne: Hormonal imbalances in PCOS often cause severe acne, typically affects the lower parts of your face
Obesity: Can cause obesity or make it harder to lose weight
Dark patches of the skin: Dark or darkish-red, velvety skin patches are a result of insulin resistance; they are called acanthosis nigricans
Hirsutism: Unusual growth of hair on the women's body compared to typical women's body hair growth

should exacerbate many PCOS problems, producing a vicious circle of symptoms. Lifestyle changes, pharmacotherapy, and control of associated diseases are usually necessary to properly control PCOS and to decrease risks and improve quality of life.

9.5 Challenges in Nutritional Management of PCOS

Table 9.3 highlights several challenges in nutritional management of PCOS.

9.5.1 The Use of AI in Healthcare

The introduction of AI to the healthcare sector has resulted in many modifications in patient care and management, as well as nutrition. AI allows you to process and analyze large datasets, identifying patterns and insights that may go unnoticed by humans. AI is particularly useful in complex diseases such as PCOS as it can draw data from multiple sources and provide a comprehensive care solution [34]. As AI continues to mature, its potential to enhance outcomes for patients, personalize treatment plans, and improve diagnostic accuracy are expanding, ushering in a new age of healthcare in which technology and medicine collaborate to give the best possible care.

9.5.2 Utilizing Data Analytics to Provide Nutritional Advice

AI and data analytics have immensely transformed the nutritional science arena through the possibility of personalized nutrition. AI systems, as previously

Table 9.3 Showing various challenges in nutritional management of PCOS

Challenge	Explanation
Variability in dietary needs	Wide diversity of possible dietary needs. As previously mentioned, nutrition is among the main challenges of PCOS management due to the need for a highly individualized approach. It has to be based on the level of the patient's body weight, the extent of insulin resistance, and other comorbidities [30]. For example, low-glycemic index diet may be useful for a patient with insulin resistance syndrome or captured pro-inflammatory state; at the same time, another patient would have benefited from such dietary approach as a diet high in omega-3 fatty acids regulating inflammation [31]. Such diversity in dietary patterns outlines the importance of relying on a personalized plan, to be developed in collaboration with nutritionists and endocrinologists, to increase the effectiveness of symptom treatment and lower the risk of other health hitches
Limitations of conventional dietetics	Previous dietary strategies were mostly based on minimizing weight and reducing calories, which is insufficient for a person with PCOS. Due to the inherent metabolic and hormonal disorders associated with PCOS, a proper diet should address not only weight and calorie level but also micronutrient assimilation, hormone regulation, and metabolic health [32]. A vague diet that did not fully target the precise issues of PCOS control can be condensed due to insufficient and incomplete knowledge and understanding of the disease-specific dietary requirements. Research and education remain important in raising modern dietary recommendations for successful PCOS management

mentioned, can provide customized nutritional recommendations based on various features that can then be harnessed to meet the PCOS patient's exact needs. The recommendations can be based on the eating behavior, genome information, and the patient's metabolic state. This precision nutritional communication powered by AI might be able to reduce signs, improve metabolic health, and possibly decrease long-term PCOS exposure. As data analytics develops, so will the recommendations, offering a more precise and nuanced approach to health and nutrition.

9.6 Personalizing PCOS Care with AI

The utilization of artificial intelligence for PCOS diagnosis and treatment is a significant achievement in the development of personalized medicine. Physicians and other healthcare personnel may lead to the delivery of tailored care plans to satisfy patient-found physiological and metabolism requirements by taking advantage of AI that processes data. Artificial intelligence algorithms may be evaluated against many factors, including hormone levels, insulin sensitivity, and eating cravings, to provide tailored food suggestions and treatment. This individualized method aims to enhance the effectiveness of treatments while also increasing patient compliance, resulting in better health and quality of life for women suffering with PCOS.

Figure 9.2 illustrates the four image processing stages applied to the medical ultrasound scans to enhance the quality and detail level of image data with a clearer clinical value. The sequence starts with the first ultrasound picture, panel A, which, like most first ultrasound pictures, has an unprocessed grainy and still slightly blurry appearance afforded by the ultrasound image approach characteristics.

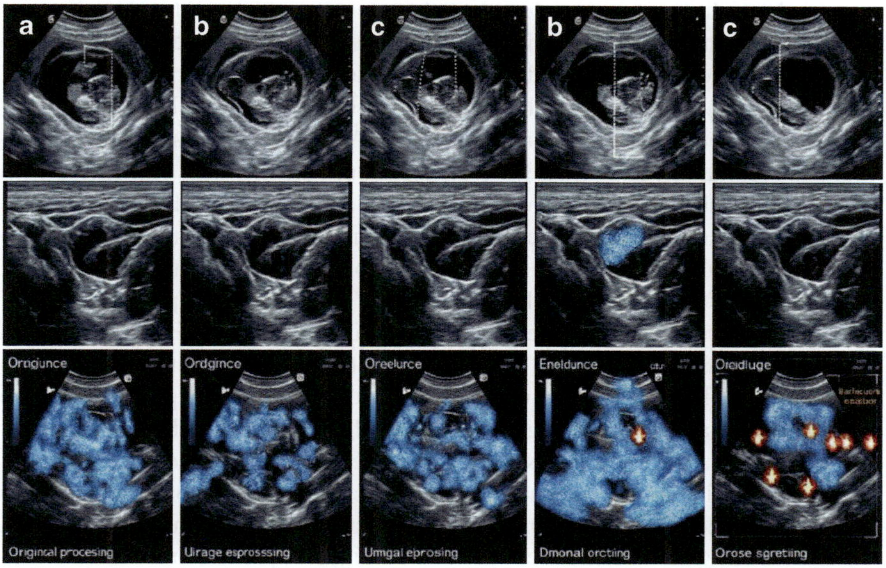

Fig. 9.2 Progressive steps in ultrasound image processing. Panel (**a**) shows the original grayscale ultrasound image. Panel (**b**) displays the image after applying the first level of enhancement to increase contrast and sharpness. Panel (**c**) demonstrates the final processed image with additional texture smoothing for improved interpretability

Several processing steps then follow. The first processing step is the earliest enhancement applied, panel B, which increased the contrast and sharpness of the same image, resulting in differentiated and clarified interior structures more visible and easier to distinguish and interpret.

Next is processing which is used as a noise reduction technique to remove unnecessary visual noise, which might mask delicate details from the eye, again increasing the image's sharpness. In the later sequence stages, the morphological processing was used to highlight the structural features of the tissues, organs, or pathologies displayed on the ultrasound images. This is particularly important for increasing the edges' visibilities and their correlation to each other to help medical doctors differentiate between multiple tissue types or localize pathologic growths. The next panel uses the OTSU process for picture segmentation. The process allows for the accurate separation of the regions of interest from the background as it can automatically determine the optimal threshold levels for differentiating them, resulting in clearly separated image sections. This technique is very useful for detecting a prominent feature in a complex and busy visual field. The last panel feature extraction uses the ORB process, which highlights critical points of interest in the picture. These afford crucial diagnostic insight points are sites where there are major differences in tissue densities, which may indicate the presence of disease.

AI has revolutionized the identification and care of disorders including PCOS. Artificial intelligence techniques such as machine learning algorithms and deep learning networks, have facilitated the creation of automated systems that can diagnose heart disease sex reproducibly and, it more accurately artificial intelligence techniques can interpret medical data like drug levels to differentiate individuals who suffer from polycystic ovary syndrome results in an increase in clinical competence at an early stage, and all patients benefit from these accurate overall results. In addition, an expert once said, monitoring patients to AI-driven systems capable of continuous observation can explain the patient's requirements to the clinician, which entails additional essential information for potential therapy and allows faster, more accurate treatments. Much maybe significantly simpler and more effective improvement could result from existing or newly developed technology using various AI insights. Feature selection is a technique to reduce the number of input variables that you need to consider while developing a predictive model. Feature selection approaches in machine learning aim to select only the most suitable features to develop a model that can make reliable predictions of observed patterns. Feature selection is the automatic strategy of selecting the most useful characteristics for your machine learning model based on the problem you need to solve. We accomplish this by including or eliminating significant characteristics from our data without modifying them. It can help with data that has a lot of noise or incoming data that requires reducing. A hybrid model can be a technique, approach, or framework mix of two or more dissimilar kinds of models or methodologies used to address a single issue or accomplish one objective. In machine learning, a hybrid model is utilized to improve performance and accuracy by integrating multiple approaches or methodologies. In this context, a hybrid model can boost the predicted utility and precision of neural networks and decision trees by combining the most valuable attributes of each. For instance, combining statistical and rule-based models is a hybrid model.

A model creates a consistent trade-off between the complexity of a model and how well it generalizes. A simple model such as a linear regression model may predict more generalizable and understandable conclusions compared to complex machine learning and deep learning models. Therefore, providing a clear and understandable explanation of such a complex model is vital in boosting trust in a generated model for this reason. This question reasoning arises for the inadequacy of complicated models. The black-box model shows an inability to maintain model faith without proper explanation. Explainable AI approaches aim at improving the understanding, interpretability, and credibility of model predictions. There is a two-level categorization of explainability, which includes local explainability and global explainability. A global explanation provides a description of a final decision that touches every data point. The informal analysis exists in relation to the global accuracy. This point of this paper was to clarify the employment of the local level; as demonstrated by reference, the idea of local commitment can be broken down in reference to all samples. It entails providing a more accurate informal explanation.

9.6.1 Case Studies: AI-Driven Nutritional Interventions

Examining real-world examples of AI-driven dietary recommendations demonstrates the usefulness of this technology in PCOS management. An AI system might, for example, examine data from a cohort of PCOS patients, finding patterns and trends that result in effective dietary modifications. AI can assist in creating more efficient, individualized meal plans by analyzing how various food ingredients impact symptoms and the course of a disease. These case studies highlight how AI has the power to change PCOS treatment as it now exists, making it more patient-centered and responsive.

9.6.2 Adapting AI to Individual Physiological Profiles

With disorders like PCOS, where patient responses to treatment vary greatly, AI's capacity to adjust to unique physiological profiles is especially advantageous. With the assistance of AI systems, to identify the most effective interventions for each patient, vast datasets might be taken; these might include metabolic rates and genetic information [36]. This method benefits a broader patients' aspect of PCOS care, such as diet, weight management, hormone balance, and fertility problems, while also allowing for more accurate dietary recommendations. Recommendations are based on artificial intelligence. AI may produce recommendations that are designed to change with the patient. This is frequently accomplished by allowing the AI to learn from additional data over time.

9.7 Integrating AI with Micronutrient Optimization

Individual metabolism and hormonal health thus adapt nutrition even more effectively to one's personal needs. This would combat micronutrient shortages while also allowing for a more precise calculation of nutrient amounts, when correctness can ensure the proper hormonal and metabolic levels and ideal influences on PCOS treatment, hence radically advancing patient outcomes. Based on the principles of personalized nutrition [35], it has the potential to radically expand the spectrum of nutritional intervention customized to the specific health blueprint of everyone.

9.7.1 AI Algorithms for Diet Optimization

One of the most promising developments in the realm of precision nutrition has been the development of AI algorithms that optimize diets [33]. Based on an individual's diet, health data, and preferences, it gives effective, data-informed nutritional recommendations. As with all AI start-ups, these platforms utilize the intelligence factor—it improves as people use it more and more. This implies that each person's diet and health journey is distinct, and the suggestions from the AI platform get more personalized with continuous use.

9.7.2 The Future of AI in Dietary Planning

When used to its full potential, these products will bring about a new era of precision nutrition that won't be the same for everyone but rather one-of-a-kind recommendations based on the individual's body and metabolism. This has the potential to pave the path for AI-powered platforms that can continuously learn, adapt, and personalize dietary suggestions in real time based on the out-of-the-new health data. This is especially useful in complex diseases like PCOS, where such technologies can alter public health nutrition programs by providing custom yet scalable solutions for each person.

9.8 Implications for Healthcare Providers

The ramifications for healthcare professionals of incorporating artificial intelligence (AI) are extensive and diverse. AI technologies have the potential to greatly improve patient outcomes, increase efficiency, and lower healthcare costs. As they develop, they will equip healthcare providers with previously unheard-of capabilities for detecting, treating, and managing diseases as shown in Table 9.4.

Table 9.4 Showing various implications for healthcare providers

Type of implication	Explanation
Constant improvement and learning	An updated knowledge is created from AI with all interactions with respect to various skills. This helps all the medical professional to get updated with this; this was recently found with the collection information and the new approaches used for patient care
Improved diagnostic accuracy	AI's ability to process enormous volumes of medical data quickly enables healthcare professionals to spot trends and abnormalities that conventional analysis could miss. This can result in more precise and timely diagnoses, especially in complex conditions like PCOS where treatment outcomes and symptoms can vary greatly
Personalized treatment plans	AI's ability to assess patient information in the context of large datasets enables more nuanced and prosperous treatments. In yet another example, AI can help tailor meal plans and drug therapies based on individual health data of PCOS patients, which may improve the conditions under which the syndrome and its comorbidities are controlled
Ethical and training issues	AI in healthcare raises, among other things, ethical considerations, including but not limited to the protection of data and confidentiality of the patient. Using AI equipment would also necessitate customized instruction for healthcare employees to fully comprehend the advantages and shortcomings of such technology
Cost implications	It is true that while AI technology may help alleviate healthcare costs over time in the long term, including through boosting productivity and success, there will also be a substantial expense involved in investing in AI technology. Healthcare costs implications should be considered with regard to the use of such resources

9.8.1 AI Integration in Practice

The above use of AI in healthcare procedures can shift the patient management and care delivery paradigm. Nowadays, medical professionals have access to systems that can provide high-level diagnostic capabilities, therapy recommendations tailored to the patient, and predictive analysis. In nutritional research, for example, artificial intelligence can analyze data on a patient and suggest types of dietary modifications depending on their unique metabolic profiles and genetic predisposition that are more likely to be successful. However, healthcare professionals must learn new skills to fully utilize this trend. Professionals need to learn how to interpret AI-generated data and effectively communicate it to the patients. As a result, healthcare workers will likely need further continuing education and training on AI trends as they evolve to be aware of breakthroughs and harness the full potential of these technologies in clinical environments.

9.8.2 Improving Patient Results Using Technology

By providing more precise, tailored, and timely solutions, artificial intelligence (AI) can improve patient outcomes in the healthcare industry, particularly in the area of nutrition. AI-driven solutions can customize dietary programs that adjust to the patient's changing health status and preferences, leading to better health outcomes and greater adherence for illnesses like PCOS, where dietary control plays a critical role. Furthermore, by enabling real-time feedback and remote monitoring, these technologies enable patients to actively participate in their health management. AI technologies have the potential to revolutionize healthcare by boosting its efficiency, effectiveness, and patient-centeredness, as they become more widely used.

9.9 Conclusion

The integration of artificial intelligence into diet seems to be a possibility to enhance PCOS/PCOD management. Artificial intelligence-powered platforms may assess large-scale data of individual food habits, metabolic attributes, and genetic susceptibility to provide individualized nutritional recommendations. It could fully alter the way diet programs are created, doing away with dated, single-size diet program methods of making diet formulas that meet the unique needs of those suffering from PCOS/PCOD. Dietitians, too, may improve patient outcomes and compliance with dietary standards using artificial intelligence to make more reliable and effective dietary recommendations. Eventually, research may focus on developing and validating AI algorithms that could accurately predict and satisfy the nutritional needs of women with PCOS/PCOD. Dietitians and endocrinologists, working together with data scientists, may use predictive modelling to create algorithms for artificial intelligence that account for the complexity of PCOS/PCOD. Additionally, clinical trials would be required to assess the efficiency of artificial intelligence-powered meal plans relative to conventional meal plans. With advances in artificial intelligence, the management of disorders such as PCOS/PCOD can be completely changed, which might suggest the future of more tailored and efficient treatments. Based on the current improvements, "real time" could incorporate real-time biometric data like glucose and hormone levels, continuously shifting nutritional guidelines as people develop the situation. New improvement that could offer help is global collaborative databases with equal treatment results over the world that might significantly boost the learning sequence behind the AI models, making approaches to managing PCOS/PCOD everywhere more efficient and effective.

References

1. Revised 2003 consensus on diagnostic criteria and long-term health risks related to polycystic ovary syndrome (PCOS). Hum Reprod. 2004;19(1):41–7.
2. Azziz R, Carmina E, Dewailly D, Diamanti-Kandarakis E, Escobar-Morreale HF, Futterweit W, Janssen OE, Legro RS, Norman R, Taylor AE, et al. The Androgen Excess and PCOS Society criteria for the polycystic ovary syndrome: the complete task force report. Fertil Steril. 2009;91:456–88.
3. Ndefo UA, Eaton A, Green MR. Polycystic ovary syndrome: a review of treatment options with a focus on pharmacological approaches. Pharm Ther. 2013;38:336.
4. Mohan V, Mehreen TS, Ranjani H, Kamalesh R, Ram U, Anjana RM. Prevalence of polycystic ovarian syndrome among adolescents and young women in India. J Diabetol. 2021;12:319–25.
5. Rojhani E, Rahmati M, Firouzi F, Saei Ghare Naz M, Azizi F, Ramezani Tehrani F. Polycystic ovary syndrome, subclinical hypothyroidism, the cut-off value of thyroid stimulating hormone; is there a link? Findings of a population-based study. Diagnostics. 2023;13:316.
6. Mcdonald TW, Malkasian GD, Gaffey TA. Endometrial cancer associated with feminizing ovarian tumor and polycystic ovarian disease. Obstet Gynecol. 1977;49:654–8.
7. Diamanti-Kandarakis E, Christakou CD. Insulin resistance in PCOS. In: Diagnosis and management of polycystic ovary syndrome. Springer; 2009. p. 35–61.
8. Legro RS, Arslanian SA, Ehrmann DA, Hoeger KM, Murad MH, Pasquali R, Welt CK. Diagnosis and treatment of polycystic ovary syndrome: an Endocrine Society clinical practice guideline. J Clin Endocrinol Metabol. 2013;98(12):4565–92.
9. Azziz R, Carmina E, Dewailly D, et al. Criteria for defining polycystic ovary syndrome as a predominantly hyperandrogenic syndrome: an androgen excess society guideline. J Clin Endocrinol Metab. 2006;91(11):4237–45.
10. Legro RS, Arslanian SA, Ehrmann DA, et al. Diagnosis and treatment of polycystic ovary syndrome: an Endocrine Society clinical practice guideline. J Clin Endocrinol Metab. 2013;98(12):4565–92.
11. Unfer V, Carlomagno G, Dante G, Facchinetti F. Effects of myo-inositol in women with PCOS: a systematic review of randomized controlled trials. Gynecol Endocrinol. 2012;28(7):509–15.
12. Wehr E, Pilz S, Schweighofer N, et al. Association of hypovitaminosis D with metabolic disturbances in polycystic ovary syndrome. Eur J Endocrinol. 2009;161(4):575–82.
13. Phelan N, O'Connor A, Kyaw Tun T, et al. Hormonal and metabolic effects of polyunsaturated fatty acids in young women with polycystic ovary syndrome: results from a cross-sectional analysis and a randomized, placebo-controlled, crossover trial. Am J Clin Nutr. 2011;93(3):652–62.
14. Jamilian M, Asemi Z. The effects of soy isoflavones on metabolic status of patients with polycystic ovary syndrome. J Clin Endocrinol Metab. 2016;101(9):3386–94.

15. Asemi Z, Esmaillzadeh A. DASH diet, insulin resistance, and serum hs-CRP in polycystic ovary syndrome: a randomized controlled clinical trial. Horm Metab Res. 2015;47(3):232–8.
16. McKeown NM, Meigs JB, Liu S, Saltzman E, Wilson PW, Jacques PF. Carbohydrate nutrition, insulin resistance, and the prevalence of the metabolic syndrome in the Framingham offspring cohort. Diabetes Care. 2004;27(2):538–46.
17. Ni Y, Nagashimada M, Zhuge F, Zhan L, Nagata N, Tsutsui A, et al. Astaxanthin prevents and reverses diet-induced insulin resistance and steatohepatitis in mice: a comparison with vitamin E. Sci Rep. 2015;5:17192.
18. Tinggi U. Selenium: its role as antioxidant in human health. Environ Health Prev Med. 2008;13(2):102–8.
19. Coskun A, Arikan T, Kilinc M, Arikan DC, Ekerbicer HC. Plasma selenium levels in Turkish women with polycystic ovary syndrome. Eur J Obstet Gynecol Reprod Biol. 2013;168(2):183–6.
20. Jamilian M, Razavi M, Fakhrie Kashan Z, Ghandi Y, Bagherian T, Asemi Z. Metabolic response to selenium supplementation in women with polycystic ovary syndrome: a randomized, double-blind, placebo-controlled trial. Clin Endocrinol (Oxf). 2015;82(6):885–91.
21. Zulet MA, Puchau B, Hermsdorff HH, Navarro C, Martinez JA. Dietary selenium intake is negatively associated with serum sialic acid and metabolic syndrome features in healthy young adults. Nutr Res (New York, NY). 2009;29(1):41–8.
22. Zagrodzki P, Krzyczkowska-Sendrakowska M, Nicol F, Wietecha-Posluszny R, Milewicz T, Kryczyk-Koziol J, et al. Selenium status parameters in patients with polycystic ovary syndrome. J Trace Elem Med Biol. 2017;44:241–6.
23. Mohammad Hosseinzadeh F, Hosseinzadeh-Attar MJ, Yekaninejad MS, Rashidi B. Effects of selenium supplementation on glucose homeostasis and free androgen index in women with polycystic ovary syndrome: a randomized, double blinded, placebo controlled clinical trial. J Trace Elem Med Biol. 2016;34:56–61.
24. Obeid O, Elfakhani M, Hlais S, Iskandar M, Batal M, Mouneimne Y, et al. Plasma copper, zinc, and selenium levels and correlates with metabolic syndrome components of Lebanese adults. Biol Trace Elem Res. 2008;123(1–3):58–65.
25. Sy C, Dangles O, Borel P, Caris-Veyrat C. Interactions between carotenoids from marine bacteria and other micronutrients: impact on stability and antioxidant activity. Mar Drugs. 2015;13(11):7020–39.
26. Teede HJ, Misso ML, Costello MF, Dokras A, Laven J, Moran L, Piltonen T, Norman RJ. Recommendations from the international evidence-based guideline for the assessment and management of polycystic ovary syndrome. Fertil Steril. 2018;110:364–79.
27. Arksey H, O'Malley L. Scoping studies: towards a methodological framework. Int J Soc Res Methodol. 2005;8:19–32.
28. Salek M, Clark CCT, Taghizadeh M, Jafarnejad S. Inositol treatment of anovulation in women with polycystic ovary syndrome: a meta-analysis of randomised trials. BJOG Int J Obstet Gynaecol. 2019;126(3):299–308.
29. Sales CH, Pedrosa LF. Magnesium and diabetes mellitus: their relation. Clin Nutr. 2006;25(4):554–62.
30. Broadhurst CL, Domenico P. Clinical studies on chromium picolinate supplementation in diabetes mellitus—a review. Diabetes Technol Ther. 2006;8(6):677–87.
31. Moran LJ, Ko H, Misso M, Marsh K, Noakes M, Talbot M, et al. Dietary composition in the treatment of polycystic ovary syndrome: a systematic review to inform evidence-based guidelines. J Acad Nutr Diet. 2013;113(4):520–45.
32. Phelan N, O'Connor A, Tun TK, Correia N, Boran G, Roche HM, Gibney J. Hormonal and metabolic effects of polyunsaturated fatty acids in young women with polycystic ovary syndrome: results from a cross-sectional analysis and a randomized, placebo-controlled, crossover trial. Am J Clin Nutr. 2011;93(3):652–62.

33. Douglas CC, Gower BA, Darnell BE, Ovalle F, Oster RA, Azziz R. Role of diet in the treatment of polycystic ovary syndrome. Fertil Steril. 2006;85(3):679–88.
34. Jeanes YM, Reeves S, Gibson EL, Piggott C, May VA, Hart KH. Binge eating behaviours and food cravings in women with polycystic ovary syndrome. Appetite. 2017;109:24–32.
35. Zeevi D, Korem T, Zmora N, Israeli D, Rothschild D, Weinberger A, et al. Personalized nutrition by prediction of glycemic responses. Cell. 2015;163(5):1079–94.
36. Shaheen MY. Applications of artificial intelligence (AI) in healthcare: a review. ScienceOpen Preprints; 2021.

Supplements and Herbal Remedies: An Exploration of Nutritional Supplements and Herbal Remedies for PCOS and AI's Role in Personalized Recommendations

10

Anshika Gupta and Kalpana Katiyar

10.1 Introduction

PCOS is a complex problem categorized by abnormal testosterone levels, irregular menstrual periods, and cysts on one or both ovaries [1]. It is classified as a complicated endocrine illness with unclear origins and a complex underlying mechanism [2]. According to the World Health Organization (WHO), PCOS afflicted approximately 117 million females worldwide in 2012, with one out of every five Indian females suffering from the disorder [3]. Between 2007 and 2017, 1.55 million instances of PCOS were reported among females aged 15 to 49 globally, indicating a 4.47% increase [4]. A comprehensive research conducted throughout India in late 2020 revealed that around 16.1% of female individuals between the ages of 20 and 39 had been identified as having PCOS [5].

PCOS is a complicated sickness categorized by hormonal imbalances, irregular menstruation periods, and ovarian cysts [6]. Common symptoms include acne, excessive hair growth, and weight gain. While the specific reason is unknown, lifestyle variables like food, exercise, and stress management are becoming recognized as important [6]. This transition has resulted in a more comprehensive approach to therapy, including lifestyle and dietary therapies alongside medicines. The work of Begum et al. [7] delves into the complex link between lifestyle choices, diet, and PCOS to empower readers to manage their health more successfully. It discusses issues such as the consequence of diet on insulin resistance and the significance of stress reduction in PCOS therapy [8].

A. Gupta · K. Katiyar (✉)
Dr. Ambedkar Institute of Technology for Divyangjan, Kanpur, Uttar Pradesh, India
e-mail: kalpna@aith.ac.in

R. Kumar et al. (eds.), *AI-Based Nutritional Intervention in Polycystic Ovary Syndrome (PCOS)*, https://doi.org/10.1007/978-981-96-2120-0_10

Over the last span of time, females' use of complementary medicine (CM) has increased significantly, with percentages ranging from 26% to 91% [9]. Herbal medicine is one of the most widely practiced types of Chinese medicine [10]. Herbal treatments are known to include bioactive components that might affect female endocrinology, potentially reducing the possibility of breast cancer, osteoporosis, and cardiovascular disease [11]. However, herbal medicines are complicated treatments because they include a variety of active ingredients that might interact synergistically or antagonistically. Furthermore, their impacts on the body can be complex, requiring simultaneous interactions with many metabolic pathways and organ functions [9].

In recent years, technology, particularly machine learning (ML), has transformed healthcare, providing insights and support with illness detection. The capacity of machine learning (ML) to interpret massive volumes of data holds promise for improving the analysis and supervision of illnesses such as PCOS [12]. Despite multiple research investigating ML's potential in PCOS diagnosis, constraints such as limited sample numbers and diverse criteria prevent a thorough understanding [13]. To address this, Barrera et al. [14] conducted a systematic assessment of relevant research through January 1, 2022, to give a concise synopsis of AI/ML applications in PCOS diagnosis. Authors reviewed 135 studies that used AI/ML treatments for PCOS diagnosis. These treatments used a variety of data sources and approaches, with encouraging outcomes showing high accuracy and efficacy when compared to clinical diagnosis. The AI/ML models performed well across several assessment measures, indicating their potential for improving PCOS diagnosis and therapy.

Organization of Chapter

The rest of the chapter is organized as follows: Section 10.2 illustrates origin of PCOS followed by onset of PCOS in Sect. 10.3. Section 10.4 highlights nutritional supplements for PCOS. Section 10.5 enlightens herbal remedies for PCOS. Section 10.6 discusses AI's role in personalized recommendations followed by lifestyle modification discussion in Sect. 10.7. Finally, Sect. 10.8 concludes the chapter.

10.2 Origin of PCOS

PCOS origin is impacted by both environmental and genetic factors as described in Fig. 10.1.

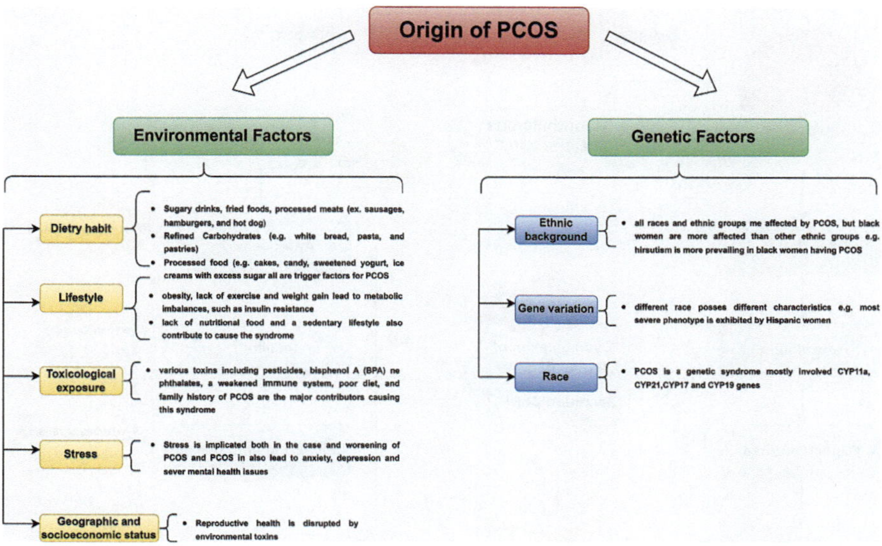

Fig. 10.1 Origin of PCOS

10.3 Onset of PCOS

The onset of this illness involves several major hormones, as illustrated in Fig. 10.2.

PCOS is mostly caused by genetics. Women with PCOS have increased GnRH release and hyperandrogenism, which are key to the condition's symptoms [15]. Hyperandrogenism, defined by increased androstenedione, testosterone, and occasionally DHEA levels, is present in 50% of patients [16].

Increased GnRH frequency causes excessive LH release and decreased FSH release, with some patients reporting hyperactive LH-producing cells that raise LH levels. This imbalance in hormones prevents follicular growth, resulting in insufficient estrogen production. Insufficient FSH-mediated granulosa cell growth causes thecal cells, which are responsible for androgen synthesis, to overproduce androgens, causing hyperandrogenism. Elevated 5α-reduced androgens lead to decreased aromatase activity, which further inhibits estrogen production. As a result, inadequate ovulation, along with hyperandrogenism-induced follicular abnormalities, increases AMH levels, aggravating FSH inhibition [17].

PCOS symptoms are exacerbated by comorbidities including obesity and insulin resistance. Obesity increases testosterone conversion to estrogen via adipose tissue aromatase. Insulin resistance, caused by increased free fatty acids and adipokines, exacerbates inflammation and impairs insulin signaling. Hyperandrogenism can cause insulin resistance, and high insulin levels exacerbate hyperandrogenism by promoting androgen synthesis in thecal cells [18].

Elevated androgen levels and insulin resistance limit SHBG synthesis, which amplifies androgen effects. Adipose tissue aromatase in obese PCOS individuals

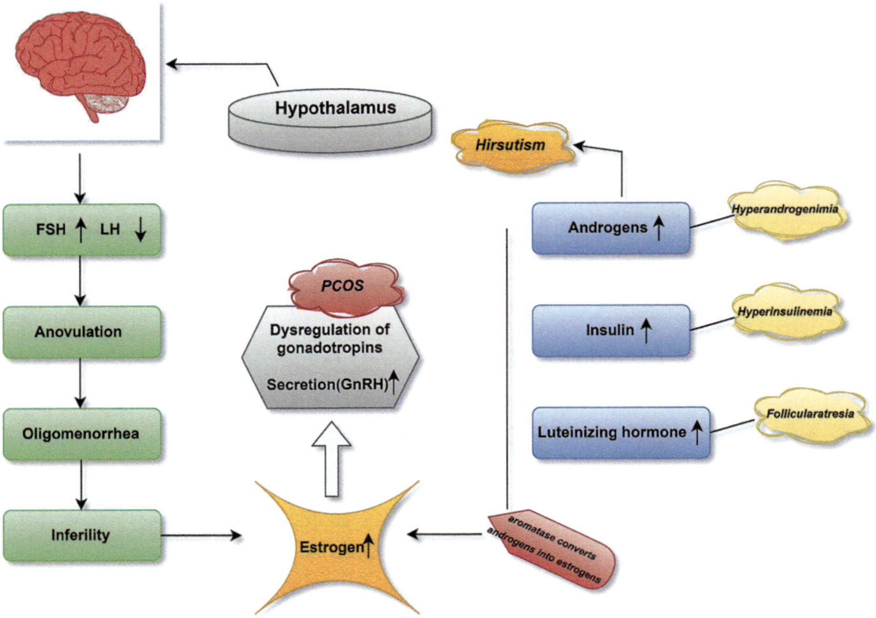

Fig. 10.2 Onset of PCOS

produces estrogens, increasing hypoestrogenism. Hyperandrogenism produces hirsutism, whereas hypoestrogenism causes endometrial hyperplasia. Insulin resistance and obesity raise cardiovascular and diabetes risk in PCOS patients [19, 20].

10.4 Nutritional Supplements for PCOS

According to studies, motherly consumption of high-fat and high-sugar meals during gestation might influence brain circuits connected to reward in children, perhaps leading to a liking for comparable foods [21]. Hormonal alterations in PCOS patients may affect appetite control circuits, resulting in greater satiety points and increased appetite compared to individuals without the disease. Normal-weight women with PCOS consume fewer calories per day, but they eat more carbs [22]. Furthermore, many PCOS patients have insufficient nutritional and physical activity levels. Surprisingly, even adopting a diet similar to the Mediterranean style, which is typically considered healthy, PCOS women may still have increased hunger and calorie consumption, perhaps contributing to weight gain [23, 24]. Table 10.1 summarizes the supplements examined in this study.

10.4.1 Inositol

Inositol, a carbocyclic sugar present abundantly in mammalian organs such as the brain, kidney, and liver, controls cell signaling in response to neurotransmitters,

Table 10.1 Summary of supplement's effects in PCOS

S. no.	Supplements	Effects in PCOS
1	Inositol	Multifaceted roles in cellular pathways, hormone regulation
2	Curcumin	Powerful inflammatory, antioxidant, improves insulin sensitivity
3	Calciferol	Increases insulin sensitivity, helps with hair loss, reduces inflammation
4	N-acetylcysteine	Balances hormone, reduces oxidative stress and inflammation
5	D-chiro-inositol	Improves body mass index, FSH, LH, and blood insulin levels
6	Tocopherol	Antioxidant, neutralizes free radicals, anticoagulant, improves the endometrial lining in infertile women
7	Folate	Increases insulin sensitivity, reduces inflammation
8	Omega-3 fatty acids	Antioxidant, improve glucose metabolism

growth factors, and hormones. It can exist in nine stereoisomeric forms via epimerization, the most clinically significant of those being myoinositol and D-chiro-inositol (DCI) [24, 25].

Myoinositol, in particular, is required for a variety of physiological processes, notably in endocrine diseases such as insulin resistance and diabetes [26]. It serves as a secondary messenger for insulin, promoting glucose absorption into cells. Because of its critical role, myoinositol is frequently regarded as semi-essential, with shortage linked to a variety of clinical diseases [27].

Myoinositol has been shown to be useful in treating illnesses such as in PCOS, reducing both procreative and metabolic abnormalities linked with the syndrome. Its supplementation has demonstrated promise reducing the incidence of gestational diabetes, particularly in high-risk individuals [28].

Furthermore, supplementing with myoinositol has been shown to be both safe and advantageous to male and female reproductive health [29]. It restores ovarian function in PCOS patients and improves results in hyperinsulinemia illnesses such as metabolic syndrome. Its regulatory role includes hormone regulation, which affects insulin, follicle-stimulating hormone (FSH), and thyroid-stimulating hormone (TSH), as well as pathways involved in anti-Müllerian hormone synthesis in granulosa cells.

10.4.2 Curcumin

Curcumin, derived from turmeric, is a potent antioxidant that boosts the activity of key enzymes including glutathione peroxidase, superoxide dismutase, and catalase. It also scavenges free radicals and modulates the Keap1-Nrf2/ARE signaling pathway, hence increasing cleansing and antioxidant gene expression. Furthermore, curcumin has been revealed to promote ovulation and recover the metabolic profile of individuals with PCOS [30, 31].

PCOS, a significant cause of female infertility, is distinguished by insulin resistance and hyperandrogenism [32]. Curcumin appears to reduce hyperandrogenism by inhibiting the activity of cytochrome P450c17, decreasing LH levels. It also downregulates ovarian androgen receptor proteins, which may help in anovulation in PCOS. Curcumin has anti-inflammatory capabilities, decreasing stages of provocative issues such as TNF-α and IL-6 [33]. It can help reduce insulin resistance, promote ovulation, regulate body weight, and address lipid abnormalities in PCOS patients [34, 35].

A meta-analysis found that curcumin supplement improves glycemic control in PCOS patients by controlling indicators such abstaining insulin, fast glucose, the HOMA-IR score, and the measurable insulin sensitivity check index. Despite its potential advantages, the therapeutic use of curcumin is limited by a variety of inherent and extrinsic characteristics associated with herbal medications, such as differences in organ specialization, chemical ingredients, and production procedures [30, 33].

10.4.3 Calciferol

Calciferol most commonly known as vitamin D insufficiency has been found as a key donor to insulin resistance and metabolic syndrome in females with PCOS. According to research, vitamin D insufficiency is mutual among females with PCOS, with rates fluctuating from 67% to 85% [36]. This deficit is linked to a variation of diseases, including insulin resistance, type 2 diabetes, cardiovascular disease, and metabolic conditions. Vitamin D receptors, which govern a large section of the human genome, including genes crucial for glucose metabolism, play an important role in this situation. Polymorphisms in vitamin D-related genes, DHCR7 and Cdx2, are connected with insulin sensitivity and resistance. Variations in the vitamin D receptor α-I gene are tied with testosterone stages in females with PCOS [37].

Calciferol affects glucose-insulin balance by activating insulin receptors of pancreatic β cells and skeletal muscle, resulting in increased insulin synthesis and release [38]. As a result, vitamin D supplementation is advised for women with PCOS to correct low levels. Supplementing with low dosages (<4000 IU/d) or larger doses (≥4000 IU/d) for at slightest 12 weeks will improve insulin compassion, glucose levels, hormonal function, and hyperlipidemia in PCOS patients.

Vitamin D helps to treat reproductive and metabolic difficulties in PCOS by reducing insulin resistance and regulating ovarian androgen production. It also improves pregnancy outcomes by increasing endometrial receptivity and implantation. When combined with myoinositol and melatonin, vitamin D supplementation boosts pregnancy rates [39]. Furthermore, it possesses progesterone-like action, promoting follicular growth and progesterone generation in granulosa cells, which are essential from the luteal phase forward in the reproductive cycle [15].

10.4.4 N-Acetylcysteine

N-acetylcysteine (NAC), generated from cysteine, functions as an acetylated version of both L-cysteine and glutathione's reduced form. It has insulin-stimulating effects, modulates insulin receptors, and is an effective antioxidant. NAC's sulfhydryl group increases glutathione-S-transfer enzyme activity, providing cellular protection from oxidative stress. It also promotes detoxification by lowering blood homocysteine levels. NAC supplementation in women through PCOS has been proven to improve fertility, ovulation, lipid profile, and insulin resistance [40–42]. In a 12-week medical trial of 108 females with PCOS, those treated with NAC exhibited substantial reductions in hirsuteness and blood sugar stages compared to those treated with metformin.

10.4.5 D-Chiro-Inositol (DCI)

DCI is generated after breakdown of phytic acids present in foods such as fruits, legumes, nuts, and cereals. It has critical involvement in cell membrane development, intracellular signaling, and reproductive processes. DCI supplementation had been proven to enhance menstrual regularity and insulin resistance in PCOS-affected females [43, 44].

In a trial of overweight females with PCOS, daily oral administration of 1200 mg of DCI condensed serum-free testosterone, plasma lipid levels, and blood pressure [45]. Another study found that combining myoinositol with DCI successfully improved PCOS symptoms and the jeopardy of metabolic syndrome in overweight females with insulin resistance [44]. There were also substantial improvements in body weight, FSH, LH, and plasma insulin levels.

10.4.6 Tocopherol, Folate, and Omega-3 Fatty Acids

Tocopherol, commonly known as vitamin E, scavenges free radicals, balancing the oxidant-antioxidant equilibrium. Its anticoagulant and antioxidant qualities have been shown in studies to improve the endometrial lining in infertile women [46].

Folate supplementation (5 mg/day) has been demonstrated to lower plasma homocysteine (Hcy), increase insulin sensitivity, and reduce inflammatory indicators while raising antioxidant levels when compared to a placebo [47].

In females with PCOS, combining omega-3 fatty acid and tocopherol supplementation has been demonstrated to reduce gene activity associated with lipid metabolism and cholesterol levels. In addition, it boosts antioxidant capacity and lowers oxidative stress indicators as compared to a placebo [48]. In comparison to a placebo, 12 weeks of flaxseed oil omega-3 supplementation was linked to lower insulin resistance and inflammatory indicators, as well as improved lipid profiles [49]. However, there were no discernible changes in hormonal profiles or nitric oxide levels.

In comparison to a placebo, omega-3 fatty acid consumption had been demonstrated to lessen insulin levels, insulin resistance, and hirsutism, as well as to decrease tenderness and oxidative stress indicators and increase antioxidant levels [47, 50].

10.5 Herbal Remedies for PCOS

The demand for herbal medications is increasing owing to rising economic prices and the various side effects connected with allopathic treatments. Herbal plants have long been used to make medical remedies [9]. Despite significant advances in pharmaceuticals, particularly in the early twentieth century, which allowed for the synthesis of various medicinal compounds and the treatment of beforehand untreatable illnesses, thousands of therapeutic plants with potent effects on PCOS symptoms are still used worldwide [51]. This tendency is especially prominent in developing nations, as indicated by the growing popularity of herbal treatments [52]. Table 10.2 summarizes the specifications of the herbal florae examined in this study.

Table 10.2 Specifications of the herbal plants and their influence on PCOS

S. no.	Medicinal plants	Family	Effective compound	Influence on PCOS
1	*Aloe arborescens* (aloe vera)	Liliaceae	Polysaccharide, anthraquinones, saponins, salicylic acid, plant sterols, amino acids, enzymes, vitamins, and minerals	Beneficial impact on the tissue of ovaries and folliculogenesis
2	*Matricaria chamomilla* (chamomile)	Compositae	Gallic acid, kamazelin, farnesene, matricin, coumarin derivatives, apigenin, and choline, apigenin, bisabolol, coumarins	Reducing indications of PCOS in the tissue of ovaries, expanding uterine follicles, and improving LH secretion
3	*Cinnamomum verum* (cinnamon)	Lauraceae	Phosphatidylinositol 4-kinase, polyphenols, eugenol, terpenoids, cinnamaldehyde	Raising glucose absorption, increasing glycogen synthesis, and stimulating insulin receptor phosphorylation can all boost the sensitivity of insulin, resulting in lower lipid and blood sugar concentrations
4	*Panax ginseng* (ginseng)	Araliaceae	Glutathione, polyacetylenes superoxide dismutase, and ginsenosides	It controls corticotropin and the amount of cortisol, immune response, antioxidant generation, neuroendocrine functioning, and carbohydrate and fat metabolism
5	*Foeniculum vulgare* (fennel)	Apiaceae	Dianetholes embrace fenchone, trans-estragole and p-anisaldehyde	Reduces estrogen and uterine lining while boosting progesterone and endometrial width
6	*Glycyrrhiza glabra* (licorice)	Fabaceae	Glycyrrhiza	Preventing the negative consequences of PCOS-related diabetes

10.5.1 *Aloe arborescens* (Aloe Vera)

Aloe vera, formally identified as *Aloe arborescens* is a perennial herbaceous shrub from the family of Liliaceae. This shrub comprises vital vitamins A, C, and E, as well as antioxidants that aid to decrease lipid peroxidation. Aloe vera gel is typically composed of water and polysaccharides such as pectins, cellulose, hemicellulose, glucomannan, skyman, and mannose derivatives. Both the gel and the leaves include active components such as aloe, asmodin, aloe asmodine, barbaloin, and poly-monosaccharides such as sterols and organic acids [53].

The polysaccharide components in aloe gel include anti-inflammatory, antibacterial, and antimicrobial activities, which help with inflammation reduction and healing [54]. Aloe vera has been demonstrated in studies to normalize the amount of primary germ cells in the ovary, potentially promoting ovarian tissue and folliculogenesis [55].

Aloe vera gel treatment produced good effects in PCOS rats. Letrozole administration to female rats elicited PCOS-like symptoms, which were alleviated by subsequent treatment with aloe vera gel. This therapy regimen restored ovarian steroid grade and modulated steroidogenic bustle, which was linked to substances found in aloe vera gel such as phytosterols and phytophenol. Aloe vera gel has been shown to directly affect important enzymes such as 3β HSD, which influences estradiol production [56].

Another research on PCOS rats found that administering aloe vera hydroalcoholic extract improved fertility and reduced PCOS symptoms. Treatment with various dosages of aloe vera extract in addition to estradiol valerate resulted in substantial decreases in estrogen concentrations compared to the PCOS group, as well as improvements in progesterone levels [57]. These data imply that aloe vera may have a therapeutic function in PCOS management and reproductive improvement.

10.5.2 *Matricaria chamomilla* (Chamomile)

Chamomile, properly known as *Matricaria chamomilla*, is an annual plant in the family of Asteraceae. Its extract comprises flavonoid components and antioxidants such as gallic acid, kamazelin, farnesene, matricin, coumarin derivatives, apigenin, and choline, all of which have strong anti-inflammatory activities [58]. Chamomile's antispasmodic qualities help to reduce period cramps and minimize the risk of premature labor in women. It also treats skin disorders and eczema because of its capacity to excite leukocytes such as macrophages and B lymphocytes [59, 60].

Research on the impact of chamomile in PCOS used 30 adult Wistar rats. These rats were placed into two groups: a control group and one in which PCOS was persuaded by estradiol valerate. For 10 days, rats with PCOS were given intraperitoneal injections of chamomile alcoholic extract at various levels (25, 50, and 75 mg/kg). Tissue and hormonal trials demonstrated that chamomile successfully reduced PCOS symptoms in ovarian tissue, increased the amount of uterine follicles, and enhanced LH production [60]. These data highlight chamomile's potential medicinal significance in reducing PCOS problems.

10.5.3 *Cinnamomum verum* (Cinnamon)

Cinnamon, technically known as *Cinnamomum zeylanicum* and an associate of the Lauraceae native, is one of the traditional medicine's primogenital and most valuable herbal treatments. Various components of the cinnamon plant, especially the bark, have several therapeutic effects, which are mostly attributable to the volatile oil. Cinnamaldehyde, eugenol, and safrole are key components. These essential oil has insulin-like effects [61]. Cinnamon extract has been demonstrated to improve glucose uptake, glycogen synthesis, and insulin receptor phosphorylation, thus enhancing insulin sensitivity [62]. It also helps to reduce blood fat and glucose levels, which improves general metabolic health [63]. Furthermore, its powerful antioxidant qualities aid to prevent the oxidation of organic materials.

Beyond its metabolic advantages, cinnamon has stood and shown to help regulate the menstrual cycle and treat gynecological difficulties, as well as respiratory and digestive illnesses [64].

A study of 15 females with PCOS who took 333 mg of cinnamon extract tablets on three occasions a day for a period of 8 weeks resulted in substantial increases in insulin sensitivity. Patients' insulin levels fell significantly 2 h after consuming cinnamon extract, which was ascribed to enhanced phosphatidylinositol 4-kinase activity [65]. These data support cinnamon's use as a treatment agent for PCOS-related insulin resistance.

10.5.4 *Panax ginseng* (Ginseng)

Ginseng is a medicinal herb noted for its potent antioxidant activity. It upsurges the movement of essential antioxidant enzymes similar to glutathione and superoxide dismutase, which help scavenge damaging free radicals and prevent lipid peroxidation in cell membranes [66].

Ginseng has been shown in studies to reduce plasma LH levels, improve endocrine status, and address ovulation abnormalities in PCOS patients [67]. This demonstrates ginseng's potential therapeutic significance in treating PCOS-related hormonal imbalances and problems.

10.5.5 *Foeniculum vulgare* (Fennel)

Fennel, technically known as *Foeniculum vulgare*, is a herbaceous shrub from the family of Apiaceae that is well-known for its estrogenic qualities. It has a long history of usage in traditional medication to treat digestive, endocrine, reproductive, and menstrual issues. Fennel and its components have a variety of therapeutic properties, including antibacterial, antifungal, antioxidant, antithrombotic, antidiabetic, and antitumor actions, with trans-anethole being the most active molecule [68, 69]. In a study of PCOS rats, fennel was shown to reduce estrogen levels and uterine epithelial thickness while boosting progesterone levels and uterine endometrial width. This shows that fennel might preserve uterine tissue in PCOS rats [70, 71].

10.5.6 *Glycyrrhiza glabra* (Licorice)

Licorice, technically known as *Glycyrrhiza glabra L.*, belongs to the family of Fabaceae and has been rummage sale in traditional remedy for a variety of purposes, including wound healing, pain treatment, and cough and gastritis alleviation. Its roots contain vital therapeutic ingredients including as flavonoids, sterols, gums, starches, and essential oils. Notably, glycyrrhizin, the main active ingredient in licorice root, has a mineralocorticoid-like effect, increasing glucocorticoid levels in the blood, stimulating insulin secretion and lowering blood sugar levels [67, 72, 73].

In a study of rats with polycystic ovary syndrome (PCOS), administering licorice root hydroalcoholic extract resulted in a drop in blood glucose levels associated with the group treated with letrozole alone; however, the effect was not statistically significant. However, there were no noteworthy alterations in blood triglyceride and cholesterol levels across the study groups. These data show that licorice root extract may help to alleviate the negative consequences of PCOS-related diabetes [72].

10.6 AI's Role in Personalized Recommendations

AI, with its combination of thinking, learning, problem-solving, vision, and language comprehension, ushers in a watershed moment, opening the way for robots with cognitive capacities similar to human nature. Its extensive use resolves real-world challenges quickly and correctly. Because of a lack of long-term cohort studies, the course of polycystic ovary syndrome (PCOS) across different life stages is still unknown. However, longitudinal investigations have revealed age-related changes such as increased menstrual cycle frequency, lower testosterone levels, and enhanced insulin resistance. PCOS' pathophysiology is mostly caused by genetic susceptibility and prenatal/postnatal environmental factors. High androgen levels during intrauterine development may boost glucocorticoid production, resulting in epigenetic changes and increased PCOS risk. Noninvasive ultrasound technology plays a vital role in diagnosing PCOS by identifying ovarian anomalies, particularly follicle count [74].

Chen et al. [75] created a technique for reliably counting follicles in 3D ultrasound pictures of the ovary that incorporates both local and global data. Authors solution includes using this data to predict follicular sizes and locations, as well as adopting a grouped bordering space learning strategy to solve the difficulty of identifying many items in a high-dimensional space. In addition, they used a database-guided graph-cut division approach for follicle identification. While this study adds to our understanding of follicular development in the human ovary, it is also found to have rather high rates of missed detection (19.7%) and erroneous detection (22.5%).

Ultrasound imaging is critical for finding follicles in PCOS patients [76]. Manual follicle detection takes time and is prone to concerns like inter- and intra-observer variability, which can have a negative influence on female's health. Thus, there is an urgent demand for strategies and technologies to automate follicle identification operations [77].

Faghih et al. [78] suggested a cellular neural networks (CNN)-based approach with four consecutive phases. Initially, the approximate location of follicles is determined in the first phase of CNN. The second phase involves the expansion of follicles to their boundary sites. The final step is to determine the location of recessive follicles. Finally, in the final stage of CNN, actual and phantom follicles are mixed to distinguish between impacted follicles.

Soni and Vashisht [79] devised a technique that takes grayscale ultrasound pictures as input. The image quality and brightness are improved via histogram equalization. The background and object classes are then separated using two threshold methods: global basic threshold and Otsu threshold. Binarization is then used to differentiate between background and foreground photos. The image's foreground and background are differentiated using region-based and watershed approaches. Finally, a cellular neural network (CNN) is used to divide the picture into two classes: PCOS and non-PCOS.

Lv et al. [80] investigated an automated deep learning strategy for identifying PCOS based on scleral abnormalities. They used a collection of full-eye pictures from 721 Chinese females, 388 of whom had PCOS. The approach employed a promoted U-Net to segregate scleral and full-eye pictures, which were subsequently processed using a ResNet model to obtain deep features. A multi-instance classification model was then developed. To assess the effectiveness of their technique, they employed a range of outcome metrics, including area under the curve (AUC), classification accuracy, precision, recall, and the F1-score. The results indicated a precision for classification of 0.929 with a mean AUC of 0.979, suggesting the significant possible of deep learning in PCOS detection.

In this work, Barrera et al. [14] emphasized the significance of improving methodological quality in future AI/ML studies on PCOS and other disorders to ensure the validity of results. They recommended five critical strategies to increase the usefulness of AI/ML in detecting and managing PCOS:

1. Encourage collaboration among physicians, researchers, and computational biologists to capitalize on their various knowledge.
2. Create integrated registries for PCOS patients that include comprehensive data such as clinical, radiological (including pictures), and laboratory data, as well as standardized reference values.

3. Use standardized criteria for training machine learning models, and conduct rigorous training and validation experiments on PCOS patient datasets.
4. Evaluate the consistency of model performance over time, taking into account any alterations in the data used for model development.
5. Integrate population-based research by electronic health information to uncover risk features and enhancers of PCOS, hence improving understanding of the disorder.

In addition, they called for adding routinely cast-off biochemical tests, such as anti-Müllerian hormone (AMH), gonadal hormones, and insulin struggle indicators, into AI/ML algorithms to discover valid biomarkers for PCOS diagnosis. These methods are intended to boost the accuracy and reliability of AI/ML apps for PCOS diagnosis and treatment.

10.7 Lifestyle Modifications

A lack of activity combined with a diet rich in fried meals, processed meats, sugary snacks, and carbonated beverages can cause obesity and disturb insulin and hormone levels, leading to PCOS by overstimulating androgen receptors separate the ovaries. Changes in lifestyle such as regular exercise, a nutritious diet, and a reduction in dairy besides fast food consumption can help PCOS patients lose weight and recover their insulin sensitivity. However, these alterations sometimes produce only brief advantages, necessitating lifetime dedication for long-term weight loss [81].

For people who are severely obese, bariatric surgery is a possible option for long-term weight loss. Current National Institutes of Health standards promote weight loss surgery for persons having a BMI higher than 40 or those with a BMI better than 35 and major health problems. Because PCOS is connected with hormonal and endocrine difficulties, bariatric surgery has demonstrated significant reductions in symptoms and may even result in remission of the disorder [82, 83].

10.8 Conclusion

In conclusion, PCOS is a predominant hormonal condition in females with a variety of difficulties, including infertility and metabolic problems. While synthetic drugs are effective, their long-term usage is limited due to negative side effects. Herbal remedies are a viable alternative for treating problems such as hyperandrogenism and insulin sensitivity. Personalized advice may be adjusted to each patient's specific genetic composition, metabolic profile, and lifestyle variables by using the power of artificial intelligence and machine learning algorithms. This personalized strategy has tremendous promise for increasing therapeutic efficacy, reducing side effects, and improving overall patient outcomes. Further study into natural chemicals and herbs may improve PCOS therapy.

References

1. Ndefo UA, Eaton A, Green MR. Polycystic ovary syndrome: a review of treatment options with a focus on pharmacological approaches. Pharm Ther. 2013;38(6):336.
2. Bharathi RV, et al. An epidemiological survey: effect of predisposing factors for PCOS in Indian urban and rural population. Middle East Fertil Soc J. 2017;22(4):313–6.
3. Yadav K, Ghadge P, Langeh A, Kalbhare S, Phadtare P, Bhoite R. A review on herbal medicinal plant for treatment of polycystic ovarian syndrome (PCOS). Asian J Pharm Res Dev. 2020;8(4):83–7.
4. Liu J, et al. Measuring the global disease burden of polycystic ovary syndrome in 194 countries: Global Burden of Disease Study 2017. Hum Reprod. 2021;36(4):1108–19.
5. Abasian Z, Rostamzadeh A, Mohammadi M, Hosseini M, Rafieian-Kopaei M. A review on role of medicinal plants in polycystic ovarian syndrome: pathophysiology, neuroendocrine signaling, therapeutic status and future prospects. Middle East Fertil Soc J. 2018;23(4):255–62.
6. Zuo M, Liao G, Zhang W, Xu D, Lu J, Tang M, et al. Effects of exogenous adiponectin supplementation in early pregnant PCOS mice on the metabolic syndrome of adult female offspring. J Ovarian Res. 2021;14(1):1–12.
7. Begum MS, Areen S. Optimizing polycystic ovarian disorder (PCOD) treatment with personalized lifestyle and nutrition strategies. J Clin Med Res. 2023;2(cc):1–8. https://doi.org/10.46889/jcmr.2023.4306.
8. Szczuko M, Zapałowska-Chwyć M, Maciejewska D, Drozd A, Starczewski A, Stachowska E. Significant improvement selected mediators of inflammation in phenotypes of women with PCOS after reduction and low GI diet. Mediat Inflamm. 2017;2017:5489523.
9. Arentz S, Abbott J, Smith C. Herbal medicine for the management of polycystic ovary syndrome (PCOS). BMC Complement Altern Med. 2014;14:511–30.
10. Smith CA, Bateson DJ, Weisberg E. A survey describing the use of complementary therapies and medicines by women attending a family planning clinic. BMC Complement Altern Med. 2013;13:1–8.
11. Wei W, Zhao H, Wang A, Sui M, Liang K, Deng H, et al. A clinical study on the short-term effect of berberine in comparison to metformin on the metabolic characteristics of women with polycystic ovary syndrome. Eur J Endocrinol. 2012;166(1):99–105.
12. Choi RY, Coyner AS, Kalpathy-Cramer J, Chiang MF, Campbell JP. Introduction to machine learning, neural networks, and deep learning. Transl Vis Sci Technol. 2020;9(2):14.
13. Silva IS, Ferreira CN, Costa LBX, Sóter MO, Carvalho LML, de C. Albuquerque J, et al. Polycystic ovary syndrome: clinical and laboratory variables related to new phenotypes using machine-learning models. J Endocrinol Investig. 2022;45(3):497–505.
14. Barrera FJ, Brown ED, Rojo A, Obeso J, Plata H, Lincango EP, et al. Application of machine learning and artificial intelligence in the diagnosis and classification of polycystic ovarian syndrome: a systematic review. Front Endocrinol. 2023;14:1106625. https://doi.org/10.3389/fendo.2023.1106625.
15. Witchel SF, Oberfield SE, Peña AS. Polycystic ovary syndrome: pathophysiology, presentation, and treatment with emphasis on adolescent girls. J Endocr Soc. 2019;3(8):1545–73.
16. Soni T, Prabhakar PK. Pathophysiology of poly cystic ovarian syndrome. IntechOpen; 2022.
17. Fujibe Y, Baba T, Nagao S, Adachi S, Ikeda K, Morishita M, et al. Androgen potentiates the expression of FSH receptor and supports preantral follicle development in mice. J Ovarian Res. 2019;12:1–8.
18. Unluhizarci K, Karaca Z, Kelestimur F. Role of insulin and insulin resistance in androgen excess disorders. World J Diabetes. 2021;12(5):616.
19. Spritzer PM, Marchesan LB, Santos BR, Fighera TM. Hirsutism, normal androgens and diagnosis of PCOS. Diagnostics. 2022;12(8):1922.
20. Hill MA, Yang Y, Zhang L, Sun Z, Jia G, Parrish AR, Sowers JR. Insulin resistance, cardiovascular stiffening and cardiovascular disease. Metabolism. 2021;119:154766.
21. Gugusheff J, Ong Z, Muhlhausler B. The early origins of food preferences: targeting the critical windows of development. FASEB J. 2015;29:365.

22. Moran LJ, Pasquali R, Teede HJ, Hoeger KM, Norman RJ. Treatment of obesity in polycystic ovary syndrome: a position statement of the Androgen Excess and Polycystic Ovary Syndrome Society. Fertil Steril. 2009;92(6):1966–82.
23. Moran LJ, Grieger JA, Mishra GD, Teede HJ. The association of a Mediterranean-style diet pattern with polycystic ovary syndrome status in a community cohort study. Nutrients. 2015;7(10):8553–64.
24. Kiani AK, Donato K, Dhuli K, Stuppia L, Bertelli M. Dietary supplements for polycystic ovary syndrome. J Prev Med Hyg. 2022;63(2):E206–13. https://doi.org/10.15167/2421-4248/jpmh2022.63.2S3.2762.
25. Kiani AK, Paolacci S, Calogero AE, Cannarella R, Di Renzo GC, Gerli S, et al. From Myo-inositol to D-chiro-inositol molecular pathways. Eur Rev Med Pharmacol Sci. 2021;25(5):2390–402.
26. Facchinetti F, Espinola MSB, Dewailly D, Ozay AC, Prapas N, Vazquez-Levin M, et al. Breakthroughs in the use of inositols for assisted reproductive treatment (ART). Trends Endocrinol Metab. 2020;31(8):570–9.
27. Pacchiarotti A, Carlomagno G, Antonini G, Pacchiarotti A. Effect of myo-inositol and melatonin versus myo-inositol, in a randomized controlled trial, for improving in vitro fertilization of patients with polycystic ovarian syndrome. Gynecol Endocrinol. 2016;32(1):69–73.
28. Cirillo F, Catellani C, Lazzeroni P, Sartori C, Tridenti G, Vezzani C, et al. HMGB1 is increased in adolescents with polycystic ovary syndrome (PCOS) and decreases after treatment with MYO-inositol (MYO) in combination with alpha-lipoic acid (ALA). Gynecol Endocrinol. 2020;36(7):588–93.
29. Santamaria A, Di Benedetto A, Petrella E, Pintaudi B, Corrado F, D'Anna R, et al. Myo-inositol may prevent gestational diabetes onset in overweight women: a randomized, controlled trial. J Matern Fetal Neonatal Med. 2016;29(19):3234–7.
30. Abdelazeem B, Abbas KS, Shehata J, Baral N, Banour S, Hassan M. The effects of curcumin as dietary supplement for patients with polycystic ovary syndrome: an updated systematic review and meta-analysis of randomized clinical trials. Phytother Res. 2022;36(1):22–32.
31. Sohrevardi SM, Heydari B, Azarpazhooh MR, Teymourzadeh M, Simental-Mendía LE, Atkin SL, et al. Therapeutic effect of curcumin in women with polycystic ovary syndrome receiving metformin: a randomized controlled trial. Adv Exp Med Biol. 2021:1308:109–17.
32. Dennett CC, Simon J. The role of polycystic ovary syndrome in reproductive and metabolic health: overview and approaches for treatment. Diabetes Spectr. 2015;28(2):116–20.
33. Chien Y-J, Chang C-Y, Wu M-Y, Chen C-H, Horng Y-S, Wu H-C. Effects of curcumin on glycemic control and lipid profile in polycystic ovary syndrome: systematic review with meta-analysis and trial sequential analysis. Nutrients. 2021;13(2):684.
34. Gao XY, Liu Y, Lv Y, Huang T, Lu G, Liu HB, Zhao SG. Role of androgen receptor for reconsidering the 'true' polycystic ovarian morphology in PCOS. Sci Rep. 2020;10(1):8993.
35. Sahebkar A, Cicero AFG, Simental-Mendía LE, Aggarwal BB, Gupta SC. Curcumin downregulates human tumor necrosis factor-α levels: a systematic review and meta-analysis of randomized controlled trials. Pharmacol Res. 2016;107:234–42.
36. Wehr E, Trummer O, Giuliani A, Gruber H-J, Pieber TR, Obermayer-Pietsch B. Vitamin D-associated polymorphisms are related to insulin resistance and vitamin D deficiency in polycystic ovary syndrome. Eur J Endocrinol. 2011;164(5):741–9.
37. Filipe J, Bessa RJ, Reis M, Alves R, Póvoa P. Data-driven predictive energy optimization in a wastewater pumping station. Appl Energy. 2019;252:113423. https://doi.org/10.1016/j.apenergy.2019.113423.
38. Wdowiak A, Filip M. The effect of myo-inositol, vitamin D3 and melatonin on the oocyte quality and pregnancy in in vitro fertilization: a randomized prospective controlled trial. Eur Rev Med Pharmacol Sci. 2020;24(16):8529–36.
39. Pittas AG, Lau J, Hu FB, Dawson-Hughes B. The role of vitamin D and calcium in type 2 diabetes. A systematic review and meta-analysis. J Clin Endocrinol Metab. 2007;92(6):2017–29.

40. Lak TB, Hajshafiha M, Nanbakhsh F, Oshnouei S. N-acetyl cysteine in ovulation induction of PCOS women underwent intrauterine insemination: an RCT. Int J Reprod Biomed. 2017;15(4):203.
41. Shivani N, Anitha R, Rajeshkumar S, Lakshmi T, Sciences T, Chennai TS. Anti-inflammatory activity of nutmeg oleoresin mediated silver nanoparticles- an *in-vitro* study. Biomedicine. 2019;39(2):234–8.
42. Shirani M, Nouri M, Askari G. Effect of N-acetylcysteine supplementation on polycystic ovary syndrome (PCOS) in infertile women: a systematic review of clinical trials. Clin Excell. 2019;8(3):1–10.
43. Saito B, Nakashima H, Abe M, Murai S, Baba Y, Arai N, et al. Efficacy of palonosetron to prevent delayed nausea and vomiting in non-Hodgkin's lymphoma patients undergoing repeated cycles of the CHOP regimen. Support Care Cancer. 2018;26:269–74. https://doi.org/10.1007/s00520-017-3845-y.
44. Nordio M, Proietti E. The combined therapy with myo-inositol and D-chiro-inositol reduces the risk of metabolic disease in PCOS overweight patients compared to myo-inositol supplementation alone. Eur Rev Med Pharmacol Sci. 2012;16(5):575–81.
45. Nestler JE, Jakubowicz DJ, Reamer P, Gunn RD, Allan G. Ovulatory and metabolic effects of D-chiro-inositol in the polycystic ovary syndrome. N Engl J Med. 1999;340(17):1314–20.
46. Cicek N, Eryilmaz OG, Sarikaya E, Gulerman C, Genc Y. Vitamin E effect on controlled ovarian stimulation of unexplained infertile women. J Assist Reprod Genet. 2012;29(4):325–8. https://doi.org/10.1007/s10815-012-9714-1.
47. Amini M, Bahmani F, Foroozanfard F, Vahedpoor Z, Ghaderi A, Taghizadeh M, et al. Retracted article: The effects of fish oil omega-3 fatty acid supplementation on mental health parameters and metabolic status of patients with polycystic ovary syndrome: a randomized, double-blind, placebo-controlled trial. J Psychosom Obstet Gynaecol. 2024;45(1):1508282. https://doi.org/10.1080/0167482X.2018.1508282.
48. Rahmani E, Samimi M, Ebrahimi FA, Foroozanfard F, Ahmadi S, Rahimi M, et al. The effects of omega-3 fatty acids and vitamin E co-supplementation on gene expression of lipoprotein(a) and oxidized low-density lipoprotein, lipid profiles and biomarkers of oxidative stress in patients with polycystic ovary syndrome. Mol Cell Endocrinol. 2017;439:247–55. https://doi.org/10.1016/j.mce.2016.09.008.
49. Mirmasoumi G, Fazilati M, Foroozanfard F, Vahedpoor Z, Mahmoodi S, Taghizadeh M, et al. The effects of flaxseed oil omega-3 fatty acids supplementation on metabolic status of patients with polycystic ovary syndrome: a randomized, double-blind, placebo-controlled trial. Exp Clin Endocrinol diabetes. 2018;126(4):222–8. https://doi.org/10.1055/s-0043-119751.
50. Dubey P, Reddy S, Boyd S, Bracamontes C, Sanchez S, Chattopadhyay M, Dwivedi A. Effect of nutritional supplementation on oxidative stress and hormonal and lipid profiles in PCOS-affected females. Nutrients. 2021;13(9):2938. https://doi.org/10.3390/nu13092938.
51. Swiglo BA, Cosma M, Flynn DN, Kurtz DM, LaBella ML, Mullan RJ, et al. Antiandrogens for the treatment of hirsutism: a systematic review and metaanalyses of randomized controlled trials. J Clin Endocrinol Metab. 2008;93(4):1153–60.
52. Iqbal SM, Hussain L, Hussain M, Akram H, Asif M, Jamshed A, et al. Nephroprotective potential of a standardized extract of *Bambusa arundinacea*: *in vitro* and *in vivo* studies. ACS omega. 2022;7(21):18159–67.
53. Akbar S. Aloe vera (L.) Burm. f. (Asphodelaceae/Xanthorrhoeaceae) (Syns.: A. barbadensis Mill.; A. chinensis Steud. ex Baker; A. elongata Murray; A. vulgaris Lam.). In: Handbook of 200 medicinal plants: a comprehensive review of their traditional medical uses and scientific justifications. Springer; 2020. p. 187–206.
54. Mezzetti M, Minuti A, Bionaz M, Piccioli-Cappelli F, Trevisi E. Effects of Aloe arborescens whole plant homogenate on lipid metabolism, inflammatory conditions and liver function of dairy cows during the transition period. Animals. 2020;10(5):917.
55. Yagi A. Putative prophylaxes of Aloe vera for age-related diseases. J Gastroenterol Hepatol Res. 2015;4(1):1407–24.

56. Maharjan R, Nagar PS, Nampoothiri L. Effect of Aloe barbadensis Mill. formulation on letrozole-induced polycystic ovarian syndrome rat model. J Ayurveda Integr Med. 2010;1(4):273.
57. Hemayatkhah-Jahromi V, Rahmanian-Koushkaki M. Effect of hydro-alcoholic extract of Aloe vera L. on polycystic ovary syndrome in rat. KAUMS J. 2016;20(3):221–7.
58. Srivastava JK, Pandey M, Gupta S. Chamomile, a novel and selective COX-2 inhibitor with anti-inflammatory activity. Life Sci. 2009;85(19–20):663–9.
59. McKay DL, Blumberg JB. A review of the bioactivity and potential health benefits of peppermint tea (Mentha piperita L.). Phyther Res. 2006;20(8):619–33.
60. Farideh ZZ, Bagher M, Ashraf A, Akram A, Kazem M. Effects of chamomile extract on biochemical and clinical parameters in a rat model of polycystic ovary syndrome. J Reprod Infertil. 2010;11(3):169–74.
61. Singh G, Maurya S, DeLampasona MP, Catalan CAN. A comparison of chemical, antioxidant and antimicrobial studies of cinnamon leaf and bark volatile oils, oleoresins and their constituents. Food Chem Toxicol. 2007;45(9):1650–61.
62. Uslu GA, Gelen V, Uslu H, Özen H. Effects of *Cinnamomum cassia* extract on oxidative stress, immunreactivity of iNOS and impaired thoracic aortic reactivity induced by type II diabetes in rats. Braz J Pharm Sci. 2018;54(3):e17785.
63. Sheng X, Zhang Y, Gong Z, Huang C, Zang YQ. Improved insulin resistance and lipid metabolism by cinnamon extract through activation of peroxisome proliferator-activated receptors. PPAR Res. 2008;2008:581348.
64. Heshmati J, Sepidarkish M, Morvaridzadeh M, Farsi F, Tripathi N, Razavi M, Rezaeinejad M. The effect of cinnamon supplementation on glycemic control in women with polycystic ovary syndrome: a systematic review and meta-analysis. J Food Biochem. 2021;45(1):e13543.
65. Wang JG, Anderson RA, Graham III, GM, Chu MC, Sauer MV, Guarnaccia MM, Lobo RA. The effect of cinnamon extract on insulin resistance parameters in polycystic ovary syndrome: a pilot study. Fertil Steril. 2007;88(1):240–3.
66. Attele AS, Wu JA, Yuan C-S. Ginseng pharmacology: multiple constituents and multiple actions. Biochem Pharmacol. 1999;58(11):1685–93.
67. Andhalkar S, Chaware V, Redasani V. A review on medicinal plants of natural origin for treatment of polycystic ovarian syndrome (PCOS). Asian J Pharm Res Dev. 2021;9(3):76–81.
68. Ghavi F, Taghizadeh M, Taebi M, Abdolahian S. Effect of *Foeniculum vulgare* essence on symptoms of polycystic ovarian syndrome (PCOS): a randomized double-blind, Placebo-Controlled Trial. J Herb Med. 2019;17:100277.
69. Parandin R, Yousofvand N. In utero and lactational effects of aqueous *Foeniculum vulgare* (fennel) seed extract on puberty timing, estrus cycle and sexual behavior in mice. J Arak Uni Med Sci. 2018;20:1–12.
70. Meena DM, Sharma DM, Dhakar A, Singh C, Sharma L, Purvia RP. Role of *Foeniculum vulgare* in PCOS—a review article. World J Pharm Res. 2019;8:344–50.
71. Fozalaee SS, Farokhi F, Khaneshi F. The effect of metformin and aqueous extract *Foeniculum vulgare* (fennel) on endometrial histomorphometry and the level of steroid hormones in rats with polycystic ovary syndrome. Qom Univ Med Sci J. 2015;8(5 Suppl):12–9.
72. Barazesh F, Mirzaei A, Abbasian Z, Ghavami Zadeh M. The effect of hydroalcoholic extract of *Glycyrrhizaglabra L.* (licorice) root on serum level of glucose, triglyceride and cholesterol in polycystic ovary syndrome induced by letrozole in rats. Armaghane Danesh. 2016;21(2):148–59.
73. Batiha GES, Alkazmi LM, Wasef LG, Beshbishy AM, Nadwa EH, Rashwan EK. *Syzygium aromaticum* L. (myrtaceae): traditional uses, bioactive chemical constituents, pharmacological and toxicological activities. Biomol Ther. 2020;10(2) https://doi.org/10.3390/biom10020202.
74. Hande AH, Chaudhary MS, Gadbail AR, Zade PR, Gawande MN, Patil SK. Role of hypoxia in malignant transformation of oral submucous fibrosis. J Datta Meghe Inst Med Sci Univ. 2018;13(1):38–43. https://doi.org/10.4103/jdmimsu.jdmimsu.

75. Chen T, Zhang W, Good S, Zhou KS, Comaniciu D. Automatic ovarian follicle quantification from 3D ultrasound data using global/local context with database guided segmentation. In: 2009 IEEE 12th International Conference on computer vision. IEEE; 2009. p. 795–802.
76. Deepika V. Applications of artificial intelligence techniques in polycystic ovarian syndrome diagnosis. J Adv Res Technol Manag Sci. 2019;1(3):59–63.
Al-Qahtani WH, Dinakarkumar Y, Arokiyaraj S, Saravanakumar V, Rajabathar JR, Arjun K, et al. Phyto-chemical and biological activity of *Myristica fragrans*, an ayurvedic medicinal plant in southern India and its ingredient analysis. Saudi J Biol Sci. 2022;29(5):3815–21. https://doi.org/10.1016/j.sjbs.2022.02.043.
77. Faghih RT, Styer AK, Brown EN. Automated ovarian follicular monitoring: A novel real-time approach. In: 2017 39th Annual International Conference of the IEEE Engineering in Medicine and Biology Society (EMBC). IEEE; 2017. p. 632–5.
78. Soni P, Vashisht S. Image segmentation for detecting polycystic ovarian disease using deep neural networks. Int J Comput Sci Eng. 2019;7(3):534–7.
79. Lv W, Song Y, Fu R, Lin X, Su Y, Jin X, et al. Deep learning algorithm for automated detection of polycystic ovary syndrome using scleral images. Front Endocrinol. 2022;12:789878.
80. Zeng LH, Rana S, Hussain L, Asif M, Mehmood MH, Imran I, et al. Polycystic ovary syndrome: a disorder of reproductive age, its pathogenesis, and a discussion on the emerging role of herbal remedies. Front Pharmacol. 2022;13:874914. https://doi.org/10.3389/fphar.2022.874914.
81. Cowan S, Lim S, Alycia C, Pirotta S, Thomson R, Gibson-Helm M, et al. Lifestyle management in polycystic ovary syndrome—beyond diet and physical activity. BMC Endocr Disord. 2023;23(1):14. https://doi.org/10.1186/s12902-022-01208-y.
82. Hoeger KM. Role of lifestyle modification in the management of polycystic ovary syndrome. Best Pract Res Clin Endocrinol Metab. 2006;20(2):293–310.

Ethical Aspects of AI Nutrition: Discussion of Ethical Considerations Related to AI-Based Nutritional Guidance in Terms of Privacy, Data Security, and Potential Biases

11

Kanchan Naithani, Y. P. Raiwani, Shrikant Tiwari, and Alok Singh Chauhan

11.1 Introduction: AI in Nutritional Guidance

The intersection of artificial intelligence (AI) and nutritional guidance has heralded a transformative era in healthcare, offering personalized and data-driven approaches to dietary recommendations. Harnessing the power of machine learning algorithms, AI systems analyze vast datasets encompassing individual health metrics, dietary habits, and genetic information. This synthesis of information allows for the tailoring of nutritional advice to meet the unique needs of individuals, promising more effective and targeted health outcomes [1].

However, as AI penetrates the nutritional landscape, ethical considerations emerge as pivotal factors in shaping the responsible deployment of these technologies. This book chapter sets the stage for a comprehensive exploration of the ethical aspects surrounding AI in nutritional guidance, focusing on privacy, data security, and the potential biases inherent in these systems.

K. Naithani (✉) · Y. P. Raiwani
Department of Computer Science and Engineering, Hemvati Nandan Bahuguna Garhwal University (A Central University), Srinagar, Uttarakhand, India

S. Tiwari · A. S. Chauhan
School of Computing Science and Engineering, Galgotias University, Greater Noida, Uttar Pradesh, India

R. Kumar et al. (eds.), *AI-Based Nutritional Intervention in Polycystic Ovary Syndrome (PCOS)*, https://doi.org/10.1007/978-981-96-2120-0_11

11.1.1 Technical Advancements in AI for Nutritional Guidance Systems

The integration of artificial intelligence into nutritional guidance systems as shown in Fig. 11.1 has been propelled by significant technical advancements. Machine learning algorithms, a subset of AI, have played a pivotal role in transforming the landscape of personalized nutrition. The advent of sophisticated models, such as deep learning and neural networks, has empowered these systems to analyze vast and diverse datasets with unprecedented accuracy [2].

One key technical breakthrough is the ability of AI to process intricate biological and health-related data, including genetic information, metabolic markers, and individual dietary patterns. This allows for a more nuanced understanding of each user's unique nutritional requirements, moving beyond one-size-fits-all recommendations. Furthermore, natural language processing (NLP) capabilities enable AI to interpret and contextualize complex dietary information from sources such as food diaries, enabling more precise and personalized guidance. AI algorithms can adapt and learn from user feedback, continuously refining their recommendations based on real-time data, fostering a dynamic and evolving approach to nutritional support [3, 4].

The seamless integration of AI into wearable devices and mobile applications as shown in Fig. 11.2 has also democratized access to personalized nutritional guidance. These technologies facilitate real-time monitoring of dietary habits, physical activity, and health metrics, creating a feedback loop that enhances the accuracy of AI-driven recommendations. In essence, the technical prowess of AI, marked by advancements in machine learning, NLP, and user-centric interfaces, has paved the way for a new era in nutritional guidance. As these technologies continue to evolve,

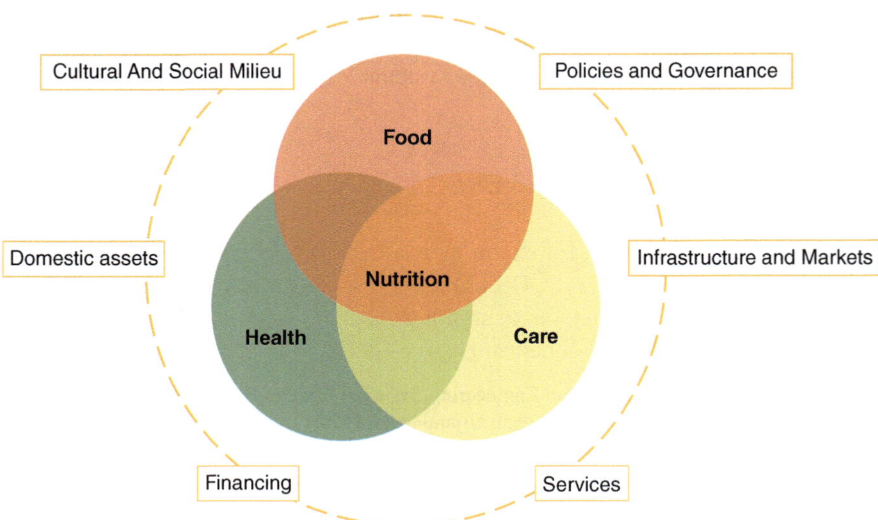

Fig. 11.1 AI into nutritional guidance systems

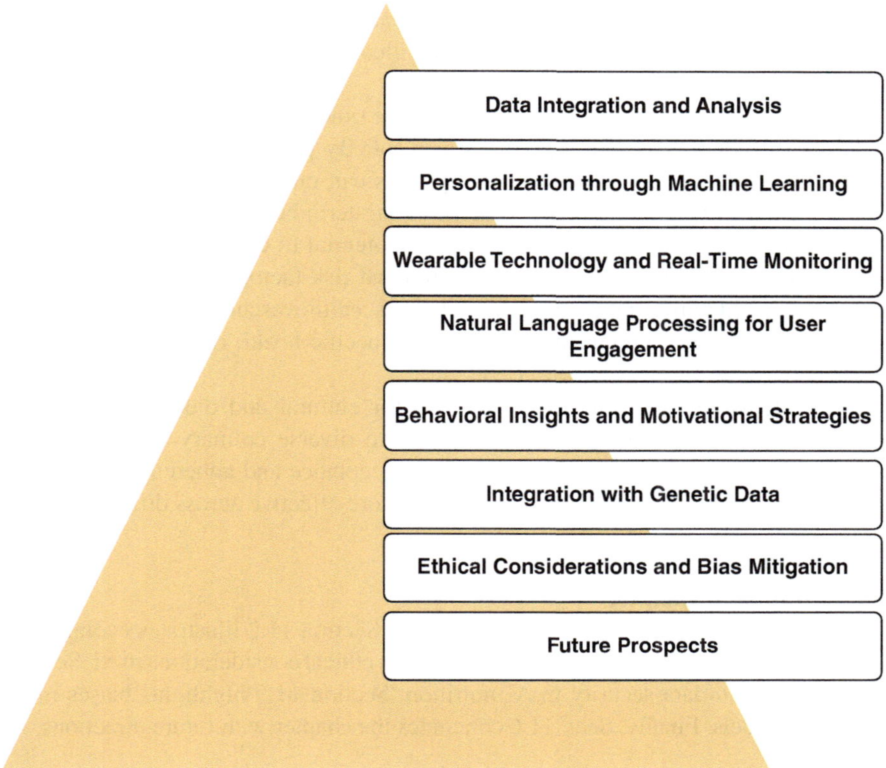

Fig. 11.2 Evolution of AI in nutritional guidance

the potential for more precise, accessible, and individualized nutrition interventions holds promise for improving public health outcomes on a global scale [5, 6].

11.1.2 Potential Benefits of AI-Driven Nutritional Guidance in Promoting Healthier Dietary Practices

AI-driven nutritional guidance holds significant promise in promoting healthier dietary practices, offering a range of potential benefits that can positively impact individual well-being and public health.

AI leverages advanced algorithms to analyze diverse datasets, including personal health metrics, genetic information, and dietary habits. This enables the creation of highly personalized nutritional recommendations, tailored to meet the unique needs of individuals. This level of precision ensures that dietary advice aligns with specific health goals, considering factors such as allergies, sensitivities, and lifestyle choices.

The integration of AI into mobile applications and wearable devices provides users with accessible and convenient tools for monitoring and improving their dietary practices. Real-time tracking of nutritional intake, coupled with instant feedback and recommendations, empowers individuals to make healthier choices on a day-to-day basis [7].

AI algorithms can analyze user behavior over time, offering insights into dietary patterns and identifying areas for improvement. By providing personalized feedback and positive reinforcement, these systems can motivate individuals to adopt and sustain healthier eating habits, fostering long-term behavioral change.

Personalized nutritional guidance has the potential to contribute to the prevention of chronic diseases by addressing individual risk factors. AI can identify patterns associated with conditions such as diabetes, cardiovascular disease, or obesity, offering targeted recommendations to reduce specific health risks through dietary modifications [8, 9].

AI systems can be designed to account for cultural and dietary preferences, ensuring that recommendations are sensitive to diverse culinary traditions. This adaptability enhances the likelihood of user acceptance and adherence to the suggested dietary changes, making the guidance more effective across different demographic groups.

Organization of Chapter

The rest of the chapter is organized as follows: Section 11.2 illustrates evolution of AI in nutritional guidance. Section 11.3 discusses ethical considerations in AI. Section 11.4 focuses on data security in AI nutrition. Section 11.5 highlights biases in AI nutrition models. Finally, Sect. 11.6 concludes the chapter with future directions.

11.2 Evolution of AI in Nutritional Guidance

The evolution of artificial intelligence (AI) in nutritional guidance represents a dynamic journey marked by technological advancements and a growing understanding of the intricate relationship between diet and health. Over the years, several key milestones as shown in Fig. 11.2 have shaped the progression of AI applications in this field [10, 11]:

(a) **Data Integration and Analysis**: Early stages of AI in nutritional guidance involved the integration of diverse datasets, including nutritional information, health records, and lifestyle factors. Basic algorithms were employed to analyze this data, providing generalized dietary recommendations.
(b) **Personalization Through Machine Learning**: As machine learning algorithms gained sophistication, the focus shifted toward personalized nutrition. AI began to factor in individual variations, such as genetics, metabolic rates, and personal preferences, leading to more tailored dietary advice. This marked a significant leap from one-size-fits-all approaches.
(c) **Wearable Technology and Real-Time Monitoring**: The integration of AI into wearable devices revolutionized nutritional guidance by enabling real-time

monitoring of dietary habits. Users could track their nutritional intake, physical activity, and health metrics, allowing AI algorithms to offer instantaneous feedback and personalized suggestions.

(d) **Natural Language Processing for User Engagement**: The incorporation of natural language processing (NLP) enhanced user engagement with AI-driven nutritional guidance. Interactive interfaces and chatbots equipped with NLP capabilities enabled users to communicate more intuitively with the system, fostering a better understanding of individual needs and preferences.

(e) **Behavioral Insights and Motivational Strategies**: Advanced AI algorithms started incorporating behavioral science principles to understand and influence user habits. By providing insights into dietary patterns and employing motivational strategies, AI became a powerful tool for encouraging positive behavior change and long-term adherence to healthier lifestyles.

(f) **Integration with Genetic Data**: The inclusion of genetic data in AI models further refined personalized nutritional guidance. Analyzing genetic information allowed AI to predict individual responses to specific dietary components, offering insights into optimal nutritional choices based on an individual's genetic predispositions.

(g) **Ethical Considerations and Bias Mitigation**: The evolving landscape of AI in nutritional guidance brought attention to ethical considerations, including privacy, data security, and biases. Ongoing efforts have been made to address these concerns through transparent algorithms, robust security measures, and continuous monitoring to mitigate biases in recommendations.

(h) **Future Prospects**: The future of AI in nutritional guidance holds the promise of even greater integration with emerging technologies, such as blockchain for enhanced data security and explainable AI to improve transparency. As research progresses and technological capabilities expand, AI is poised to play an increasingly pivotal role in shaping personalized, effective, and ethical nutritional guidance for individuals worldwide.

The evolution of AI in nutritional guidance reflects a transformative journey from generalized recommendations to highly personalized, technology-driven solutions. This trajectory continues to unfold, with ongoing innovations poised to further refine and optimize the intersection of AI and nutrition for improved health outcomes.

11.2.1 Examine the Evolution of Machine Learning Algorithms Specifically Tailored for Nutritional Analysis

The evolution of machine learning algorithms as tailored for nutritional analysis has been a remarkable journey characterized by continuous refinement and adaptation to the complexities of dietary data. Key milestones in this evolution have significantly enhanced the precision and scope of nutritional analysis [12]:

(a) **Early Rule-Based Systems**: In the initial stages, rule-based systems were employed to interpret nutritional data. These systems relied on predefined rules and heuristics to categorize foods and calculate nutritional content. While useful, they lacked the adaptability and learning capabilities crucial for handling the intricacies of diverse dietary patterns.
(b) **Transition to Statistical Models**: The progression toward statistical models marked a shift in nutritional analysis. Machine learning algorithms, particularly linear regression and clustering models, were introduced to uncover patterns and relationships within large datasets. These statistical approaches allowed for more nuanced insights into the nutritional composition of foods and dietary habits.
(c) **Emergence of Feature Engineering**: As machine learning advanced, the focus shifted toward feature engineering, where algorithms could automatically identify relevant features in nutritional datasets. This enabled the extraction of meaningful patterns and relationships, enhancing the accuracy of nutritional analysis by considering a broader set of variables.
(d) **Integration of Neural Networks**: The integration of neural networks, especially deep learning architectures, revolutionized nutritional analysis. Neural networks, with their ability to learn hierarchical representations, proved effective in handling complex and high-dimensional nutritional data. This facilitated more accurate predictions and the discovery of intricate relationships between different dietary components.
(e) **Personalized Nutrition Through Recommender Systems**: Tailoring nutritional recommendations to individual preferences and requirements became a priority with the advent of recommender systems. Machine learning algorithms began to leverage user-specific data, including dietary preferences, health goals, and cultural considerations, to provide personalized nutritional guidance.
(f) **Integration of Natural Language Processing (NLP)**: The incorporation of natural language processing into machine learning algorithms enhanced their ability to analyze unstructured data, such as textual information from food diaries and recipes. NLP enabled algorithms to understand and interpret user-generated content, contributing to more comprehensive and context-aware nutritional analysis.
(g) **Real-Time Monitoring and IoT Integration**: The evolution of machine learning algorithms parallel to the increasing adoption of real-time monitoring is facilitated by its integration with the Internet of Things (IoT) devices and wearables. This facilitated continuous data collection, enabling algorithms to adapt and provide instant feedback on dietary habits, fostering a more dynamic approach to nutritional analysis.
(h) **Advances in Explainable AI (XAI)**: The ongoing evolution of machine learning algorithms in nutritional analysis includes a focus on explainability. As ethical considerations gain prominence, efforts are directed toward developing models that provide clear and interpretable insights, ensuring transparency in how recommendations are generated.

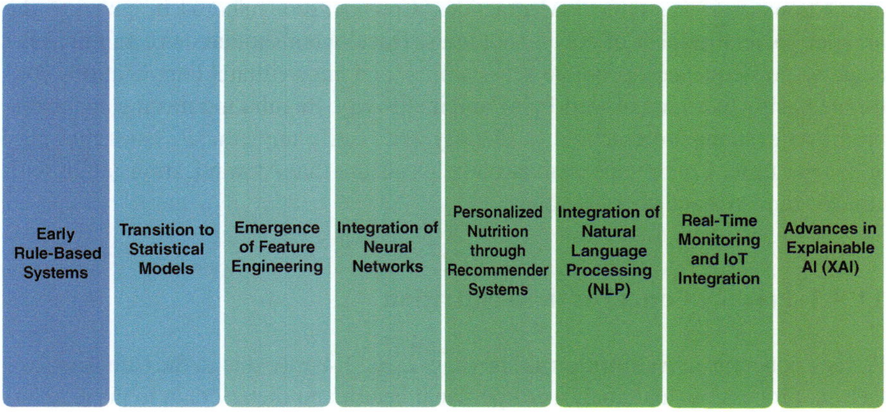

Fig. 11.3 Evolution of machine learning algorithms for nutritional analysis

The evolution of machine learning algorithms for nutritional analysis as shown in Fig. 11.3 showcases a progression from rule-based systems to sophisticated, adaptive models capable of handling diverse and personalized dietary data. This trajectory continues to evolve, with ongoing innovations aimed at further enhancing the accuracy, personalization, and ethical considerations of AI-driven nutritional analysis.

11.3 Ethical Considerations in AI

Ethical considerations in artificial intelligence (AI) have become paramount as AI technologies increasingly permeate various aspects of society. These considerations encompass a range of principles and guidelines aimed at ensuring responsible and fair deployment of AI systems. Ensuring fairness in AI systems is crucial to prevent biases that may lead to discriminatory outcomes. Developers must actively address biases in training data and algorithms to avoid perpetuating or exacerbating existing social inequalities. AI often relies on vast amounts of data for training and decision-making. Protecting individuals' privacy is paramount, necessitating robust data protection measures, informed consent, and transparent data usage policies to prevent unauthorized access or misuse.

Establishing clear lines of accountability is essential in AI development and deployment. Developers, organizations, and users must be aware of their respective responsibilities to mitigate risks and address any unintended consequences of AI applications. AI systems should be designed with security in mind to prevent vulnerabilities and potential exploitation. Ensuring the robustness of AI technologies is crucial to prevent malicious uses or unintended consequences that may compromise safety and well-being. Users interacting with AI systems should be provided with clear information about how their data will be used and have the ability to provide informed consent. Empowering users with control over their data and AI interactions promotes ethical AI practices. Considerations should be given to the broader societal impact of AI technologies. Developers should strive to minimize negative consequences, promote accessibility, and ensure that AI applications contribute positively to social well-being and inclusivity. Regular monitoring and auditing of AI systems are essential to identify and rectify any ethical issues that may arise over time. Continuous evaluation helps ensure that AI applications align with ethical standards and societal values.

11.3.1 Privacy Concerns in AI Nutrition

Privacy concerns in AI nutrition as shown in Fig. 11.4 arise due to the extensive collection, processing, and analysis of personal health and dietary data to provide tailored recommendations. The intersection of AI and nutrition, while promising for personalized guidance, necessitates careful consideration of the following privacy-related challenges [13]:

(a) **Sensitivity of Health Data**: AI nutrition systems often require access to sensitive health information, including medical history, dietary habits, and genetic data. The compilation and analysis of such personal health data raise worries about potential misuse or unauthorized access highlighting the importance of strong privacy safeguards.
(b) **Informed Consent and User Awareness**: Obtaining informed consent from users is a critical aspect of privacy protection. Users should be fully aware of how their data will be used, the purpose of AI-driven nutritional analysis, and

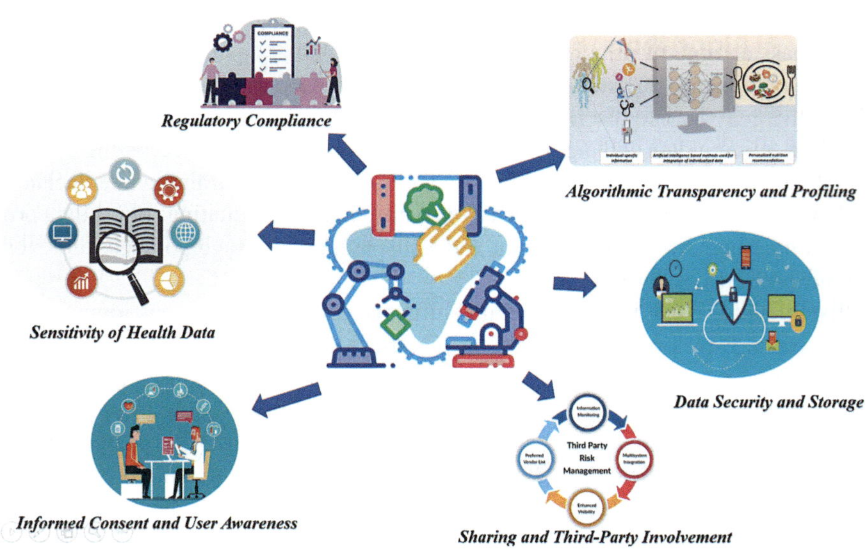

Fig. 11.4 Privacy concerns in AI nutrition

the extent to which their information will be shared. Transparent communication is essential to empower users to make informed decisions about participating in AI nutrition programs.

(c) **Data Security and Storage**: The storage and security of personal health and dietary data present significant privacy challenges. Ensuring secure data storage, transmission, and processing is essential to prevent unauthorized access, data breaches, or cyberattacks. Robust encryption and adherence to data security best practices are imperative to safeguard user privacy.

(d) **Sharing and Third-Party Involvement**: Collaborations or data sharing with third-party entities, such as healthcare providers or food suppliers, may introduce additional privacy risks. It is crucial to establish clear guidelines and limitations on data sharing, ensuring that users have control over the dissemination of their health information and that it aligns with ethical standards and legal requirements.

(e) **Algorithmic Transparency and Profiling**: The opacity of AI algorithms can lead to concerns about profiling and unintended consequences. Users may worry about how their data is used to create personalized profiles and whether these profiles can be misused. Promoting algorithmic transparency and explaining how profiles are generated can help address these concerns and build user trust.

(f) **Regulatory Compliance**: Adherence to privacy regulations and standards, such as GDPR in Europe or HIPAA in the United States, is crucial for AI nutrition systems. Compliance ensures that user rights are protected and privacy measures align with legal requirements, minimizing the risk of regulatory penalties and safeguarding user privacy.

As the integration of AI in nutrition continues to evolve, it is essential to prioritize privacy considerations to build and maintain user trust. Striking a balance between the benefits of personalized nutritional guidance and robust privacy protections is key to fostering responsible and ethical AI deployment in the realm of nutrition.

11.3.2 Differential Privacy and Federated Learning as Technical Solutions for Preserving User Privacy in AI-Based Nutritional Guidance

Differential privacy and federated learning are robust technical solutions that play a pivotal role in preserving user privacy in AI-based nutritional guidance applications. These techniques address concerns related to the confidentiality and protection of sensitive personal dietary information, ensuring that individuals can benefit from personalized recommendations without compromising their privacy [14, 15].

Differential privacy is a privacy-preserving mechanism that introduces controlled noise to individual data points, preventing the extraction of specific information about any single user. In the context of AI-based nutritional guidance, differential privacy allows for the secure aggregation of dietary data from multiple users. The noise injected into individual data points ensures that the contribution of any single user does not significantly impact the overall analysis, protecting their privacy. Users can have confidence that their dietary information is included in the overall analysis without being individually identifiable. Differential privacy provides a strong privacy guarantee, assuring users that their specific dietary choices remain confidential during the analysis process. AI models trained using differentially private techniques strike a balance between personalization and privacy. Users receive tailored nutritional guidance without the risk of their specific dietary information being exposed, fostering trust in the AI system [16].

Federated learning is a decentralized machine learning approach where the model is trained across multiple devices or servers without the need for centralizing raw data. In AI-based nutritional guidance, federated learning offers distinctive advantages. Individual user data remains on their devices, and the AI model is trained collaboratively across these devices. This decentralized approach ensures that personal dietary information does not leave the user's device, enhancing privacy. During the federated learning process, only model updates, rather than raw data, are shared among devices. This minimizes the risk of exposing personal dietary details and ensures that users contribute to model improvement without compromising their privacy. Federated learning enables the creation of personalized AI models for each user without centralizing their data. This adaptive personalization ensures that users receive tailored nutritional guidance based on their dietary habits while maintaining the privacy of their information [17].

When used together, differential privacy and federated learning offer a powerful combination for preserving user privacy in AI-based nutritional guidance. Differential privacy provides robust protection for individual data points, while federated learning ensures that raw data remains decentralized. The combination of these techniques adds an extra layer of security, reinforcing user privacy throughout the entire process. Users benefit from personalized nutritional guidance tailored to their dietary needs without compromising the confidentiality of their specific dietary choices. This ensures that individuals can make informed decisions about their nutrition without sacrificing their privacy.

The differential privacy and federated learning are instrumental in addressing privacy concerns in AI-based nutritional guidance. By incorporating these techniques, developers can create systems that provide personalized recommendations while upholding the highest standards of user privacy, fostering trust and user acceptance in the AI-driven nutritional guidance landscape.

11.4 Data Security in AI Nutrition

Data security is a critical aspect of AI applications in nutrition, where the processing and analysis of sensitive health and dietary data are central to providing personalized recommendations. Ensuring robust data security measures is imperative to safeguard individuals' privacy and maintain trust in AI nutrition systems [18]. The key considerations for data security in AI nutrition comprise of implementing strong encryption protocols that ensures that data, both in transit and at rest, remains secure. End-to-end encryption protects user data during transmission between devices and servers, while data stored in databases should be encrypted to prevent unauthorized access [19]. Then utilizing secure and compliant data storage solutions is crucial. Access controls, encryption, and regular security audits should be applied to databases storing health and dietary information. Compliance with industry standards and regulations, such as HIPAA for healthcare data, is essential. Implementation of robust authentication mechanisms to ensure that only authorized personnel have access to sensitive AI nutrition data plays a major role in data security in AI nutrition. Multifactor authentication adds an extra layer of security. Authorization protocols should restrict access based on roles, granting permissions only to those who require specific data for their responsibilities.

Conducting regular security audits and implementing continuous monitoring systems help detect and address potential vulnerabilities promptly. Automated tools and manual reviews should be employed to identify unusual patterns or potential security threats in real time—adopting a principle of data minimization by collecting only the necessary information for AI nutrition analysis. Reducing the amount of stored data mitigates the impact of a potential breach and aligns with privacy best practices. If AI nutrition systems integrate with external applications or data sources, ensure that APIs (application programming interfaces) and integrations follow secure coding practices. This includes validating input data, securing communication channels, and regularly updating API security measures. Keeping all software components, including operating systems, databases, and AI frameworks, up-to-date with the latest security patches is essential. Regular updates help address known vulnerabilities and enhance the overall security posture of AI nutrition systems [20].

Training employees involved in handling AI nutrition data on security best practices and raising awareness about potential security risks are another key considerations in establishing clear guidelines for handling sensitive data and conducting regular training sessions to keep staff informed about evolving cybersecurity threats.

Integrating privacy and security measures from the inception of AI nutrition system development lays a foundation for data security in AI nutrition. By adopting a privacy-by-design approach, developers can proactively address potential security risks and ensure that user data is protected throughout the system's life cycle—adhering to relevant data protection regulations, such as GDPR, HIPAA, or other regional and industry-specific standards. Compliance ensures that AI nutrition systems meet legal requirements for the protection of user data and avoids potential legal consequences [21].

By implementing a comprehensive data security strategy encompassing these considerations, developers and organizations can create AI nutrition systems that not only deliver personalized and accurate recommendations but also prioritize the privacy and security of user health and dietary data.

By adopting these best practices and technologies, health technology systems can significantly enhance data security, protecting patient information and maintaining the integrity of healthcare processes. Regularly updating security measures and staying informed about emerging threats are essential components of a robust and proactive security strategy.

11.5 Biases in AI Nutrition Models

Biases in AI nutrition models represent a significant challenge that can impact the accuracy, fairness, and effectiveness of personalized dietary recommendations. These biases can arise from various sources, including the data used for model training, algorithmic design, and societal preconceptions. Understanding and addressing biases in AI nutrition models are crucial for ensuring equitable and reliable outcomes [22].

Biases often stem from the data used to train AI nutrition models. If the training dataset is not diverse and representative of various demographics, cultural backgrounds, and dietary habits, the model may develop biases favoring certain groups while neglecting others [23]. Dataset biases can perpetuate existing health disparities and limit the applicability of dietary recommendations across diverse populations.

AI nutrition models might exhibit biases related to cultural preferences and regional dietary habits. Cultural variations in food choices, preparation methods, and nutritional priorities may not be adequately captured in models trained on data biased toward specific cultural norms. This can result in recommendations that are less relevant or appropriate for individuals from different cultural backgrounds.

Socioeconomic factors influence dietary choices, accessibility to certain foods, and lifestyle behaviors. If AI nutrition models are trained on data that primarily represents certain socioeconomic groups, the recommendations may not be suitable for individuals with different economic backgrounds. This can exacerbate health disparities related to nutrition and well-being.

AI nutrition models may inadvertently develop biases related to prevalent health conditions in the training data. For example, if the dataset is skewed toward individuals with specific health issues, the model might provide recommendations that prioritize those health concerns, potentially neglecting preventive or holistic approaches to nutrition [24]. AI models may exhibit biases based on the representation of certain dietary preferences in the training data. If the dataset disproportionately includes or excludes specific dietary trends, the model may not provide balanced and unbiased recommendations, potentially favoring or discouraging certain eating patterns. Gender-related biases can emerge if the training data reflects gender-based dietary stereotypes or if the model is not adequately designed to account for diverse dietary needs across genders. Biases may lead to recommendations that are not inclusive or considerate of varying nutritional requirements. Biases can be embedded in the algorithms themselves. If the algorithmic design favors certain features or attributes over others, it may inadvertently introduce biases into the decision-making process. Additionally, biases may be present in the selection of features that influence dietary recommendations. Biases in AI nutrition models may arise from the limited diversity in research studies that inform the development of dietary guidelines. If studies predominantly include specific demographics, the resulting recommendations may not be applicable or beneficial for individuals with different characteristics.

11.5.1 Algorithm Transparency and Explainability

Algorithm transparency and explainability are critical aspects of responsible AI development, particularly in applications like nutritional guidance, where the recommendations directly impact individuals' health and well-being. Ensuring that AI algorithms are transparent and explainable enhances user trust, facilitates accountability, and allows users and stakeholders to understand the reasoning behind the model's decisions [25]. Here is an exploration of the importance of algorithm transparency and explainability in the context of AI nutritional guidance:

(a) **User Trust and Acceptance**

Importance: Transparent and explainable algorithms foster user trust by providing insight into how recommendations are generated. Users are more likely to accept and follow advice when they understand the underlying processes, leading to increased engagement and positive outcomes.

Application in Nutrition Models: In AI nutritional guidance, users are more likely to adopt dietary recommendations if they can comprehend why certain suggestions are made. Transparency assures users that the model considers their unique dietary preferences, health conditions, and cultural factors.

(b) **Accountability and Ethical Considerations**

Importance: Transparency is essential for holding developers and organizations accountable for the performance and impact of AI algorithms. It allows stakeholders to identify and rectify biases, errors, or ethical concerns that may arise during the algorithm's life cycle.

Application in Nutrition Models: Accountability is crucial in nutritional guidance as biased or inaccurate recommendations may have significant health implications. Transparent algorithms enable continuous scrutiny and adjustment to ensure ethical, unbiased, and culturally sensitive dietary advice.

(c) **User Empowerment and Informed Decision-Making**

Importance: Explainable algorithms empower users to make informed decisions about their health. When users understand the factors influencing recommendations, they are better equipped to assess and adjust their dietary choices according to their preferences and values.

Application in Nutrition Models: In the realm of nutrition, users benefit from understanding why certain foods are recommended or discouraged. Transparent explanations empower users to make dietary choices aligned with their health goals and cultural or personal preferences.

(d) **Identification and Mitigation of Biases**

Importance: Transparent algorithms facilitate the identification of biases in the training data or algorithmic decision-making processes. This transparency is essential for mitigating biases and ensuring that recommendations are fair and unbiased across diverse demographic groups.

Application in Nutrition Models: Identifying and mitigating biases in nutritional guidance are crucial for providing equitable recommendations. Transparent models enable developers to address biases related to cultural, socioeconomic, or health factors, promoting inclusivity.

(e) **Compliance with Regulations and Standards**

Importance: Many regulations, such as GDPR and industry-specific standards, emphasize the need for transparency in AI systems. Compliance with these standards is critical to protect user privacy, prevent discrimination, and adhere to ethical guidelines.

Application in Nutrition Models: Transparency is essential for compliance with regulations in the healthcare and nutrition domains. Clearly explaining how user data is used and ensuring fairness in recommendations help meet legal and ethical obligations.

(f) **Building User Confidence**

Importance: Transparent algorithms build user confidence in the technology. When users have visibility into the decision-making process, they are more likely to trust and rely on the AI system for personalized guidance.

Application in Nutrition Models: Building confidence in nutritional guidance models is vital for user engagement. Transparent explanations assure users that the model considers their individual characteristics, making the recommendations more trustworthy and user-friendly.

(g) **Educational Value**

Importance: Algorithm transparency provides educational value by helping users understand the principles of nutrition and health. Users can gain insights into the relationships between various dietary factors and their impact on well-being.

Application in Nutrition Models: Transparent explanations in nutritional guidance models serve as educational tools, fostering a deeper understanding of nutrition principles. Users can learn about the nutritional benefits and potential drawbacks of different dietary choices.

(h) **Iterative Model Improvement**

Importance: Transparency facilitates iterative model improvement by allowing developers to analyze model performance and user feedback. Understanding how the model behaves in real-world scenarios enables continuous refinement and enhancement.

Application in Nutrition Models: In nutritional guidance, transparent models support ongoing improvements based on user feedback, emerging nutritional research, and changing dietary guidelines. This iterative approach ensures the model remains relevant and effective over time.

Algorithm transparency and explainability are essential components of responsible AI deployment, particularly in applications like nutritional guidance where user health is at stake. Prioritizing these aspects not only enhances user trust and acceptance but also enables developers to address biases, promote accountability, and continuously improve the model's performance.

11.5.2 Explore Technical Methodologies for Algorithm Transparency

Exploring technical methodologies for algorithm transparency is crucial in building trust and understanding the decision-making processes of complex AI models. Model interpretability techniques, such as LIME (local interpretable model-agnostic explanations), offer effective ways to make machine learning models more transparent and explainable [26]. Here is an exploration of various technical methodologies for algorithm transparency, with a focus on model interpretability techniques like LIME shown in Table 11.1.

Incorporating these technical methodologies, especially model interpretability techniques like LIME, SHAP, and others, enhances the transparency of AI models in nutritional guidance. These approaches empower users to comprehend the decision-making process and make informed choices based on personalized and explainable recommendations.

11.5.3 Responsible Deployment of AI in Nutrition

The responsible deployment of AI in nutrition is paramount to ensuring the ethical, accurate, and user-centric utilization of technology in promoting health and well-being. As AI-driven nutritional guidance systems become increasingly prevalent, it is essential to address key considerations to mitigate potential risks and maximize the positive impact on individuals and communities [27]. Here is a comprehensive overview of the principles and practices for the responsible deployment of AI in nutrition:

(a) **Ethical Considerations**

User Autonomy and Informed Consent: Prioritize user autonomy by ensuring individuals have the right to control their personal dietary information and receive transparent information about how AI algorithms will be used to provide nutritional guidance.

Fairness and Equity: Design AI systems to be unbiased and avoid perpetuating existing health disparities. Consider diverse demographic factors to ensure that nutritional recommendations are fair, equitable, and inclusive of various cultural, socioeconomic, and health contexts.

Privacy Protection: Implement robust privacy measures to safeguard sensitive dietary and health information. Adhere to data protection regulations and provide clear information about data collection, storage, and usage practices.

Table 11.1 Techniques for algorithm transparency with concept and applications

Technique	Concept	Application
Model-agnostic techniques	Model-agnostic techniques, such as LIME, are designed to provide explanations for the predictions of any machine learning model, irrespective of its underlying architecture	Model-agnostic techniques are versatile and can be applied to a wide range of models, including complex deep learning models used in nutritional guidance. This flexibility is crucial for transparency across diverse algorithmic implementations
LIME (local interpretable model-agnostic explanations)	LIME produces explanations that are faithful to local contexts by altering input data points and analyzing the model's reactions. Subsequently, it constructs an interpretable, localized model (such as a linear model) to offer understanding into how the model makes decisions	In nutritional guidance models, LIME can be used to explain specific recommendations for an individual by generating interpretable insights into the model's reasoning for that particular case. This helps users understand why certain dietary suggestions are made
SHAP (SHapley additive exPlanations)	SHAP values allocate contributions of each feature to the model's output in a cooperative game theory framework. This technique provides a unified measure of feature importance, enhancing interpretability	SHAP values can be applied to nutritional guidance models to quantify the impact of different dietary features on the recommendations. This allows users to understand which factors contribute most significantly to the model's decision
Tree-based models and decision paths	Decision trees and tree-based models inherently offer interpretability by representing decision paths. Visualizing decision trees or extracting rules from tree-based models allows users to understand the logic behind specific predictions	Rule-based systems are valuable for creating transparent nutritional guidance models with explicit rules that users can understand and follow easily
Explanation dashboards	Visualization tools and dashboards can aggregate various interpretability techniques to provide a comprehensive, user-friendly overview of the model's decision factors	Explanation dashboards in nutritional guidance can present a holistic view of how different interpretability techniques align, allowing users to explore and understand the model's recommendations in a user-friendly interface

(b) **Transparency and Explainability**

Model Transparency: Strive for transparency in algorithmic decision-making. Provide users with understandable explanations of how AI models generate nutritional recommendations, enabling them to comprehend the reasoning behind specific dietary suggestions.

Explainable AI Techniques: Utilize explainable AI techniques, such as LIME (local interpretable model-agnostic explanations) or SHAP (SHapley Additive exPlanations), to enhance the interpretability of complex models and make their outputs more accessible to users.

(c) **User-Centric Design**

Personalization with User Input: Involve users in the decision-making process by allowing them to provide feedback, preferences, and goals. Enable personalization based on individual dietary habits, preferences, and health conditions to enhance user engagement.

User Education: Implement educational components within the AI-driven nutrition systems to inform users about the principles of nutrition, health benefits, and potential risks associated with dietary choices. Encourage users to make informed decisions about their well-being.

(d) **Accuracy and Evidence-Based Recommendations**

Continuous Validation: Regularly validate and update AI models based on the latest nutritional science, dietary guidelines, and emerging research. Ensure that recommendations align with evidence-based practices and stay current with evolving knowledge in the field of nutrition.

Clinical Collaboration: Collaborate with healthcare professionals, nutritionists, and dietitians to validate AI recommendations against clinical guidelines. This collaboration ensures that the AI system aligns with professional expertise and contributes to the overall health of users.

(e) **Security and Data Integrity**

Data Security Measures: Put in place strong security protocols to safeguard user data from unauthorized access, breaches, or malicious activities. Encrypt sensitive information, ensure secure data transmission, and adhere to industry standards for data security.

Data Accuracy and Quality: Regularly audit and validate the quality of dietary data used for training AI models. Minimize the impact of inaccurate or biased data on model performance, ensuring that nutritional recommendations are reliable and aligned with real-world dietary patterns.

(f) **Inclusivity and Cultural Sensitivity**

Diverse Representation: Ensure that AI models are trained on diverse datasets that represent various demographic groups, cultural backgrounds, and dietary habits. This promotes inclusivity and prevents biased recommendations that may disproportionately affect certain populations.

Cultural Adaptability: Design AI systems to be adaptable to diverse cultural preferences and dietary practices. Consider regional variations and cultural nuances to provide recommendations that resonate with users from different backgrounds.

Within the realm of AI-driven nutritional guidance, ethical considerations play a pivotal role in ensuring user autonomy, fairness, and privacy protection. Transparency and explainability are essential for users to comprehend algorithmic decision-making processes. User-centric design focuses on personalization and education to engage users effectively. Accuracy is maintained through continuous validation and clinical collaboration. Security measures safeguard data integrity, while inclusivity and cultural sensitivity promote diverse representation. Regulatory compliance and accountability frameworks ensure ethical deployment, with continuous monitoring and improvement mechanisms enhancing user feedback loops. Social responsibility underscores community engagement and public awareness campaigns to address health challenges responsibly.

The responsible deployment of AI in nutrition requires a holistic and multidimensional approach that encompasses ethical considerations, transparency, user-centric design, security, inclusivity, and ongoing accountability. By prioritizing these principles, developers and organizations can contribute to the creation of AI systems that positively impact individuals' health while respecting their autonomy and well-being.

11.6 Conclusion and Future Directions

The chapter underscored the importance of prioritizing user autonomy, providing individuals with the right to control their dietary information and make informed decisions about their well-being. Informed consent mechanisms and user education were highlighted as crucial elements in this regard. The exploration of ethical considerations brought to the forefront the imperative of fairness and inclusivity in AI-driven nutritional guidance. Acknowledging diverse cultural, socioeconomic, and health contexts is essential to avoid biases and ensure equitable recommendations for users from various backgrounds. Robust privacy measures, including cryptographic techniques, secure computation methods, and adherence to data protection regulations, were identified as fundamental in safeguarding sensitive dietary and health information. Users must be able to comprehend the rationale behind nutritional recommendations, fostering trust and understanding in the AI-driven guidance process. Techniques like LIME and SHAP were presented as valuable tools in achieving transparency. The incorporation of user feedback loops and adaptive learning mechanisms emerged as essential for the continuous monitoring and improvement of AI-driven nutritional guidance systems. This iterative approach ensures responsiveness to user experiences and evolving dietary trends.

In conclusion, this chapter has delved into the intricate landscape of AI-driven nutritional guidance systems, shedding light on the pivotal role of ethical considerations in their development and deployment. As we navigate the evolving intersection of technology and health, several key findings and insights have emerged, emphasizing the significance of ethical frameworks in shaping the trajectory of these innovations.

As AI continues to evolve, the field of nutritional guidance is poised for transformative advancements. The integration of multimodal data, personalized behavioral interventions, collaboration with healthcare professionals, and explainable AI are crucial aspects for the future development of AI systems in nutrition. Real-time monitoring and feedback, addressing socioeconomic disparities, predicting long-term health outcomes, fostering global collaboration for diverse datasets, establishing ethical guidelines and standards, and promoting continuous learning and adaptation are essential for the evolution of AI in nutritional guidance. These recommendations aim to enhance personalization, user trust, healthcare collaboration, real-time feedback, socioeconomic inclusivity, predictive capabilities, global applicability, ethical standards, and ongoing learning within AI-driven nutritional systems. As the landscape of AI in nutritional guidance evolves, these future directions and recommendations aim to guide the development of responsible, effective, and user-centric applications. By embracing innovation, collaboration, and ethical considerations, the future of AI in nutrition holds the promise of revolutionizing how individuals approach and maintain healthy dietary practices.

References

1. Misra SC, Mukhopadhyay K. Data harnessing to nurture the human mind for a tailored approach to the child. Pediatr Res. 2023;93(2):357–65.
2. Zhang A, Wu Z, Wu E, Wu M, Snyder MP, Zou J, Wu JC. Leveraging physiology and artificial intelligence to deliver advancements in health care. Physiol Rev. 2023;103(4):2423–50.
3. Amugongo LM, Kriebitz A, Boch A, Lütge C. Operationalising AI ethics through the agile software development lifecycle: a case study of AI-enabled mobile health applications. AI and Ethics. 2023; https://doi.org/10.1007/s43681-023-00331-3.
4. Hassan M, Malhotra K, Firdaus M. Application of artificial intelligence in IoT security for crop yield prediction. ResearchBerg Rev Sci Technol. 2022;2(1):136–57.
5. Sharma A, Sharma V, Jaiswal M, et al. Recent trends in AI-based intelligent sensing. Electronics. 2022;11(10):1661.
6. Sodiya EO, Amoo OO, Umoga UJ, Atadoga A. AI-driven personalization in web content delivery: a comparative study of user engagement in the USA and the UK. World J Adv Res Rev. 2024;21(2):887–902.
7. Suryadevara CK. Revolutionizing dietary monitoring: a comprehensive analysis of the innovative mobile app for tracking dietary composition. Int J Innov Eng Res Technol. 2023;10(8):44–50.
8. Brouwer ID, van Liere MJ, de Brauw A, Dominguez-Salas P, Herforth A, Kennedy G, et al. Reverse thinking: taking a healthy diet perspective towards food systems transformations. Food Secur. 2021;13(6):1497–523.
9. Alowais SA, Alghamdi SS, Alsuhebany N, Alqahtani T, Alshaya AI, Almohareb SN, et al. Revolutionizing healthcare: the role of artificial intelligence in clinical practice. BMC Med Educ. 2023;23(1):689.
10. Dave S, Dave A, Radhakrishnan S, Das J, Dave S. Biosensors for healthcare: an artificial intelligence approach. In: Biosensors for emerging and re-emerging infectious diseases. Academic Press; 2022. p. 365–83.
11. Liu Z, Wang S, Zhang Y, Feng Y, Liu J, Zhu H. Artificial intelligence in food safety: a decade review and bibliometric analysis. Food Secur. 2023;12(6):1242.
12. Rolnick D, Donti PL, Kaack LH, et al. Tackling climate change with machine learning. ACM Comput Surv. 2022;55(2):1–96.
13. Quach S, Thaichon P, Martin KD, Weaven S, Palmatier RW. Digital technologies: tensions in privacy and data. J Acad Mark Sci. 2022;50(6):1299–323.
14. Rahman A, Hossain MS, Muhammad G, Kundu D, Debnath T, Rahman M, et al. Federated learning-based AI approaches in smart healthcare: concepts, taxonomies, challenges and open issues. Clust Comput. 2023;26(4):2271–311.
15. Qian C, Liu Y, Barnett-Neefs C, Salgia S, Serbetci O, Adalja A, et al. A perspective on data sharing in digital food safety systems. Crit Rev Food Sci Nutr. 2023;63(33):12513–29.
16. Hassan MU, Rehmani MH, Chen J. Differential privacy techniques for cyber physical systems: a survey. IEEE Commun Surv Tutor. 2019;22(1):746–89.

17. Imteaj A, Thakker U, Wang S, Li J, Amini MH. A survey on federated learning for resource-constrained IoT devices. IEEE Internet Things J. 2021;9(1):1–24.
18. Ahmad K, Maabreh M, Ghaly M, Khan K, Qadir J, Al-Fuqaha A. Developing future human-centered smart cities: critical analysis of smart city security, data management and ethical challenges. Comput Sci Rev. 2022;43:100452.
19. Ahmed A, Parveen I, Abdullah S, Ahmad I, Alturki N, Jamel L. Optimized data fusion with scheduled rest periods for enhanced smart agriculture via blockchain integration. IEEE Access. 2024;12:15171–93.
20. Neethirajan S. Artificial intelligence and sensor innovations: enhancing livestock welfare with a human-centric approach. Hum-Centric Intell Syst. 2024;4:77–92.
21. Tariq MU. Revolutionizing health data management with blockchain technology: enhancing security and efficiency in a digital era. In: Emerging technologies for health literacy and medical practice. IGI Global; 2024. p. 153–75.
22. Gichoya JW, Thomas K, Celi LA, et al. AI pitfalls and what not to do: mitigating bias in AI. Br J Radiol. 2023;96(1150):20230023.
23. Mehrabi N, Morstatter F, Saxena N, Lerman K, Galstyan A. A survey on bias and fairness in machine learning. ACM Comput Surv. 2021;54(6):1–35.
24. Kaur D, Uslu S, Rittichier KJ, Durresi A. Trustworthy artificial intelligence: a review. ACM Comput Surv. 2022;55(2):1–38.
25. Khosravi H, Shum SB, Chen G, Khosravi H, Shum SB, Chen G, Conati C, Tsai YS, Kay J, et al. Explainable artificial intelligence in education. Comput Educ AI. 2022;3:100074.
26. Parisineni SR, Pal M. Enhancing trust and interpretability of complex machine learning models using local interpretable model agnostic shap explanations. Int J Data Sci Anal. 2024;18:457–66.
27. Wang X, Oussalah M, Niemilä M, Ristikari T, Petri V. Towards AI-governance in psychosocial care: a systematic literature review analysis. J Open Innov: Technol Mark Complex. 2023;9(4):100157.

Mobile Applications and Wearable in PCOS Nutrition: mHealth Solutions and Personalized Health Monitoring

12

Bhupinder Singh and Anand Nayyar

12.1 Introduction and Background

Polycystic ovary syndrome (PCOS) is a multifaceted condition characterized by increased androgen levels, irregular menstrual cycles, and the presence of small cysts on one or both ovaries [1]. This disorder can manifest as either morphological with the appearance of polycystic ovaries or predominantly biochemical, involving elevated androgen levels [2, 3]. Hyperandrogenism, a key clinical feature of PCOS, can lead to the inhibition of follicular development, the formation of microcysts in the ovaries, anovulation, and alterations in the menstrual cycle [4, 5]. As an integral aspect of managing PCOS, nutrition plays a crucial role in alleviating symptoms and improving overall health [6, 7]. In this case, the technology is used to empower people in their pursuit of health and to usher in a new age of all-encompassing, patient-centered care [8]. Also, essentially, the incorporation of mobile health tools signifies a dedication to use technology to improve personal health and wellness, stressing the significance of customized treatments and comprehensive health tracking in PCOS treatment [9].

According to the National Institutes of Health Office of Disease Prevention, five million American women of reproductive age are affected with PCOS, a complex illness that affects at least 7% of adult women [10, 11]. In the US healthcare system, the yearly cost of diagnosing and treating PCOS is estimated to be $4 billion [12]. Research shows that PCOS is the most common endocrine condition among American women of reproductive age, affecting 5–10% of females between the ages of 18 and 44 [13, 14]. PCOS is frequently diagnosed to women who seek

B. Singh (✉)
Sharda University, Greater Noida, Uttar Pradesh, India

A. Nayyar
School of Computer Science, Duy Tan University, Da Nang, Vietnam
e-mail: anandnayyar@duytan.edu.vn

R. Kumar et al. (eds.), *AI-Based Nutritional Intervention in Polycystic Ovary Syndrome (PCOS)*, https://doi.org/10.1007/978-981-96-2120-0_12

medical attention for issues including obesity, acne, amenorrhea, excessive hair growth, and infertility. PCOS is classified as an oligogenic condition, meaning that its varied clinical and biochemical phenotype is caused by a confluence of several genetic and environmental variables [15, 16]. Even though the genetic cause of PCOS is unknown, there is a definite indication that the disorder runs in families, albeit it is unclear exactly which relatives are affected [17, 18]. A formal segregation study is impeded by the lack of comprehensive phenotypic data, but the research that is currently available suggests that PCOS clusters within families in a manner akin to an autosomal dominant pattern [19].

12.1.1 Polycystic Ovary Syndrome (PCOS): Overview and Its Impact on Women's Health

Women who have PCOS are more likely to develop type 2 diabetes mellitus, dyslipidemia, cardiovascular disease, and endometrial cancer [20]. Environmental variables can aggravate PCOS; they include bad food choices, sedentary lifestyles, and the possible presence of pollutants and infectious agents [21]. This issue is obesity as the reproductive and metabolic features of PCOS may be reversible with lifestyle changes including exercise and weight loss [22, 23]. The disorder known as polycystic ovary syndrome (PCOS) is typified by an overabundance of androgens which are male sex hormones that are normally present in women in trace amounts [24, 25]. Numerous tiny cysts, or sacs filled with fluid, seen in the ovaries are referred to as "polycystic ovary syndrome." It is interesting to note that while some women with PCOS may not develop cysts, others without the disorder may [26]. A developed egg being released from the ovary during ovulation is essential for possible male sperm fertilization. During menstruation, the unfertilized egg is released from the body if fertilization is unsuccessful [27].

It is possible that women don't create enough of the hormones needed for ovulation [28]. The ovaries may develop many little cysts as a result of this inability to ovulate, which release androgens [29]. In women with PCOS, high testosterone levels can interfere with the menstrual cycle and exacerbate a number of the condition's symptoms [30]. The usual method of treating PCOS is with medication. Although there isn't a cure for PCOS, medication can help manage symptoms and reduce the risk of health issues [31].

Objectives of the Chapter

The objectives of the chapter are:

- To examine the role of mHealth solutions in PCOS nutrition;
- To explore the integration of wearables for personalized health monitoring;
- And, to assess the effectiveness of these technologies in improving PCOS outcomes.

Organization of the Chapter

The rest of the chapter is organized as follows: Section 12.2 highlights the significance of nutrition in managing PCOS symptoms. Section 12.3 illustrates the emergence of mobile applications and wearables in healthcare, specifically to PCOS. Section 12.4 discusses PCOS nutrition: nutritional considerations for managing PCOS symptoms. Section 12.5 enlightens mHealth solutions in PCOS, overview of mobile applications in healthcare, followed by discussion on wearables in PCOS health monitoring, wearable technologies for continuous health monitoring in Sect. 12.6. Finally, Sect. 12.7 concludes the chapter with future scope.

12.2 Significance of Nutrition in Managing PCOS Symptoms

PCOS (polycystic ovary syndrome) is a common disorder that affects women who are fertile and has consequences for metabolism, reproduction, and mental health. As the main treatment for PCOS, current worldwide evidence-based guidelines place a high priority on weight and lifestyle control which includes nutrition, exercise, and behavioral therapies [32]. Although these guidelines support following dietary and physical activity guidelines at the general population level, research is still being done to determine whether adding psychological and sleep interventions along with different traditional, complementary, and integrative medicine (TCIM) approaches can improve PCOS management [33].

Though lifestyle changes are advised, there isn't much data to back up the suggestion of a particular dietary composition for PCOS [34, 35]. Modifications to the quantity or quality of protein, carbohydrates, or fat often have comparable impacts on PCOS presentations [36]. In terms of physical activity, rigorous aerobic exercise has been linked to changes in insulin resistance, body composition, and cardiorespiratory fitness, according to encouraging research [37]. Considering the fact that women with PCOS frequently have low emotional well-being and high rates of sleep problems, psychological and sleep issues are also quite important [38]. These elements could make it more difficult for them to make healthy lifestyle adjustments. While improving sleep and mental health may help control PCOS symptoms, further study is required to determine how beneficial treatment therapies [39].

Although the exact etiology of PCOS is still unknown, insulin resistance as a disease in which the body finds it difficult to use insulin is a common feature in women who have the disorder [40]. Increased androgen levels might be attributed to elevated insulin levels. Insulin levels can be made worse by obesity which makes PCOS symptoms worse. PCOS runs in the family and is frequently seen in sisters or in relationships between moms and daughters [41, 42]. Obesity, insulin resistance, and a family history of PCOS may all raise the risk of the condition. PCOS is associated with various symptoms which include missed, irregular, or very light periods; enlarged ovaries or the presence of multiple cysts; excessive body hair, known as hirsutism, on the chest, stomach, and back; weight gain, particularly around the abdomen; acne or oily skin; male-pattern baldness or hair thinning; infertility; skin tags, small pieces of excess skin on the neck or armpits; and dark or thick skin patches on the back of the neck, in the armpits, and under the breasts [43, 44].

12.2.1 Data Analysis and Results

Women with PCOS are becoming more and more accustomed to using TCIM methods, especially when it comes to taking vitamins and using herbal remedies. There are studies on inositol supplementation that have produced encouraging results, such as decreased hyperandrogenism and better metabolic profiles. The results for acupuncture, yoga, herbal remedies, and other supplements are still erratic. It should concentrate on certain PCOS groups with defined age and BMI ranges and use standardized methods for the administration, duration, and comparators of interventions [45]. Figure 12.1 highlights various data analysis and health.

Although there are potential benefits for people with PCOS from several lifestyle components than typical food and physical exercise guidelines, strong clinical trials

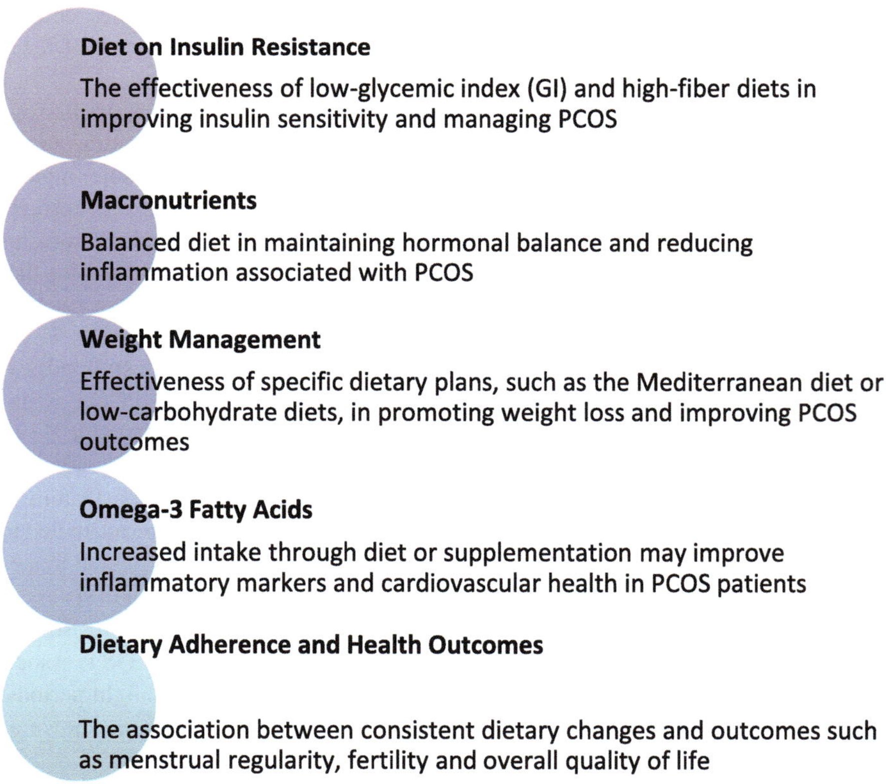

Fig. 12.1 Data analysis and results

are required to increase the relatively small body of data on holistic lifestyle therapy [46]. Healthcare professionals will need to expand their expertise in order to safely and effectively integrate these therapies as supplements to traditional medical management, as public interest in holistic healthcare continues to grow [47].

12.3 Emergence of Mobile Applications and Wearables in Healthcare: Specifically to PCOS

Smartphones and wearable technologies are bringing in a revolutionary age for patient monitoring and individualized care in modern healthcare [47, 48]. Wearables with a variety of sensing technologies built in, such as optics for heart rate and accelerometers for movement, are becoming more and more acknowledged for their extensive potential in remote patient monitoring, diagnostics, and therapeutic applications [45]. This raises the possibility of a change to a healthcare system that is more decentralized. Wearable technology is being embraced by patients and healthcare professionals more and more, opening up new possibilities for continuous health monitoring outside of typical clinical settings. Concurrently, cellphones which are increasingly useful for more than just communication are essential for health monitoring [34].

Their improved sensing capacities and Internet of Things (IoT) connection allow for a reasonably smooth shift from traditional healthcare methods to a more digitally linked era as shown in Fig. 12.2 [36]. But there are drawbacks to this changing environment such as worries about security, privacy, and equitable access to digital innovations. It is essential to realize the full potential of these technologies and guarantee their ethical and fair deployment as we get more and more engrossed in digital healthcare. In the future, according to this vision, healthcare will be effortlessly incorporated into everyday life rather than being limited to hospitals [49].

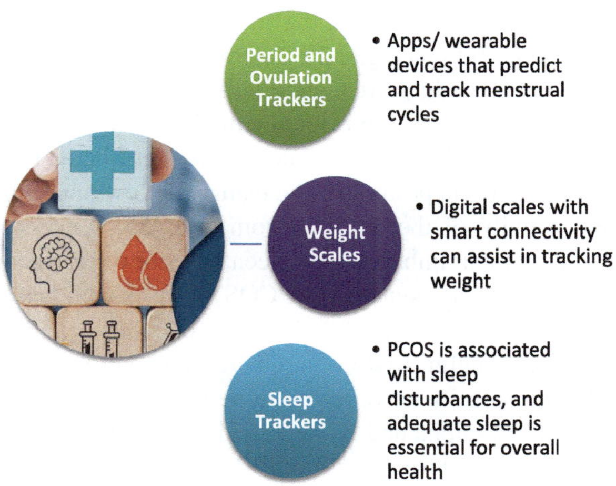

Fig. 12.2 PCOS wearable sensors

Mobile devices such as smartphones (like iPhone or Android), tablets (like iPad), and smartwatches (like Apple Watch or FitBit) are commonly used for health apps. Wearable technology includes smartwatches, which are wrist-worn gadgets that can run applications. Apps for healthcare are customized for certain end users. Patient-facing applications provide information about particular medical issues or overall well-being to help users better manage their own health [48, 50]. Clinician-facing applications help with things like clinical medication information or illness diagnosis by providing medical education or information from a therapeutic viewpoint. Certain healthcare applications function as intermediaries, enabling clinician-patient contact by capturing and sending vital signs measured by the patient. The increasing need for digital healthcare will probably spur innovation in the design of healthcare apps, resulting in more advanced goods. The Food and Drug Administration (FDA) of the United States contributes to patient safety by regulating healthcare applications [51]. The FDA may classify applications intended for medical use as medical devices even if they are not incorporated into a physical device; this classification is known as software as a medical device (SaMD). The software in a medical device (SiMD) refers to programs that are incorporated into medical equipment or smart medical devices. The FDA's guidelines for creating healthcare apps are always changing to keep up with the latest developments in technology [44, 52].

12.4 PCOS Nutrition: Nutritional Considerations for Managing PCOS Symptoms

The hypothalamic-pituitary-ovarian system's hormonal control mechanisms function via negative feedback axes, which comprise long, short, and ultrashort feedback. Gonadotropin-releasing hormone (GnRH) is produced by neurons in the suprachiasmatic nucleus of the hypothalamus and released into the pituitary portal circulation in the median eminence [53]. Interconnected neurons control the release of GnRH in a complex way, resulting in pulsatile secretion. The kind of gonadotropin produced depends on the frequency of this pulsatile rhythm; a low frequency causes the pituitary gland's anterior lobe to secrete follicle-stimulating hormone (FSH), while a high frequency causes it to secrete luteinizing hormone (LH) [54].

The process of corpus luteum luteinization which turns granulosa cells into progesterone-producing theca lutein cells is attributed to LH. FSH converts androgens to estrogens via promoting the maturity of ovarian follicles, production of estrogen, and activity of the enzyme aromatase [55]. Excessive androgen production can result from an imbalance between LH and FSH concentrations in diseases such as polycystic ovary syndrome (PCOS) [56]. Insulin has a direct and indirect effect in the pathophysiology of PCOS by reducing hepatic synthesis of sex hormone-binding globulin (SHBG) and increasing androgen production in concert with LH, which results in active testosterone circulation. With releasing inflammatory cytokines (TNF-alpha and IL-beta) and hormones like leptin and resistin, excess body fat aids in the development of PCOS [57].

Adipose tissue secretes leptin, which modifies GnRH, LH, and FSH production and may lead to an excess of androgen synthesis in the hypothalamus-pituitary gland-ovary axis. Because of hyperglycemia, adipose tissue causes inflammation and an increase in free radicals in PCOS through cytokine release [58]. Many metabolic pathways including insulin secretion and activity, steroidogenesis genes, cytochrome P450 activity, and genes linked to androgenic receptor, LH receptor, leptin, and follistatin are involved in the many clinical manifestations of PCOS. A low-glycemic index (GI), low-fat, somewhat adherent anti-inflammatory diet pattern seems to offer protection against PCOS development [59].

12.4.1 Role of Diet in Regulating Hormonal Imbalances

There are a number of things to take into account while considering a diet to resolve hormone imbalances. Hormones such as cortisol, thyroid, progesterone, estrogen, and insulin function as chemical messengers in the body. For these hormones to support mental and physical health, they must function in unison [60]. In women, symptoms like mood swings, fogging of the mind, low energy, and weight gain are frequently indicative of hormone abnormalities. Hormones are not typically the first thing that comes to mind when choosing what to eat to fuel our body [61]. Hormones are the essential chemical messengers in our bodies; they affect a variety of bodily processes, including development, metabolism, digestion, reproduction, stress, and mood. In the event that these chemical messengers are malfunctioning, an imbalance in hormones may result. An excess or shortage of any hormone, abnormalities in signaling pathways, or a breakdown in the efficient exchange of hormones among themselves can all lead to imbalances. Problems including blood sugar dysregulation, insulin resistance, weight gain, and acne may be preceded by this imbalance [6].

Hormonal imbalances can be caused by a number of things such as an unhealthy diet, insufficient sleep, allergies, stress, and exposure to pollutants in the environment [7]. Nonetheless, there are practical methods for assisting with hormone balance. A nutrient-dense, well-balanced diet that includes fresh produce, lean meats, healthy fats, and fruits is such strategy as shown in Fig. 12.3 [14]. A wide range of stresses can affect the endocrine system, which can result in abnormalities in the

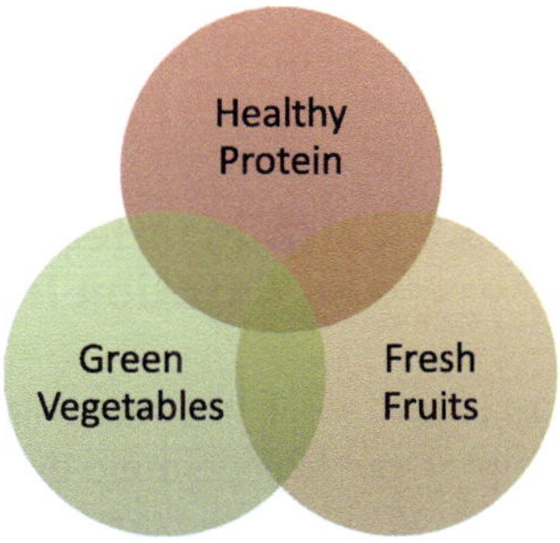

Fig. 12.3 Healthy diet: PCOS

function and balance of hormones. When signs of a hormone imbalance are identified early on, underlying problems can be addressed, and hormonal balance can be supported with the use of supplements, food, exercise, and lifestyle changes [18, 21].

12.5 mHealth Solutions in PCOS: Overview of Mobile Applications in Healthcare

The treatment of chronic illnesses like PCOS and the effective provision of healthcare services are two areas in which the use of mobile health technology is growing quickly [27]. The increasing number of Saudi Arabians utilizing the Internet and mobile phones presents a promising opportunity for remote healthcare delivery and efficient disease management through the use of mobile health systems, which might also lower costs and increase operational efficiency [29]. Clinical trials assessing the efficacy of self-managing PCOS in Saudi Arabia utilizing an integrated mobile application and text messaging system are conspicuously lacking. In order to minimize possible consequences following diagnosis, there is an urgent need to raise knowledge about PCOS management given the rising incidence of PCOS and its linked disorders [33].

An endocrine disorder called polycystic ovary syndrome (PCOS) is characterized by a wide range of symptoms brought on by hormonal imbalances. It is a common endocrine condition that has been linked to female reproductive age infertility [31, 34]. Evidence points to metabolic and reproductive abnormalities as a possible contributing factor even if the exact reason is still unknown. These abnormalities result in hormonal imbalances which in females include higher levels of androgen and estrogen [36]. This hormonal imbalance, characterized by reduced levels of normal hormone intake, shows up as a chronic condition of low progesterone and excessive luteinizing hormone (LH). PCOS which is usually diagnosed in adolescence is characterized by hyperandrogenism and malfunctioning ovarian tubes. These affected persons may face serious health risks and have a reduction in their quality of life. Overproduction of androgens, which causes anovulation, acne, and hirsutism, are common symptoms [44, 48]. PCOS can be confirmed using diagnostic techniques such as ultrasound exams for polycystic ovarian morphology, evaluation of anovulation, and assessment of androgen excess using clinical or biochemical assays. The Rotterdam criteria state that confirmation of PCOS requires fulfilling two of the three benchmarks: polycystic ovaries, clinical and/or biochemical evidence of hyperandrogenism, or oligo-ovulation or anovulation [54].

12.5.1 Existing mHealth Apps for PCOS Management and Nutrition Tracking

As part of your treatment strategy, using an app to track your symptoms might be helpful, but keep in mind that every person's experience with symptoms will be different. While some people may only have a few or minor symptoms, others may be greatly impacted by a wider variety of symptoms [60]. It's crucial to avoid self-diagnosing or relying exclusively on the app for information. Use an app to keep track of your symptoms and include it in your overall management plan [62]. Use the app's graphs and reports to help you and your healthcare practitioner have more conversations. Certain applications allow users to share their experiences in interactive features like group chat rooms or discussion boards [63]. It is important to exercise caution though, as these platforms are usually not supervised by medical experts. It's possible that the recommendations or advice given don't follow sensible or safe procedures [64].

12.5.2 User Satisfaction and Adherence to mHealth Interventions

Rapid improvements in mobile health technologies have paralleled the significant increase in mobile phone usage in developing countries [65]. Using mobile technology to promote health may be a useful strategy for improving long-term health outcomes. In low-resource environments and developing nations, mobile technology shows promise as a tool for noncommunicable illness intervention [66]. The World Health Organization's Global Action Plan (2013–2020) for poor nations is in line with the dissemination of health-related data using mobile devices. Considering that women with PCOS frequently experience symptoms at an early age, there is a chance to investigate the viability and efficacy of mobile health applications in enhancing these women's health-related behaviors [67, 68].

12.6 Wearables in PCOS Health Monitoring: Wearable Technologies for Continuous Health Monitoring

PCOS is a common medical illness that affects women and is caused by hormonal abnormalities that impact the reproductive system and cause issues in the ovaries [69]. Menstrual cycle irregularities and infertility are two problems that may result from this imbalance. Ovaries generate and release eggs during a normal menstrual cycle; however, in PCOS, these eggs may not develop normally or may be ejected prematurely during ovulation, which can lead to missing or delayed periods as well as the development of ovarian cysts [70, 71]. While each person's signs, symptoms, and risk factors for PCOS are unique, high blood sugar or diabetes are typical markers. According to the CDC, over half of PCOS-affected women will have type 2 diabetes by the time they are 40. Insulin-related problems also frequently lead to weight-related problems, such as obesity or trouble shedding weight. Other typical symptoms include thinning hair, acne, and changes in skin color as highlighted in Fig. 12.4 [72]. Menstrual cycle irregularities, such as skipped or delayed periods, are also prevalent. The useful technique for controlling PCOS-related issues is RPM (remote patient monitoring), especially those linked to diabetes and obesity. Outside of medical facilities, RPM helps women with PCOS to keep an eye on their weight and blood sugar levels. This ongoing observation gives medical professionals quick

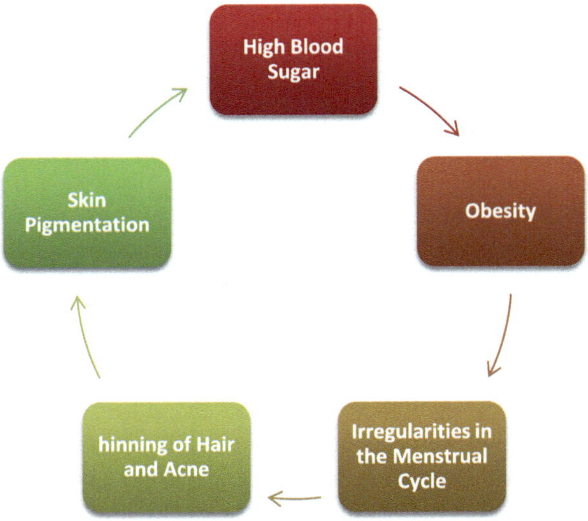

Fig. 12.4 Signs, symptoms, and risk factors of PCOS

access to vital patient information, enabling them to modify treatment regimens in a timely manner [73].

During the RPM procedure, patients take vital indicators such as blood glucose levels using a linked glucometer. The patient's mobile application receives the gathered data and uses it as a portal to a secure database. Then using their laptops or cellphones, providers may access this data, allowing them to monitor any changes in vital signs and act quickly [74]. RPM enables medical professionals to collect thorough patient data, which helps them comprehend and diagnose specific PCOS instances. Thus, more effective and individualized treatment programs that are catered to the unique requirements of every patient are made possible [75].

12.6.1 Integration of Wearables with Nutrition and Activity Tracking

Wearable technologies are smart gadgets designed to make our lives easier and improve how well our health is managed [76]. Essential health parameters like heart rate, step count, sleep quality, and even stress levels may be tracked by these gadgets. The Integro Health application's integration of key health data elements make tracking and analysis simple and effective. Setting health objectives and tracking results are made easier and more efficient by this connection [77]. With daily lives becoming more and more digitalized, the instruments available for managing and monitoring our health have changed significantly in the modern day. Wearable technology is a revolutionary development in the field of health monitoring. Via wearables like wristbands, smartwatches, and other gadgets that have become ingrained in our everyday lives, these technologies enable the seamless monitoring and evaluation of health data [78]. At Integro Health, we emphasize how our application effortlessly connects with wearable technology and see this revolutionary advancement as an opportunity to help you in closely monitoring your health. Individuals differ in what they require for optimal health. A more individualized method of measuring health is provided by the integration of wearable technology with the health application [79]. Using information from wearable technology, our app creates a personalized health profile that includes algorithm-driven recommendations based on your requirements. This guarantees that the guidance you receive is in line with your health goals which empower you to make better educated choices [80].

12.7 Conclusion and Future Scope

As compared to women without PCOS, women with PCOS have greater levels of anxiety and depressive symptoms. According to international standards, women with PCOS should manage their anxiety and depression symptoms. A 20-week diet and exercise intervention indicated that reduced depressed symptoms were only sustained for the first 10 weeks in the intervention group, despite several research suggesting that lifestyle management can lead to considerably decreased depression levels. Short-term psychological benefits were also identified in two diet-induced weight reduction trials, but they were not long-lasting. Wearable technologies comprise smart devices crafted to simplify our lives and enhance the efficient management of our health. These devices have the capability to track essential health metrics such as heart rate, step count, sleep quality, and even stress levels. The integration of these health data points with the Integro Health application allows for easy and efficient tracking and analysis. This integration facilitates the setting of health goals and monitoring progress in a more streamlined manner. For women with PCOS, maintaining health-related behavior changes over the long term might be difficult, since they frequently have low adherence to lifestyle changes in traditional face-to-face therapies. The mobile health (mHealth) application based on the transtheoretical model (TTM) affected PCOS patients' long-term health-related behavior changes, such as diet and exercise. The provision of knowledge, techniques, and motivation for lifestyle modification, as well as adaptable intervention strategies and improvements in mental health outcomes, which affect trial adherence, may be responsible for the positive effects of the TTM-based mobile health application on behavior change stages.

References

1. Subbhuraam V. FemTech solutions for advancing women's health. In: Predictive analytics in healthcare, volume 1: transforming the future of medicine. Bristol, UK: IOP Publishing; 2021. p. 3-1–3-25.
2. Costa Figueiredo M, Huynh T, Takei A, Epstein DA, Chen Y. Goals, life events, and transitions: examining fertility apps for holistic health tracking. JAMIA Open. 2021;4(1):ooab013.

3. Singh B, Kaunert C. Integration of cutting-edge technologies such as internet of things (IoT) and 5G in health monitoring systems: a comprehensive legal analysis and futuristic outcomes. GLS Law J. 2024;6(1):13–20.
4. DeNicola N, Marko K. Connected health and mobile apps in obstetrics and gynecology. Obstet Gynecol Clin. 2020;47(2):317–31.
5. Kytö M, Markussen LT, Marttinen P, et al. Comprehensive self-tracking of blood glucose and lifestyle with a mobile application in the management of gestational diabetes: a study protocol for a randomised controlled trial (eMOM GDM study). BMJ Open. 2022;12(11):e066292.
6. Kharb S, Joshi A. Multi-omics and machine learning for the prevention and management of female reproductive health. Front Endocrinol. 2023;14:358.
7. Lee VV, Vijayakumar S, Ng WY, et al. Personalization and localization as key expectations of digital health intervention in women pre-to post-pregnancy. NPJ Digit Med. 2023;6(1):183.
8. Singh B. Tele-health monitoring lensing deep neural learning structure: ambient patient wellness via wearable devices for real-time alerts and interventions. Indian J Health Med Law. 2023;6(2):12–6.
9. Kytö M, Markussen LT, Marttinen P, et al. Protocol: comprehensive self-tracking of blood glucose and lifestyle with a mobile application in the management of gestational diabetes: a study protocol for a randomised controlled trial (eMOM GDM study). BMJ Open. 2022;12(11):e066292.
10. Gandhi BH, Imani SA. Co-design and development of EndoSMS, a supportive text message intervention for individuals living with endometriosis: mixed methods study. JMIR Form Res. 2022;6(12):e40837.
11. McDonough DJ, Su X, Gao Z. Health wearable devices for weight and BMI reduction in individuals with overweight/obesity and chronic comorbidities: systematic review and network meta-analysis. Br J Sports Med. 2021;55(16):917–25.
12. Singh B. Legal dynamics lensing metaverse crafted for videogame industry and e-sports: phenomenological exploration catalyst complexity and future. J Intellect Prop Rights Law. 2024;7(1):8–14.
13. Singh B. Blockchain technology in renovating healthcare: legal and future perspectives. In: Revolutionizing healthcare through artificial intelligence and internet of things applications. IGI Global; 2023. p. 177–86.
14. Robertsson H. Facilitating behavioral change among women with polycystic ovary syndrome: a design-oriented case study. KTH Royal Institute of Technology; 2023.
15. Li K, Urteaga I, Wiggins CH, et al. Characterizing physiological and symptomatic variation in menstrual cycles using self-tracked mobile-health data. NPJ Digit Med. 2020;3(1):79.
16. Sparks JR, Ghildayal N, Hivert MF, Redman LM. Lifestyle interventions in pregnancy targeting GDM prevention: looking ahead to precision medicine. Diabetologia. 2022;65(11):1814–24.
17. Pichon A, Jackman KB, Winkler IT, Bobel C, Elhadad N. The messiness of the menstruator: assessing personas and functionalities of menstrual tracking apps. J Am Med Inform Assoc. 2022;29(2):385–99.
18. Elei FO, Ikerionwu CO, Erike AI, Mshelia YU. Transition to value-based care IoT wearable devices in maternity healthcare for low-resource countries. Int J Sci Res Comput Sci Eng. 2023;11(4):8–14.
19. Singh B. Federated learning for envision future trajectory smart transport system for climate preservation and smart green planet: insights into global governance and SDG-9 (industry, innovation and infrastructure). Natl J Environ Law. 2023;6(2):6–17.
20. Sharma A, Singh B. Measuring impact of e-commerce on small scale business: a systematic review. J Corp Gov Int Bus Law. 2022;5(1) https://doi.org/10.37591/jcgibl.v5i1.1087.
21. Su Z, Chen Y. Data-driven technology for children's health and wellbeing: a systematic review. Found Trends Hum Comput Interact. 2024;18(1):1–99.
22. Al-Turjman F. Artificial intelligence for remote patient monitoring in IoT based healthcare applications–an overview. NEU J Artif Intell IoT. 2023;2(2):75–88.
23. Saxena A, Saxena M, Deo A, Llerena AR. Transformation of mHealth in society. In: Big data and artificial intelligence for healthcare applications. CRC Press; 2021. p. 165–94.

24. Chopra S, Zehrung R, Shanmugam TA, Choe EK. Living with uncertainty and stigma: self-experimentation and support-seeking around polycystic ovary syndrome. In: Proceedings of the 2021 CHI conference on human factors in computing systems. ACM; 2021. p. 1–18.
25. Singh B. Understanding legal frameworks concerning transgender healthcare in the age of dynamism. Electron J Soc Strateg Stud. 2022;3:56–65.
26. Mishra P, Kaur R, Vikram S, Sharma P. Femtech apps and quantification of the reproductive body in India: issues and concerns. Curr Sociol. 2023;72(7):00113921231206491.
27. Islam MN, Raiyan KR, Mitra S, et al. Predictis: an IoT and machine learning-based system to predict risk level of cardio-vascular diseases. BMC Health Serv Res. 2023;23(1):171.
28. Cueto V, Sanders LM. Telehealth opportunities and challenges for managing pediatric obesity. Pediatr Clin. 2020;67(4):647–54.
29. Chew HSJ, Lim SL, Kim G, et al. Essential elements of weight loss apps for a multi-ethnic population with high BMI: a qualitative study with practical recommendations. Transl Behav Med. 2023;13(3):140–8.
30. Singh B. Relevance of agriculture-nutrition linkage for human healthcare: a conceptual legal framework of implication and pathways. Justice Law Bull. 2022;1(1):44–9.
31. Kheirmandparizi M. Perceptions of a dietary self-monitoring mobile app resembling the Canada's food guide: a qualitative study [Doctoral dissertation]. University of British Columbia; 2023.
32. Wadden TA, Tronieri JS, Butryn ML. Lifestyle modification approaches for the treatment of obesity in adults. Am Psychol. 2020;75(2):235.
33. Zhou R, Gu Y, Zhang B, et al. Digital therapeutics: emerging new therapy for nonalcoholic fatty liver disease. Clin Transl Gastroenterol. 2023;14(4):e00575.
34. Mishra P, Kaur R, Vikram S. One size (doesn't) fit all: a closer look at FemTech apps and datafied reproductive body projects in India. In: FemTech: intersectional interventions in women's digital health. Singapore: Springer Nature Singapore; 2023. p. 101–30.
35. Khamisy-Farah R, Furstenau LB, Kong JD, Wu J, Bragazzi NL. Gynecology meets big data in the disruptive innovation medical era: state-of-art and future prospects. Int J Environ Res Public Health. 2021;18(10):5058.
36. Oei K. Usability and feasibility testing of eating for wellness (E4W)–an image-recognition dietary assessment application for adolescents with obesity [Doctoral dissertation]. University of Toronto; 2023.
37. Singh B. COVID-19 pandemic and public healthcare: endless downward spiral or solution via rapid legal and health services implementation with patient monitoring program. Justice Law Bull. 2022;1(1):1–7.
38. Singh B. Global science and jurisprudential approach concerning healthcare and illness. Indian J Health Med Law. 2020;3(1):7–13.
39. Costa Figueiredo M. Data work and data tracking technologies in fertility care: a holistic approach [Doctoral dissertation]. UC Irvine; 2021.
40. Costa Figueiredo M, Chen Y. Health data in fertility care: an ecological perspective. In: Proceedings of the 2021 CHI conference on human factors in computing systems. ACM; 2021 May. p. 1–17.
41. Rozga M, Jones K, Robinson J, Yahiro A. Nutrition and physical activity interventions for the general population with and without cardiometabolic risk: a scoping review. Public Health Nutr. 2021;24(14):4718–36.
42. Singh B. Profiling public healthcare: a comparative analysis based on the multidimensional healthcare management and legal approach. Indian J Health Med Law. 2019;2(2):1–5.
43. Ensari I, Pichon A, Lipsky-Gorman S, Bakken S, Elhadad N. Augmenting the clinical data sources for enigmatic diseases: a cross-sectional study of self-tracking data and clinical documentation in endometriosis. Appl Clin Inform. 2020;11(05):769–84.
44. Seyi SE, Imaralu JO, Digban KA, John-Ugwuanya GA, Ajike SO. Improving women's health in the 21st century: current challenges, medical advancements and future prospects. J Women Health Care Issues. 2023;6(5) https://doi.org/10.31579/2642-9756/162.

45. Lin GE, Mynatt ED, Kumar N. Investigating culturally responsive design for menstrual tracking and sharing practices among individuals with minimal sexual education. In: Proceedings of the 2022 CHI conference on human factors in computing systems. ACM; 2022 April. p. 1–15.
46. Summers C, Curtis K. Novel Digital architecture of a "Low Carb Program" for initiating and maintaining long-term sustainable health-promoting behavior change in patients with type 2 diabetes. JMIR Diabetes. 2020;5(1):e15030.
47. Padhy S, Dash S, Routray S, Ahmad S, Nazeer J, Alam A. IoT-based hybrid ensemble machine learning model for efficient diabetes mellitus prediction. Comput Intell Neurosci. 2022;2022:2389636.
48. Roesler A, Butten K, Calyx C, Holmes-Truscott E, Taylor PJ. Use and preferences of health apps among women and healthcare professionals regarding Gdm postpartum care: a cross-sectional survey. Nutrients. 2023;15(15):3304.
49. Fazakis N, Kocsis O, Dritsas E, Alexiou S, Fakotakis N, Moustakas K. Machine learning tools for long-term type 2 diabetes risk prediction. IEEE Access. 2021;9:103737–57.
50. Banerjee S. A preventive medicine framework for wearable abiotic glucose detection system [Doctoral dissertation]. Old Dominion University; 2022.
51. Tuli A, Singh S, Narula R, Kumar N, Singh P. Rethinking menstrual trackers towards period-positive ecologies. In: Proceedings of the 2022 CHI conference on human factors in computing systems. ACM; 2022 April. p. 1–20.
52. Shilts MK, Horowitz M, Townsend MS. Goal setting as a strategy for dietary and physical activity behavior change: a review of the literature. Am J Health Promot. 2004;19(2):81–93.
53. McKillop M, Mamykina L, Elhadad N. Designing in the dark: eliciting self-tracking dimensions for understanding enigmatic disease. In: Proceedings of the 2018 CHI conference on human factors in computing systems. ACM; 2018 April. p. 1–15.
54. Gualtieri S. Digital innovation in home care: insights from the startup global landscape. Politecnico di Milano; 2023.
55. Hasan ST, Ahmed SI, Khan MA, Sarker SA, Ahmed T. Achieving optimal gestational weight gain, birth weight, and perinatal outcomes among pregnant women at risk of hypertension: protocol for a pilot randomized controlled trial. JMIR Res Protoc. 2020;9(6):e16676.
56. de Santiago I, Polanski L. Big data and artificial intelligence (AI) are poised to transform infertility healthcare. Preprints.org; 2020.
57. Nazir S, Nawaz M, Adnan A, Shahzad S, Asadi S. Big data features, applications, and analytics in cardiology—a systematic literature review. IEEE Access. 2019;7:143742–71.
58. Petroni ML, Brodosi L, Marchignoli F, et al. Nutrition in patients with type 2 diabetes: present knowledge and remaining challenges. Nutrients. 2021;13(8):2748.
59. Costa Figueiredo M, Su HI, Chen Y. Using data to approach the unknown: Patients' and healthcare providers? Data practices in fertility challenges. Proc ACM Hum Comput Interact. 2021;4(CSCW3):1–35.
60. Tyagi AK, editor. Privacy preservation of genomic and medical data. John Wiley & Sons; 2023.
61. Scholten M. Serious games combined with wearables in battling pediatric obesity: the medical professionals' perspective [Master's thesis]. University of Twente; 2018.
62. Al-Worafi YM, Ming LC, Dhabali AA, Al-Shami AM. Obesity in developing countries. In: Handbook of medical and health sciences in developing countries: education, practice, and research. Cham: Springer International Publishing; 2023. p. 1–42.
63. Wang W. The "N of one" method in Chinese medicine investigation: unraveling individualized treatment approaches. J Comm Med Pub Health Rep. 2023;4(6) https://doi.org/10.38207/JCMPHR/2023/AUG04060293.
64. Diallo A. The use of artificial intelligence in healthcare: cure or curse. Edward Waters Univ Undergrad Res J. 2023;1(1) https://doi.org/10.62962/001c.88333.
65. Prakash C, Singh LP, Gupta A, Kumar R, Bhardwaj A. Future consideration and challenges in women's health using AI. In: Combating women's health issues with machine learning. CRC Press; 2023. p. 215–36.
66. Dimitri P, Savage MO. Artificial intelligence in paediatric endocrinology: conflict or cooperation. J Pediatr Endocrinol Metab. 2024;37(3):209–21.

67. Min A, Miller WR, Rocha LM, Börner K, Brattig Correia R, Shih PC. Understanding contexts and challenges of information management for epilepsy care. In: Proceedings of the 2023 CHI conference on human factors in computing systems. ACM; 2023 April. p. 1–15.
68. Min A, Miller W, Rocha L, Börner K, Correia R, Shih P. Understanding contexts and challenges of information management for epilepsy care. Proc SIGCHI Conf Hum Factor Comput Syst. 2023;2023:328. https://doi.org/10.1145/3544548.3580949.
69. Brandt EJ, Tobb K, Cambron JC, et al. Assessing and addressing social determinants of cardiovascular health: JACC state-of-the-art review. J Am Coll Cardiol. 2023;81(14):1368–85.
70. Smolander N, Huuskonen A, Kunnas K, Ylistalo E. DigiCare model: digitalized healthcare and coaching of patients in an Asian context. Tampere University of Applied Sciences (TAMK); 2023.
71. Elmaleh-Sachs A, Schwartz JL, Bramante CT, Nicklas JM, Gudzune KA, Jay M. Obesity management in adults: a review. JAMA. 2023;330(20):2000–15.
72. Islam MN, Mim ST, Tasfia T, Hossain MM. Enhancing patient treatment through automation: the development of an efficient scribe and prescribe system. Inform Med Unlocked. 2024;45:101456.
73. Vicente MSPP. Evaluating patient experience when using digital healthcare services: surveys and natural language processing-based methods [Doctoral dissertation]. Faculdade de Ciências da Universidade de Lisboa; 2023.
74. Salama M, Biggs BK, Creo A, Prissel R, Al Nofal A, Kumar S. Adolescents with type 2 diabetes: overcoming barriers to effective weight management. Diabetes Metab Syndr Obes. 2023;16:693–711.
75. Ahmedani MY, El-Sayed AAA, Yousuf S. Diabetes and Ramadan fasting. In: BIDE's diabetes desk book. Elsevier; 2024. p. 359–83.
76. Collins R, Collins D, Carson HJ. Show me, tell me: an investigation into learning processes within skateboarding as an informal coaching environment. Front Psychol. 2022;13:812068. https://doi.org/10.3389/fpsyg.2022.812068.
77. Vargas-Rubilar J, Richaud MC, Balabanian C, Lemos V. Parenting, gender, and perception of changes in children's behavior during the COVID-19 pandemic. Int J Environ Res Public Health. 2023;20(15):6452; Ruan-Iu L, Pendergast LL, Liao PC, et al. Measuring depression in young adults: preliminary development of an English version of the Teate depression inventory. Int J Environ Res Public Health. 2023;20(15):6470; Lipari D, Bocci BM, Rivieri C, et al. Trend of correlations between psychological symptoms and socioeconomic inequalities among Italian adolescents: cross-sectional study from 2006 to 2018 in Tuscany region. Int J Environ Res Public Health. 2023;20(15):6473.
78. Pach D. Evaluation nichtpharmakologischer Interventionen aus der Integrativen Medizin und Digitalen Gesundheit bei chronischen Schmerzen. 2023.
79. Heredia Ciuró A. Abordaje terapéutico de supervivientes de cáncer de pulmón tras tratamiento coadyuvante. 2023.
80. Ibacache Saavedra PA. Impacto de la cirugía bariátrica sobre la condición física asociada a la salud y la variabilidad del ritmo cardiaco en adultos con obesidad severa. 2023.

Human-Artificial Intelligence Collaborations in Polycystic Ovary Syndrome (PCOS) Clinical Trials and Research

13

Wasswa Shafik

13.1 Introduction

Polycystic ovary syndrome[1] (PCOS) is a multifaceted hormonal condition that impacts many individuals globally [1]. The expression of this condition exhibits significant variation among individuals, presenting symptoms that include hormonal abnormalities, irregular menstrual cycles, insulin resistance, and fertility problems [2]. The utilization of human-artificial intelligence (HAI) technology in nutritional analysis has great potential in the management of PCOS [3]. AI algorithms analyze extensive quantities of data, considering individual health records, genetic predispositions, and lifestyle factors to produce personalized nutritional recommendations. HAI recommends a diet that is abundant in complex carbohydrates and lean proteins, which helps maintain stable blood sugar levels to address insulin[2] resistance, a prevalent problem in PCOS [4]. In addition, through the analysis of dietary patterns, HAI identifies connections between certain foods and worsened symptoms, allowing patients to make well-informed dietary decisions that ease concerns connected to PCOS. This individualized strategy caters to the varied manifestations of PCOS, as some symptoms are demonstrated in Fig. 13.1, providing specific interventions to control its complex elements effectively [5].

HAI-powered nutritional treatments are transforming conventional dietary methods by providing accurate and individualized recommendations. Machine learning algorithms utilize large datasets to analyze dietary information and health markers

[1] https://www.who.int/news-room/fact-sheets/detail/polycystic-ovary-syndrome?

[2] https://www.medicalnewstoday.com/articles/323760

W. Shafik (✉)
Dig Connectivity Research Laboratory, Kampala, Uganda

School of Digital Science, Universiti Brunei Darussalam, Gadong, Brunei

R. Kumar et al. (eds.), *AI-Based Nutritional Intervention in Polycystic Ovary Syndrome (PCOS)*, https://doi.org/10.1007/978-981-96-2120-0_13

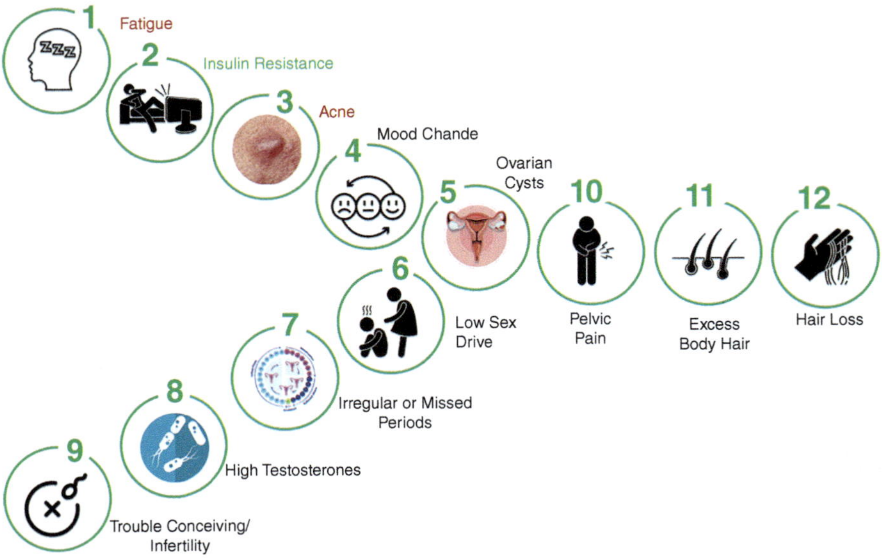

Fig. 13.1 Selected polycystic ovary syndrome symptoms

to provide personalized dietary recommendations [6]. For instance, in PCOS, HAI suggests a dietary plan that includes a high number of anti-inflammatory foods such as fruits, vegetables, and omega-3 fatty[3] acids. This is to address the inflammatory aspect commonly linked to the illness effectively. These interventions are designed to meet the specific needs of individuals, maximizing the consumption of nutrients to target health issues [2]. HAI analyzes individual nutritional data and enables the development of dietary programs that surpass generic suggestions, offering detailed advice that considers a person's health profile and objectives [7].

Precision medicine, which focuses on individualized healthcare and personalized treatment, forms a seamless alliance with HAI-driven nutritional analysis. HAI furthermore creates customized food regimens that adhere to precision medicine concepts by combining genetic markers, biomarkers, and lifestyle data [8]. Several frameworks of PCOS[4] occur depending on the cause and the effect. AI examines hormonal profiles, genetic predispositions associated with insulin resistance, and inflammatory markers to develop dietary plans that alleviate symptoms and enhance overall health [9]. This meticulous approach guarantees that dietary suggestions not only are tailored to each individual but also reflect the fundamental biological processes that contribute to illnesses [10]. The combination of HAI-driven precision and nutritional therapies enhances the capacity for efficient and focused healthcare initiatives [5].

[3] https://my.clevelandclinic.org/health/articles/17290-omega-3-fatty-acids

[4] https://twc-ms.com/about-polycystic-ovary-syndrome/

The use of HAI-driven tools in clinical practice signifies a revolutionary period in healthcare, namely, in the field of nutritional analysis. Healthcare providers equipped with HAI-powered insights acquire a more profound comprehension of patients' food patterns and nutritional needs using the current generative AI to provide quick search in disease-related responses [11, 12]. Within the field of PCOS care, practitioners who have access to AI-generated data can create customized dietary plans to target individual metabolic abnormalities and hormonal imbalances [13]. AI can examine the relationship between certain food elements and worsened PCOS symptoms, allowing clinicians to provide customized nutritional strategies. Such thorough analysis helps optimize patient treatment by providing precise interventions, thereby enhancing patient outcomes and promoting a proactive approach to managing complicated illnesses like PCOS in clinical settings [14].

The incorporation of AI into nutritional studies raises significant ethical concerns. In this technologically advanced healthcare environment, it is crucial to prioritize the protection of patient confidentiality, guarantee openness in the utilization of data, and address any potential biases in algorithms [15, 16]. HAI significantly depends on large datasets, which raises concerns over the security of data and the confidentiality of patients. Likewise, it is crucial to guarantee that HAI algorithms do not propagate biases, particularly when it comes to sensitive health issues like probiotics [17]. To achieve a harmonious integration of AI in personalized nutritional therapies, it is necessary to continuously examine and enforce strong guidelines and laws in the healthcare field while ensuring ethical standards are upheld [18, 19]. Ethical frameworks must progress alongside technological developments to guarantee the proper and fair utilization of HAI in nutritional analysis.

Hormonal data is crucial in disorders, mainly PCOS, where hormonal imbalances have a substantial effect on health. The potential of HAI to evaluate complex hormonal patterns and establish connections with dietary treatments shows great promise in optimizing nutritional strategies for maintaining hormonal balance [20–22]. HAI algorithms can assess hormonal swings and their correlation with dietary choices, therefore providing suggestions for dietary alterations that can assist in controlling hormone levels. Having a more profound comprehension of hormonal data enables persons with illnesses such as PCOS to make well-informed food choices that have a favorable impact on their hormonal well-being [23]. In addition, by integrating hormonal data into HAI-powered nutritional analysis, healthcare providers can create more accurate and focused dietary therapies designed to address hormonal imbalances. This has the potential to alleviate symptoms related to hormonal illnesses like PCOS [24].

The application of AI-driven nutritional analysis shows the potential to impact long-term health results, specifically in disorders such as PCOS. Through the utilization of HAI algorithms, patients suffering from PCOS can obtain personalized dietary suggestions that not only address current symptoms but also work toward reducing potential long-term health hazards linked to the illness [2]. HAI-power-driven analysis prioritizes dietary patterns that lower the risk of cardiovascular issues commonly associated with PCOS and fertility.[5] The continual monitoring and adaptive nature of HAI can enhance long-term health outcomes by fostering sustainable food habits and reducing the risks associated with chronic illnesses. This proactive technique redirects attention from symptom management to promoting comprehensive and long-lasting health enhancements in individuals with PCOS and other comparable health disorders in line with cannabidiol[6] (CBD) [6, 25].

Objectives of the Chapter

The objectives of the chapter are:

- To demonstrate how HAI enables users to monitor their eating patterns with precision and consistency, allowing for more accurate tracking and analysis of nutrient intake compared to traditional approaches;
- To present how HAI-enabled algorithms can be utilized to provide individualized recommendations for nutritional intake, considering individual health goals, preferences, and special dietary demands;
- To highlight that an HAI-driven examination of eating behaviors can offer useful behavioral insights, assisting individuals in identifying triggers for unhealthy eating habits or deficits to treat them effectively;
- To illustrate that customized dietary regimens, utilizing HAI analysis, can assist in the prevention and management of diseases by targeting nutrient consumption that is essential for different health conditions;
- To prove that by integrating wearable sensors, the accuracy can be improved by the monitoring of biological indicators or the analysis of sweat to obtain real-time information on nutritional levels;
- To justify the ability of HAI to process large volumes of data can simplify nutrient analysis and enhance its accessibility for those aiming to optimize their diet;
- And, to show HAI systems can provide immediate feedback and coaching, assisting users in making improved food selections or proposing alternatives in cases where their diet lacks specific nutrients, future research trends, and lessons learned.

Organization of Chapter

The rest of the chapter is organized as follows: Section 13.2 explores the utilization of human-artificial intelligence collaboration for recognizing food products and determining their nutritional content using picture analysis. It also elucidates the data processing methods employed by HAI to generate other nutritional insights. Section 13.3 examines the use of artificial intelligence in delivering customized nutrition suggestions by utilizing individualized data and the use of artificial intelligence in the supervision and enhancement of nutrient consumption to achieve improved health results. Section 13.4 assesses possible avenues for expansion and

[5] https://www.hopkinsmedicine.org/health/conditions-and-diseases/

[6] https://www.cdc.gov/marijuana/featured-topics/CBD.html

additional improvement in HAI-driven nutritional analysis. Likewise, it discusses the constraints or difficulties encountered while applying AI for nutritional analysis. Section 13.5 analyzes the ethical consequences of utilizing personal health data for AI-powered dietary analysis and examines the significance of transparency and accountability in managing confidential health-related information. Finally, Sects. 13.6 and 13.7 conclude the chapter with future scope and lessons learned.

13.2 Human-AI Collaboration in Polycystic Ovary Syndrome Trials and Research

The utilization of AI in nutritional analysis has fundamentally transformed our comprehension and enhancement of food intake to achieve superior health results, as depicted.

13.2.1 Food Recognition and Nutrient Analysis

The advanced capability of HAI in food recognition is transforming the field of nutritional analysis by precisely identifying food items and accurately evaluating their nutritional composition. Employing machine learning techniques, applications, and devices can examine photographs or descriptions of meals to offer detailed nutritional analyses [26, 27]. MyFitnessPal[7] employs artificial intelligence to identify food items from photographs supplied by users, providing comprehensive information on calorie content, macronutrients, vitamins, and minerals. The high level of accuracy in nutrient analysis enables individuals to monitor their dietary consumption precisely, promoting informed decision-making for the adoption of healthier eating habits [28]. This application provides users with up-to-date nutritional information, allowing them to maximize their nutrient consumption and effectively work toward their specific health objectives while keeping well-balanced meals.

Women with PCOS presented in Fig. 13.2 have elevated plasma renin levels and an overactive renin-angiotensin system (RAS), resulting in excessive production of Ang II. An excessive amount of Ang II leads to the dissociation of ACE2 from the angiotensin receptor 1 AT1R and its subsequent binding to AT1R. Angiotensin II binding to AT1R causes narrowing of blood vessels, heightened permeability of blood vessels, accumulation of fluid in the lungs (pulmonary edema), and the onset of acute respiratory distress syndrome (ARDS). When ACE2 separates from AT1R (as shown by the broken red arrow), it enhances the entry of SARS-CoV-2 into pneumocytes [29].

The viral infection may also be aided by the excessive production of TMPRSS2, which is caused by androgens in individuals with PCOS due to elevated androgen levels. After attaching to ACE2, the SARS-CoV-2[8] virus forms a complex with ACE2,

[7] https://www.myfitnesspal.com/

[8] https://www.cdc.gov/coronavirus/2019-ncov/variants/variant-classifications.html

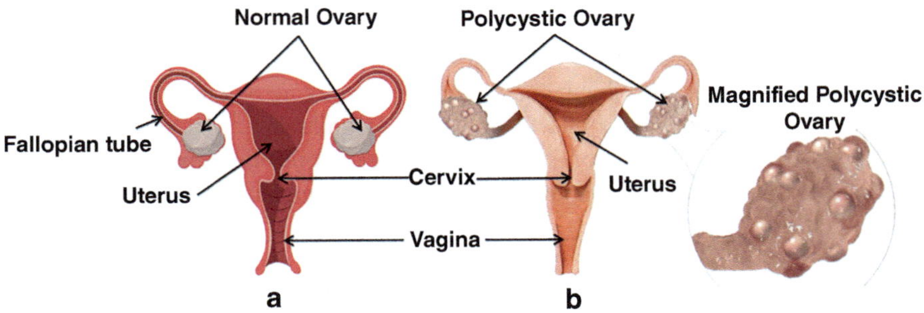

Fig. 13.2 Female reproduction system showing the PCOS: (**a**) Normal Ovary and (**b**) Polycystic Ovary

which is then taken inside the cell and undergoes proteasomal destruction of ACE2. This could potentially lead to a decrease in ACE2 expression within pulmonary cells [29]. Elevated levels of Ang II also prompt the adrenal gland to boost aldosterone production, leading to a decrease in potassium and a rise in sodium levels. Consequently, this results in elevated blood pressure. Collectively, these pathways may lead to serious consequences in women with PCOS who are infected with COVID-19,[9] as demonstrated early in the study during the high peak of the pandemic [30].

13.2.2 Personalized Dietary Recommendations

The ability of HAI to analyze large quantities of data enables the creation of personalized dietary recommendations that are specifically tailored to individual health profiles. Human-arranged AI platforms like Habit[10] utilize AI algorithms to analyze users' genetic, metabolic, and lifestyle information to create personalized meal programs [31]. These plans consider dietary preferences, nutritional requirements, and health objectives, offering precise guidance to maximize nutrient consumption. This tailored approach not only improves compliance with dietary regimens but also tackles specific nutritional shortfalls or health issues [32]. This degree of personalization in dietary suggestions results in more successful interventions and enhanced health results by addressing an individual's own nutritional needs.

13.2.3 Continuous Monitoring and Trend Analysis

The significance of AI in continuously monitoring and analyzing food behaviors enables a thorough understanding of long-term nutritional patterns. Lose It![11]

[9] https://www.who.int/health-topics/coronavirus

[10] https://aihabit.net/

[11] https://www.loseit.com/

employs HAI algorithms to monitor and analyze users' nutritional information over some time, detecting patterns such as variations in macronutrient consumption or inconsistent eating habits [33]. This analysis empowers individuals to modify their diets proactively, thus assuring a more well-rounded nutritional consumption and addressing any shortfalls. Users can achieve persistent gains in overall health by identifying patterns and trends and adjusting their food habits accordingly to match their nutritional goals [34].

13.2.4 Health Condition-Specific Dietary Plans

The versatility of AI enables the development of dietary regimens that are specifically designed for individual needs based on their health conditions. HAI-powered applications, like MySugr,[12] utilize artificial intelligence to create personalized meal plans for patients who are managing diabetes, with a specific emphasis on regulating glycemic index levels [35]. These tailored diets consider the individual nutritional needs for controlling the condition and optimizing dietary selections to minimize health risks linked with sickness. HAI-driven nutritional analysis plays a crucial role in managing chronic diseases by customizing diets to address specific health problems [36]. This approach offers individuals more precise and efficient dietary interventions.

13.2.5 Behavioral Insights and Feedback

The analysis conducted by HAI on eating behaviors and the following feedback provided by AI promote the selection of healthier food options. Rise monitor[13] users' eating patterns and offer tailored guidance and evaluation depending on their nutritional practices [37]. This HAI-powered system guides users in making conscious decisions regarding their food choices, altering their eating habits, and following nutritional guidelines [38]. AI improves users' awareness of their dietary habits by providing immediate feedback and behavioral insights, leading to healthier choices and long-term enhancements in nutrient intake.

13.2.6 Research and Data Analysis for Nutritional Science

Comprehensive dietary data analysis capabilities of AI revolutionize the field of nutritional science by revealing links between nutrient consumption and health effects. Research initiatives employ HAI algorithms to analyze extensive datasets, discerning correlations between certain nutrients and the prevention or management of diseases [39]. An example of this is when artificial intelligence is used to analyze

[12] https://www.mysugr.com/en/

[13] https://www.risescience.com/

data and determine the connection between omega-3 fatty acids[14] and cardiovascular well-being. HAI enhances nutritional research by revealing these connections, hence aiding the formulation of dietary guidelines and interventions [40]. Utilizing HAI in research improves our comprehension of the influence of nutrients on health results, facilitating the development of more efficient public health efforts and tailored dietary strategies. PCOS-increased levels of male hormones stimulate the expression of the ACE2 receptor, which is the entrance point for the SARS-CoV-2 virus. Additionally, these hormones also alter the activity of host proteases, facilitating the entry of the SARS-CoV-2 virus into various tissues. The Up arrow symbolizes growth or augmentation, whereas the lightning bolt denotes harm or physical damage.

13.2.7 Integration with Wearable Devices and Biometric Data

Wearable devices like smartwatches or fitness trackers that are equipped with artificial intelligence algorithms track and analyze physiological signs such as heart rate, sleep patterns, and activity levels [41]. These gadgets offer vital data that, when combined with nutritional information, provide comprehensive insights into an individual's overall health state. Wearable sensors that monitor glucose levels can be synchronized with data on dietary intake, allowing for a comprehensive understanding of how specific foods affect blood sugar levels [42]. This integration allows individuals, especially those with illnesses such as diabetes or metabolic disorders, to make well-informed dietary decisions in real time, thereby enhancing the management of their health by optimizing nutrient consumption.

13.3 Impact of Human-Artificial Intelligence Collaboration in Polycystic Ovary Syndrome Trials and Research

The capacity of HAI to assess this combined data assists in producing more accurate dietary suggestions, hence boosting the efficacy of nutritional interventions for enhanced health results, as illustrated below.

13.3.1 Personalized Dietary Recommendations

The influence of HAI on personalized nutrition is significant, providing customized dietary suggestions derived from individual health data, preferences, and objectives. Nutrino[15] employs artificial intelligence algorithms to examine users' health measurements, genetic data, and dietary patterns to provide personalized meal plans [43]. These plans consider aspects such as allergies, dietary limitations, and health

[14] https://my.clevelandclinic.org/health/articles/17290-omega-3-fatty-acids

[15] https://www.platejoy.com/

concerns, providing precise guidance to maximize nutritional consumption. A high degree of customization enables individuals to make well-informed nutritional decisions that are in line with their requirements, promoting better eating patterns [44]. The practical significance is in individuals receiving tailored instruction, resulting in enhanced compliance with dietary regimens and improved health outcomes.

13.3.2 Behavioral Perceptions and Reactions

The function of HAI in delivering behavioral insights and feedback has a big impact on personalized nutrition. HAI-enabled Habit utilizes AI to examine users' eating habits, providing tailored guidance and evaluations [45]. This pragmatic application empowers consumers to gain a deeper comprehension of their dietary habits and obtain personalized guidance on altering behaviors to make healthier selections. The influence manifests as enhanced consciousness and attentiveness toward dietary choices, resulting in modifications in behavior that are in line with nutritional objectives [46]. HAI promotes the adoption of tailored nutritional recommendations by offering immediate feedback, which motivates individuals to make lasting adjustments and maintain adherence over the long term. In the end, this results in healthier dietary habits and better overall health outcomes.

13.3.3 Continuous Monitoring and Adaptation

The influence of HAI on personalized nutrition encompasses the ongoing surveillance and adjustment of dietary patterns. Lose It! utilizes AI algorithms to monitor and analyze users' dietary information over a period, detecting and analyzing recurring patterns and trends in nutrient consumption [47]. Uninterrupted monitoring allows for real-time adjustments to dietary recommendations, ensuring they are in line with evolving health objectives or lifestyle changes. Essentially, this implies that individuals are provided with continuous assistance, and their food programs are adjusted according to their increasing requirements [48]. The significance is in supporting enduring dietary modifications that align with individual tastes and circumstances, so encouraging sustained adherence and overall enhancements in health.

13.3.4 Tailoring Nutritional Interventions for Health Conditions

The substantial impact of HAI's ability to customize dietary therapies for specific health issues greatly influences customized nutrition. PlateJoy[16] and similar platforms employ AI to provide personalized meal plans specifically designed to address illnesses like diabetes or cardiovascular disease [32]. AI utilizes health data and

[16] https://www.platejoy.com/

nutritional analysis to provide customized meal recommendations that address the specific dietary needs associated with these illnesses. This practical application leads to more efficient management of health issues. Individuals derive advantages from specific dietary recommendations that directly address their health issues, perhaps diminishing the dangers connected with these disorders and enhancing their entire state of being [31].

13.3.5 Integration of Biometric Data for Precision Nutrition

The combination of artificial intelligence with biometric data improves accuracy in tailored nutrition. Wearable gadgets, for instance, Fitbit,[17] when combined with AI algorithms, monitor physiological indicators like heart rate variability and sleep patterns [24]. When combined with dietary information, this data provides extensive insights into an individual's health condition [31]. This practical application allows users to make well-informed dietary decisions by considering real-time physiological reactions to meals. The benefit is evident when an individual's nutrient intake is tailored to coincide with their specific physiological reactions, resulting in improved health management and enhanced performance in daily activities [33].

13.3.6 Enhanced Accessibility and Affordability

HAI-powered tailored nutrition interventions can improve accessibility and affordability. With the advancement of HAI algorithms, there is a potential for the increased availability and affordability of apps and platforms that provide tailored dietary advice [35]. This practical significance signifies that a greater number of individuals, irrespective of their socioeconomic condition, can obtain customized nutritional suggestions. The significance lies in the democratization of customized nutrition, rendering it available to a greater demographic and potentially mitigating health inequalities by offering tailored nutritional counsel to a broader public [37].

13.4 Artificial Intelligence Challenges and Open Opportunities in Polycystic Ovary Syndrome Trials and Research

To tackle these difficulties, there are prospects for innovation and enhancement in AI-driven monitoring of nutrient intake. The objective is to develop more precise, fair, and user-friendly systems that efficiently optimize dietary patterns and foster improved health results.

[17] https://www.fitbit.com/

13.4.1 Data Accuracy and Privacy Concerns

The precision of nutritional data gathered by HAI systems can be affected by several issues, such as user input mistakes or insufficient information. Furthermore, apprehensions regarding data privacy and security emerge because of the delicate nature of health-related information [38]. Enhancing the dependability of HAI-powered nutritional analysis can be achieved by utilizing sophisticated algorithms and integrating user feedback methods to improve data accuracy. By using strong encryption and transparent safeguards, privacy issues can be effectively addressed, which in turn can enhance user trust and promote increased participation in HAI-driven nutrition platforms [9].

13.4.2 Personalization and User Engagement

The obstacle arises when attempting to customize nutritional suggestions to suit individual preferences and requirements, all the while guaranteeing consistent user involvement. Long-term compliance with individualized nutrition programs might also be a challenge [7]. Utilizing HAI algorithms to acquire knowledge and adjust according to user preferences consistently can significantly improve personalization. The implementation of gamification, incorporation of social aspects, and utilization of intuitive user interfaces have the potential to enhance user engagement, hence motivating individuals to stick to individualized dietary regimens [11]. Further possibilities exist in enhancing AI models to incorporate behavioral psychology to optimize user engagement tactics.

13.4.3 Integration with Existing Healthcare Systems

The incorporation of AI-driven nutritional analysis into current healthcare systems and processes may provide difficulties in achieving interoperability. Facilitating collaboration among diverse healthcare providers and enabling the slick incorporation of HAI technologies may face opposition or technological obstacles [13]. Standardizing interfaces and procedures for data sharing among healthcare providers helps simplify the process of integration. The collaboration between HAI developers and healthcare institutions offers a chance to create flexible systems that enhance the effectiveness of nutritional analysis in healthcare settings by integrating with existing workflows [14].

13.4.4 Algorithm Bias and Ethical Considerations

HAI algorithms have the potential to unintentionally maintain biases, which can influence the precision and impartiality of dietary advice. HAI decision-making encounters substantial obstacles due to ethical considerations, including consent, openness, and fairness [18]. By using diverse and inclusive training datasets, algorithmic bias can be mitigated in AI-driven nutrition analysis. Enforcing ethical principles and legal frameworks guarantees the transparency, equity, and responsibility of HAI systems. There are opportunities to create AI models that specifically address justice and ethical concerns, which will help build trust among users and stakeholders [11].

13.4.5 Accessibility and Equity

The availability of AI-powered nutritional analysis may be restricted due to variables such as technological obstacles, cost, or lack of digital literacy, hence exacerbating current health inequalities [34]. Creating intuitive interfaces and mobile applications can improve the accessibility of HAI-driven nutrition platforms. Partnerships with public health authorities and community organizations can facilitate the dissemination of knowledge and information regarding the advantages of HAI-powered nutritional analysis [28]. This can help bridge the gap between those who have access to digital resources and those who do not while also encouraging fairness in obtaining tailored dietary guidance. Moreover, harnessing HAI for cost-efficient solutions can enhance affordability and expand access to a wide range of socioeconomic groups [24].

13.4.6 Validity and Reliability of Artificial Intelligence Recommendations

Verifying the accuracy and dependability of HAI-generated food suggestions is difficult, particularly when addressing intricate health problems or distinctive dietary requirements. There are situations in which AI may offer recommendations that lack scientific validity or fail to address individual peculiarities appropriately [36]. Partnerships among AI developers, dietitians, and healthcare professionals can substantiate HAI-generated advice via clinical trials and scientific studies. The utilization of this cooperative method guarantees that HAI suggestions are in accordance with scientifically supported nutritional principles [40]. The development of HAI explainability approaches can enhance the transparency of HAI-driven recommendations, allowing consumers to comprehend the underlying reasoning behind the ideas. This fosters trust and confidence in the advice given [34].

13.4.7 Behavioral Change and Long-Term Adherence

Facilitating consistent modification of behavior and maintaining adherence to AI-suggested food programs are considerable obstacles. People may find it challenging to consistently follow tailored dietary recommendations due to reasons, for example, lifestyle modifications, societal pressures, or motivational obstacles [28].

Integrating behavioral science ideas into HAI-powered nutrition programs can help maintain long-term compliance. HAI algorithms can utilize user actions and preferences to provide adaptive and incremental modifications in dietary programs in accordance with the users' level of preparedness for change [31]. The integration of incentive strategies, social support elements, and habit-building techniques can promote changes in behavior and cultivate a sustained commitment to individualized dietary recommendations [49].

13.4.8 Regulatory Compliance and Standardization

Managing legal frameworks and maintaining adherence to increasing standards in the field of AI-driven nutritional analysis pose a significant problem. Divergent rules in different locations and the lack of uniform norms can impede the general implementation of HAI-driven solutions in the field of nutrition [28]. Effective collaboration between regulators, healthcare stakeholders, and AI developers may generate strong regulatory frameworks and established norms for HAI-powered nutritional analysis. Establishing industry-wide benchmarks for safeguarding data privacy, ensuring algorithm openness, and addressing ethical concerns fosters confidence and widespread acceptance [39]. Promoting collaborations between regulatory agencies and technological pioneers promotes the responsible advancement and implementation of AI applications, guaranteeing that these solutions adhere to ethical, legal, and safety criteria [45].

13.5 Behavioral Ethical Considerations and Privacy Concerns on Polycystic Ovary Syndrome Trials

This section presents the behavioral, ethical, and privacy concerns of using personal health data for HAI-driven nutritional analysis.

13.5.1 Behavioral Considerations

By incorporating these behavioral factors into HAI-power-driven interventions, platforms can effectively assist and empower individuals in making enduring and beneficial modifications to their food patterns.

13.5.1.1 Adherence and Sustainability

Promoting sustained adherence to AI-recommended dietary programs relies on the principles of sustainability and behavioral modifications. Many people find it difficult to consistently stick to anything since they are used to certain behaviors and influenced by their surroundings [24]. AI can assist by progressively implementing feasible dietary modifications that fit with individual preferences. By incorporating ideas from behavioral science, for example, habit-building and goal-setting, into

AI-driven platforms, we can encourage long-lasting dietary changes. Consistent assistance and flexible tactics guarantee that modifications are practical and adjustable, hence improving long-term compliance [27].

13.5.1.2 Motivation and Engagement

Consistent drive and involvement are essential for altering dietary patterns. HAI-driven systems can utilize gamification, incentives, and tailored feedback to enhance user involvement. Customizing suggestions according to user preferences and offering immediate feedback on progress foster a feeling of accomplishment and sustain folks' involvement [28]. By applying ideas from motivational psychology, HAI-driven platforms can create a positive and inspiring atmosphere that encourages users to participate in and follow their prescribed dietary alterations consistently.

13.5.1.3 Cultural and Social Influences

Gaining insight into the cultural and societal factors that impact eating patterns is essential for developing AI-driven suggestions that are successful. Cultural dietary practices and social conventions highly influence food choices [32]. HAI systems must consider cultural diversity and social circumstances when providing recommendations. By integrating cultural preferences and social dynamics into tailored suggestions, HAI can improve its relevance and acceptance among varied people, guaranteeing that nutritional recommendations are in line with individual cultural backgrounds and social settings [38].

13.5.1.4 Behavioral Patterns and Triggers

It is crucial to identify behavioral patterns and triggers that impact food habits to provide individualized suggestions. Artificial intelligence can examine user data to identify factors that cause unhealthy eating habits or instances of noncompliance [40]. HAI-driven platforms can provide customized tactics and interventions to assist individuals in identifying and overcoming specific triggers, hence promoting healthier eating choices and long-term adherence to prescribed nutritional regimens [46].

13.5.1.5 Lifestyle Integration and Flexibility

Ensuring long-term compliance requires the incorporation of dietary modifications into a person's daily routine while also allowing for adaptability. HAI-powered platforms should provide suggestions that cater to a wide range of lifestyles, schedules, and tastes [50]. By offering versatile meal plans that may be adjusted to different circumstances, individuals can effortlessly integrate suggested dietary modifications into their everyday schedules without experiencing limitations or excessive stress [23]. The capacity of HAI to acquire knowledge and adjust to human tastes facilitates the development of customized dietary programs that correspond to various lifestyles, promoting sustained adherence and integration into one's way of life.

13.5.2 Ethical Considerations

Ethical perspectives of HAI in relation to its application in nutritional analysis are presented.

13.5.2.1 Confidentiality Protection

Ensuring the protection of user privacy is of utmost importance in HAI-powered nutritional analysis. The ethical considerations pertain to the collection and management of delicate health data. It is crucial to guarantee strong encryption, anonymization of personal data, and obtain explicit user consent prior to collecting data [17]. It is essential to have clear and open policies on the usage of data and to comply strictly with rigorous privacy regulations. Promoting user privacy in AI applications cultivates trust, motivating users to participate in nutritional analysis platforms without apprehension regarding the mishandling or unauthorized use of their data [50].

13.5.2.2 Algorithmic Bias and Fairness

The utilization of AI algorithms for food advice gives rise to ethical considerations due to the possibility of prejudice [42]. Biases can arise from distorted datasets or intrinsic limits in algorithms. To tackle algorithmic bias, it is necessary to utilize diverse and representative datasets and conduct regular audits of algorithms to ensure fairness [46]. It is of utmost ethical importance to guarantee fairness in suggestions for people from different demographics, prevent the reinforcement of preconceptions, and consistently improve algorithms to minimize biases.

13.5.2.3 Informed Consent and Transparency

It is crucial to uphold transparency and guarantee informed consent while doing HAI-driven nutritional analysis. Users should possess a comprehensive understanding of how their data is employed and have the freedom to govern its utilization [50]. Ensuring transparency in data processing, explaining the reasoning behind suggestions, and highlighting potential risks are crucial for facilitating well-informed decision-making. Providing clear and honest information about the constraints and uncertainties of HAI-engendered suggestions enables users to make well-informed decisions regarding their food habits, relying on the knowledge supplied [48].

13.5.2.4 User Autonomy and Empowerment

Respecting user autonomy involves empowering individuals to make informed decisions about their nutrition. Ethical AI applications should prioritize user preferences and values in generating recommendations, allowing users to tailor suggestions based on personal goals and beliefs [43]. Providing a range of options and educational resources empowers users to take charge of their dietary choices while fostering a supportive environment for personalized nutrition interventions.

13.5.2.5 Accountability and Responsible Deployment

The ethical obligation is to guarantee accountability at every stage of the development and implementation of AI-driven nutritional analysis. This encompasses the responsibility for assuring the accuracy of advice, guaranteeing user safety, and minimizing potential dangers linked to dietary interventions [41]. To ensure responsible utilization of HAI in nutritional analysis and to maximize the benefits for individuals aiming to enhance their health outcomes through optimized nutrient consumption, it is crucial to establish explicit guidelines, supervision systems, and accountability frameworks [37]. These measures will help minimize any negative consequences that may arise.

13.5.3 Privacy Concerns

This subsection entails some selected privacy considerations and concerns that can be examined.

13.5.3.1 Data Security and Confidentiality

Ensuring the preservation of data security and confidentiality is of utmost importance in the context of AI-powered nutritional analysis. Users divulge confidential health information, such as food patterns and medical issues, giving rise to concerns over potential data breaches or unauthorized entry [34]. Ensuring the security of user data requires the implementation of strong encryption techniques, strict access controls, and secure protocols for data storage. Moreover, the implementation of anonymization techniques guarantees the protection of personally identifiable information while also allowing HAI systems to extract valuable insights for personalized suggestions [33].

13.5.3.2 Informed Consent and Transparency

It is crucial to guarantee that individuals provide their consent based on accurate information and that there is clear disclosure regarding the utilization of data. Users must be provided with clear information regarding the utilization of their data, including its analysis using artificial intelligence, and they should explicitly give their approval [21]. Open and clear information about the procedures of collecting, storing, and using data helps to build confidence with users. By offering easily understandable privacy regulations and transparent explanations regarding the data processing methods of HAI algorithms, users are empowered to make well-informed choices regarding the sharing of their information for nutritional analysis [15].

13.5.3.3 Minimization of Data Collection

Implementing a strategy of minimizing data collection helps to reduce privacy risks. Restricting the gathering of extra data diminishes the likelihood of its misuse or illegal retrieval. AI systems should exclusively collect pertinent data to provide customized nutritional suggestions while minimizing the exposure of sensitive user information [13]. Ensuring impartiality, equity, and responsibility in HAI decision-making is crucial to avoid prejudiced results. Conducting routine audits and ensuring openness in algorithmic processes are crucial for upholding ethical norms [5]. By prioritizing fairness, HAI-driven nutritional analysis may deliver impartial suggestions that are equally applicable to various user groups.

13.5.3.4 Third-Party Data Sharing and Partnerships

Ensuring the protection of privacy in the sharing or collaborations with third-party data is of utmost importance. Partnerships with external companies for the purpose of sharing data or developing algorithms necessitate strict privacy agreements [9]. Enforcing consistent privacy rules and procedures among third parties preserves the integrity of user data during cooperation. Regular audits and oversight are crucial for monitoring adherence to privacy protocols. Granting users the ability to exercise control over their data, like through deletion or alteration, amplifies user autonomy [7]. Providing explicit and user-friendly mechanisms for users to decline specific data gathering or HAI-based analysis honors their privacy preferences.

13.5.3.5 Continuous Monitoring and User Control

Regular surveillance of user data for nutritional analysis purposes requires consistent user oversight and openness. HAI systems frequently gather up-to-date nutritional data to provide tailored recommendations [17]. Enhancing transparency is achieved by providing consumers with easy capabilities to monitor and manage their data-sharing settings. In addition, by allowing users to assess and modify their data permissions or withdraw access, it guarantees continuous consent and user autonomy in the data-gathering procedure [18]. Integrating user-friendly interfaces that simplify data administration enhances a feeling of control, hence strengthening confidence in AI-powered nutritional analysis tools.

13.5.3.6 Cross-Border Data Transfer and Compliance

The task of overseeing the transmission of data across international borders and guaranteeing adherence to various regulatory regimes poses privacy obstacles. Given the worldwide nature of AI-driven nutritional analysis platforms, it is crucial to comply with diverse data privacy regulations in different locations [21]. By implementing measures such as standard contractual provisions or obligatory company norms, data protection can be ensured when conducting international transfers. Furthermore, implementing a privacy-by-design strategy, which involves integrating privacy safeguards into the fundamental structure of HAI systems, enables adherence to various rules [47]. Engaging in partnerships with legal professionals to negotiate global privacy regulations and customize HAI systems to various regulatory contexts guarantees the preservation of user data security regardless of geographical limitations.

13.6 Future Directions and Lessons Learned

Within this section, we present future research directions, lessons learned from the chapter, and the study's conclusion.

13.6.1 Future Research Directions

The ethical frameworks and norms governing PCOS trials and research development in nutrition will progress to give priority to user privacy, permission, and the conscientious utilization of AI technology.

13.6.1.1 Multi-Omics Integration for Comprehensive Analysis

Subsequent investigations are expected to concentrate on the incorporation of multi-omics data, encompassing genomes, metabolomics, and micro-bionics, into nutritional analysis enhanced by artificial intelligence [50]. Integrating various omics information with HAI algorithms can yield a more comprehensive comprehension of how specific genetic variants, gut microbiota, and metabolic profiles impact food metabolism and dietary responses. Investigating these connections can facilitate the development of highly customized dietary therapies designed to match an individual's distinct biological composition, hence improving the accuracy and efficacy of nutritional advice [45].

13.6.1.2 Dynamic Real-Time Monitoring and Feedback Systems

Research may explore the creation of dynamic real-time monitoring systems that consistently gather physiological, nutritional, and environmental data. The incorporation of AI algorithms into wearable devices or smart sensors allows for immediate study of physiological reactions to food consumption [43]. The development of HAI-power-driven feedback mechanisms that can adaptively change dietary recommendations in real time based on physiological responses has the potential to revolutionize personalized nutrition [40]. This approach aims to optimize nutrient consumption and improve health outcomes responsively and adaptively.

13.6.1.3 Explainable AI for Enhanced User Understanding

Ensuing investigations could prioritize the enhancement of explainable AI (XAI) methods within nutritional analysis platforms. Improving the comprehensibility and clarity of AI-generated nutritional recommendations will enable people to grasp the process by which AI algorithms develop specific suggestions [32]. Creating XAI models that offer transparent and easily understandable explanations for dietary recommendations using a wide range of data inputs can enhance user confidence and involvement, encouraging well-informed decision-making and cultivating a sustained commitment to individualized dietary programs [28].

13.6.1.4 AI-Enabled Behavioral Change Strategies

Research may investigate AI-powered methods for modifying behavior that extend beyond providing nutritional suggestions. HAI algorithms can utilize behavioral science principles to provide customized therapies that consider psychological variables, routines, and societal impacts [34]. Developing AI-driven solutions that offer customized motivational strategies, habit formation approaches, and social support networks can improve behavioral changes, making it easier to stick to personalized dietary regimens in the long term [39].

13.6.1.5 Ethical and Fair Artificial Intelligence Development

The following studies are expected to prioritize the ethical and equitable development of artificial intelligence in the field of nutritional analysis. Ensuring equitable recommendations for diverse groups necessitates addressing biases, fairness, and accountability in AI systems [41]. Investigating techniques to improve the ethical decision-making of HAI, for example, fairness-aware learning and bias detection tools, will be crucial in developing AI systems that provide impartial and culturally aware food recommendations to persons from diverse backgrounds. The ethical frameworks and norms governing HAI development in nutrition will change to promote user privacy, permission, and the responsible utilization of HAI technology to enhance nutritional results [43].

13.6.1.6 Collaborative Artificial Intelligence in Healthcare Ecosystems

The research may concentrate on promoting the development of cooperative artificial intelligence systems inside larger healthcare networks. By combining HAI-powered nutritional analysis with electronic health records, telemedicine platforms, and healthcare provider networks, a comprehensive approach to individualized nutrition can be achieved [44]. This partnership enables the effortless exchange of nutritional data across individuals, healthcare practitioners, and HAI systems, hence promoting well-informed decision-making and coordinated actions [45]. Creating HAI solutions that can work together with current healthcare systems can improve the incorporation of personalized nutrition into regular clinical practice, leading to better patient results and overall population health [50].

13.6.1.7 Longitudinal Studies on Nutritional Outcomes

Potential future research avenues could entail performing longitudinal studies to investigate the enduring effects of AI-guided tailored nutrition regimens. Long-term monitoring of individuals enables the evaluation of lasting modifications in diet and their impact on health results [48]. This research helps clarify the long-lasting effectiveness of AI-recommended food programs in preventing chronic diseases, managing weight, and enhancing general health. Long-term research findings will be used to enhance HAI algorithms, improving their capacity to produce customized recommendations that result in long-lasting enhancements in dietary habits and overall well-being [46].

13.6.2 Lessons Learned

Given the specifics presented in the study, this section offers broad insights often derived from studies in the domain of HAI-powered PCOS research and clinical trials:

- Research frequently emphasizes the importance of customized dietary suggestions obtained from artificial intelligence systems. Customizing dietary regimens based on individual health profiles, tastes, and goals typically improves compliance and efficacy in attaining nutritional targets.
- Research consistently emphasizes the importance of regularly monitoring food habits and health indicators. The continuous gathering of data allows for the examination of extended patterns, facilitating the adjustment and improvement of dietary guidelines over a period.
- The focus is on the significance of integrating behavioral science with HAI-powered dietary solutions. Approaches that consider psychological variables, the building of habits, and triggers that motivate individuals tend to promote long-lasting changes in behavior among users.
- Research frequently emphasizes the significance of addressing ethical problems in AI-powered nutritional analysis. Establishing equity, clarity, and confidentiality and minimizing prejudices in HAI algorithms are essential for fostering user confidence and approval.
- The importance of interdisciplinary collaboration among nutritionists, data scientists, healthcare providers, and technology. Collaborative endeavors can harness a range of specialized knowledge to provide AI-powered nutritional solutions that are more efficient and comprehensive.
- Research consistently emphasizes the significance of conducting long-term trials to evaluate the enduring effects of HAI-guided nutritional therapy. Longitudinal study provides valuable insights into the long-term stability and efficacy of individualized nutrition programs.
- The necessity for the smooth incorporation of HAI-driven nutritional analysis into current healthcare systems. Integrating electronic health data and healthcare provider networks enables informed decision-making and coordinated actions to improve health outcomes.

13.7 Conclusion

AI is a powerful tool that is transforming the way we monitor and control our nutritional intake, with the goal of optimizing nutrient consumption. The integration of HAI technology and nutritional analysis marks the beginning of a new age, providing tailored and accurate suggestions that address individual health profiles, preferences, and objectives. The capacity of HAI to monitor and analyze extensive quantities of dietary data enables individuals to offer customized insights into their nutritional habits. HAI enables a thorough comprehension of the complex connection between diet and health outcomes through features such as tailored dietary advice and real-time monitoring of physiological data. It functions as a reliable tool, helping to navigate the intricacies of nutritional science, and provides subtle and efficient solutions. The influence of AI goes beyond simple surveillance; it encompasses the enhancement of nutritional intake by constantly adapting and refining dietary regimens. HAI utilizes behavioral insights and real-time feedback mechanisms to promote sustainable changes in behavior, hence promoting long-term adherence to individualized dietary plans. Nevertheless, as we traverse this domain of technical progress, ethical considerations such as privacy, fairness, and openness emerge as vital foundations. It is crucial to guarantee the proper advancement and implementation of HAI-driven PCOS and nutritional analysis to gain and sustain consumer confidence while adhering to ethical principles.

References

1. Yang J, Chen C. Hormonal changes in PCOS. J Endocrinol. 2024;261(1). https://doi.org/10.1530/JOE-23-0342.
2. Pai S, Childress KJ, Dietrich JE. Mccune Albright syndrome and polycystic ovary syndrome in a single individual. J Pediatr Adolesc Gynecol. 2016;29(2):188. https://doi.org/10.1016/j.jpag.2016.01.073.
3. Tang HB, Feng X, Han CH, Wang AH. An evidence-based evaluation of efficacy of Marvelon combined with metformin for polycystic ovary syndrome. Chin Pharm J. 2012;47(11):863–7. Available from: https://pesquisa.bvsalud.org/portal/resource/pt/wpr-860715
4. Jiao X, Du Q, Du X. Vascular echo tracking in evaluating early carotid atherosclerosis in patients with polycystic ovary syndrome and insulin resistance. Chin J Med Imag Technol. 2019;35(9). https://doi.org/10.13929/j.1003-3289.201903147.
5. Franik S, Eltrop SM, Kremer JAM, Kiesel L, Farquhar C. Aromatase inhibitors (letrozole) for subfertile women with polycystic ovary syndrome. Cochrane Database Syst Rev. 2018;5(5):CD010287. https://doi.org/10.1002/14651858.CD010287.pub3.
6. Deng Y, Xue W, Wang Y-F, et al. Insulin resistance in polycystic ovary syndrome improved by Chinese medicine Dingkun Pill (定坤丹): a randomized controlled clinical trial. Chin J Integr Med. 2019;25(4):246. https://doi.org/10.1007/s11655-018-2947-1.
7. Li S, Li J, Ai Q, Liu H. Development and validation of nomograms for predicting adverse neonatal outcomes in women with polycystic ovary syndrome: a retrospective study. J Obstet Gynaecol. 2022;42(6):1922. https://doi.org/10.1080/01443615.2022.2054682.
8. Liu L, Du B, Zhang H, et al. A network pharmacology approach to explore the mechanisms of Erxian decoction in polycystic ovary syndrome. Chin Med. 2018;13(1):46. https://doi.org/10.1186/s13020-018-0201-1.
9. Franik S, Le QK, Kremer JAM, Kiesel L, Farquhar C. Aromatase inhibitors (letrozole) for ovulation induction in infertile women with polycystic ovary syndrome. Cochrane Database Syst Rev. 2022;9(9):CD010287. https://doi.org/10.1002/14651858.CD010287.pub4.
10. Yasmin A, Roychoudhury S, Paul Choudhury A, et al. Polycystic ovary syndrome: an updated overview foregrounding impacts of ethnicities and geographic variations. Life (Basel). 2022;12(12):1974. https://doi.org/10.3390/life12121974.
11. Nguyen TT, Doan HT, Quan LH, Lam NM. Effect of letrozole for ovulation induction combined with intrauterine insemination on women with polycystic ovary syndrome. Gynecol Endocrinol. 2020;36(10):860. https://doi.org/10.1080/09513590.2020.1744556.
12. Shafik W. Introduction to ChatGPT. In: Advanced applications of generative AI and natural language processing models. IGI Global; 2024a. p. 1–25. https://doi.org/10.4018/979-8-3693-0502-7.ch001.
13. Hernández-Mijares A, Bañuls C, Gómez-Balaguer M, Bergoglio M, Víctor VM, Rocha M. Influence of obesity on atherogenic dyslipidemia in women with polycystic ovary syndrome. Eur J Clin Investig. 2013;43(6):549. https://doi.org/10.1111/eci.12080.
14. Cussons AJ, Watts GF, Stuckey BGA. Dissociation of endothelial function and arterial stiffness in nonobese women with polycystic ovary syndrome (PCOS). Clin Endocrinol. 2009;71(6):808. https://doi.org/10.1111/j.1365-2265.2009.03598.x.

15. Kuang H, Duan Y, Li D, et al. The role of serum inflammatory cytokines and berberine in the insulin signaling pathway among women with polycystic ovary syndrome. PLoS One. 2020;15(8):e0235404. https://doi.org/10.1371/journal.pone.0235404.
16. Shafik W. Wearable medical electronics in artificial intelligence of medical things. In: Handbook of security and privacy of AI-enabled healthcare systems and internet of medical things. CRC Press; 2024b. p. 21–40. https://doi.org/10.1201/9781003370321-2.
17. Le NSV, Le MT, Tran NQT, Nguyen QHV, Cao TN. The value of anti-Müllerian hormone in predicting ovulation induced by aromatase inhibitors in women with polycystic ovary syndrome. J Obstet Gynaecol Can. 2023;45(11):102183. https://doi.org/10.1016/j.jogc.2023.07.003.
18. Polyzos N, Tzioras S, Badawy AM, Valachis A, Dritsas C, Mauri D. Aromatase inhibitors for female infertility: a systematic review of the literature. Reprod Biomed Online. 2009;19(4):456–71. https://doi.org/10.1016/j.rbmo.2009.06.008.
19. Shafik W. A comprehensive cybersecurity framework for present and future global information technology organizations. In: Effective cybersecurity operations for enterprise-wide systems. IGI Global; 2023a. p. 56–79. https://doi.org/10.4018/978-1-6684-9018-1.ch002.
20. Alnssyan B, Ahmad Z, Malela-Majika JC, Seong JT, Shafik W. On the identifiability and statistical features of a new distributional approach with reliability applications. AIP Adv. 2023;13(12). https://doi.org/10.1063/5.0178555.
21. Kaur R, Kumar R, Gupta M. Predicting risk of obesity and meal planning to reduce the obese in adulthood using artificial intelligence. Endocrine. 2022b;78(3):458. https://doi.org/10.1007/s12020-022-03215-4.
22. Shafik W. Artificial intelligence and blockchain technology enabling cybersecurity in telehealth systems. In: Artificial intelligence and blockchain technology in modern telehealth systems. IET; 2023b. p. 285–326. https://doi.org/10.1049/PBHE061E_ch11.
23. Sosnowski Ł, Dutta S, Szymusik I. Analysis for women's' menstrual health disorders using artificial intelligence. In: Information technology for management: approaches to improving business and society. Lecture notes in business information processing. Cham: Springer; 2023. p. 471. https://doi.org/10.1007/978-3-031-29570-6_4.
24. Nsugbe E. An artificial intelligence-based decision support system for early diagnosis of polycystic ovaries syndrome. Healthc Anal. 2023;3:100164. https://doi.org/10.1016/j.health.2023.100164.
25. Kalinaki K, Fahadi M, Alli AA, Shafik W, Yasin M, Mutwalibi N. Artificial intelligence of internet of medical things (AIoMT) in smart cities: a review of cybersecurity for smart healthcare. In: Handbook of security and privacy of AI-enabled healthcare systems and internet of medical things. CRC Press; 2024. p. 271–92. https://doi.org/10.1201/9781003370321-11.
26. Fahim KE, Kalinaki K, Shafik W. Electronic devices in the artificial intelligence of the internet of medical things (AIoMT). In: Handbook of security and privacy of AI-enabled healthcare systems and internet of medical things. CRC Press; 2024. p. 41–62. https://doi.org/10.1201/9781003370321-3.
27. Fahs D, Salloum D, Nasrallah M, Ghazeeri G. Polycystic ovary syndrome: pathophysiology and controversies in diagnosis. Diagnostics. 2023;13(9). https://doi.org/10.3390/diagnostics13091559.
28. Khanna VV, Chadaga K, Sampathila N, Prabhu S, Bhandage V, Hegde GK. A distinctive explainable machine learning framework for detection of polycystic ovary syndrome. Appl Syst Innov. 2023;6(2). https://doi.org/10.3390/asi6020032.
29. De Medeiros SF, Yamamoto MMW, de Medeiros MAS, Yamamoto AKLW, Barbosa BB. Polycystic ovary syndrome and risks for COVID-19 infection: A comprehensive review: PCOS and COVID-19 relationship. Rev Endocr Metab Disord. 2022;23(2):251–64. https://doi.org/10.1007/s11154-022-09715-y.
30. Gilbert EW, Tay CT, Hiam DS, Teede HJ, Moran LJ. Comorbidities and complications of polycystic ovary syndrome: an overview of systematic reviews. Clin Endocrinol. 2018;89(6):683–99. https://doi.org/10.1111/cen.13828.

31. Kangasniemi MH, Komsi EK, Rossi HR, et al. Artificial intelligence deep learning model assessment of leukocyte counts and proliferation in endometrium from women with and without polycystic ovary syndrome. F S Sci. 2022;3(2):174–86. https://doi.org/10.1016/j.xfss.2022.01.006.
32. Elmannai H, El-Rashidy N, Mashal I, et al. Polycystic ovary syndrome detection machine learning model based on optimized feature selection and explainable artificial intelligence. Diagnostics. 2023;13(8). https://doi.org/10.3390/diagnostics13081506.
33. Ghige P, Walkunde P. Unleashing the benefits of artificial intelligence in the management of PCOS and PCOD: a paradigm shift in women's health. Int J Adv Res Sci Commun Technol. 2023;3(1):448. https://doi.org/10.48175/ijarsct-12067.
34. Kiranmai TS, Lakshmi PV. A comprehensive and systematic literature review of computational intelligence algorithms to diagnose and predict female infertility. Ann Romanian Soc Cell Biol. 2021;25(1):5926–43.
35. Vishwakarma V, Chethan S, Datla MT, Aqib MM, Roy S, Thasni T. Prediction of severity of polycystic ovarian syndrome using artificial neural networks. In: Second international conference on image processing and capsule networks. ICIPCN 2021. Lecture notes in networks and systems, vol. 300. Cham: Springer; 2022. https://doi.org/10.1007/978-3-030-84760-9_50.
36. Silva IS, Ferreira CN, Costa LBX, et al. Polycystic ovary syndrome: clinical and laboratory variables related to new phenotypes using machine-learning models. J Endocrinol Investig. 2022;45(3):497. https://doi.org/10.1007/s40618-021-01672-8.
37. Kaur R, Kumar R, Gupta M. Food image-based diet recommendation framework to overcome PCOS problem in women using deep convolutional neural network. Comput Electr Eng. 2022a;103:108298. https://doi.org/10.1016/j.compeleceng.2022.108298.
38. Zigarelli A, Jia Z, Lee H. Machine-aided self-diagnostic prediction models for polycystic ovary syndrome: observational study. JMIR Form Res. 2022;6(3):e29967. https://doi.org/10.2196/29967.
39. Aswathy VS, Vineetha Sankar P. Comparative study on AI technology in PCOS diagnosis. Int J Res Appl Sci Eng Technol. 2023;11(5):846. https://doi.org/10.22214/ijraset.2023.51615.
40. Vats S, Sengupta A, Chaurasia A, Narad P. Combination of expression data and predictive modelling for polycystic ovary disease and assessing risk of infertility using machine learning techniques. In: Innovations in computational intelligence and computer vision: proceedings of ICICV 2021. Springer; 2022. https://doi.org/10.1007/978-981-19-0475-2_48.
41. Lee S, Arffman R, Komsi E, et al. P-625 Artificial intelligence-enabled analysis of endometrial CD138 positive plasma cells in infertility-associated conditions; polycystic ovary syndrome (PCOS) and recurrent implantation failure (RIF). Hum Reprod. 2023;38(Suppl_1). https://doi.org/10.1093/humrep/dead093.953.
42. Deepika V. Applications of artificial intelligence techniques in polycystic ovarian syndrome diagnosis. J Adv Res Technol Manag Sci. 2019;1(3) Available from: https://www.jartms.org/admin/uploads/JcgPN1.pdf
43. Agrawal A, Ambad R, Lahoti R, Muley P, Pande P. Role of artificial intelligence in PCOS detection. J Datta Meghe Inst Med Sci Univ. 2022;17(2). https://doi.org/10.4103/jdmimsu.jdmimsu_278_22.
44. Neto C, Silva M, Fernandes M, Ferreira D, Machado J. Prediction models for polycystic ovary syndrome using data mining. In: Antipova T, editor. Advances in digital Science. ICADS 2021. Advances in intelligent systems and computing, vol. 1352. Cham: Springer; 2021. https://doi.org/10.1007/978-3-030-71782-7_19.
45. Allameh F, Fallah-Karkan M, Modarres SZ, et al. Machine learning approaches to predict intra-uterine insemination success rate-application of artificial intelligence in infertility. Health Forum J. 2021; https://doi.org/10.22037/mhj.v5i1.34250.
46. Makhdoomi A, Jan N, Palak P, Goel N. Machine learning techniques for medical images in PCOS. In: AIST 2022 - 4th international conference on artificial intelligence and speech technology. IEEE; 2022. https://doi.org/10.1109/AIST55798.2022.10064817.

47. Abdul Khadar A, Shreasta MS, Vani N, Vathsala KR, Vidhya Shree VN. Diagnosis of polycystic ovary syndrome using machine learning algorithms. Int J Adv Res Sci Commun Technol. 2022;2(6):869–72. https://doi.org/10.48175/ijarsct-5174.
48. Balikçi Çiçek İ, Küçükakçali Z, Yağin FH. Detection of risk factors of PCOS patients with local interpretable model-agnostic explanations (LIME) method that an explainable artificial intelligence model. J Cognit Syst. 2021;6(2):59. https://doi.org/10.52876/jcs.1004847.
49. Nasim S, Almutairi MS, Munir K, Raza A, Younas F. A novel approach for polycystic ovary syndrome prediction using machine learning in bioinformatics. IEEE Access. 2022;10:97610–24. https://doi.org/10.1109/ACCESS.2022.3205587.
50. Ahmetasevic A, Alicelebic L, Bajric B, Becic E, Smajovic A, Deumic A. Using artificial neural network in diagnosis of polycystic ovary syndrome. In: 2022 11th Mediterranean Conference on embedded computing, MECO 2022. 2022. https://doi.org/10.1109/MECO55406.2022.9797204.

GPSR Compliance

The European Union's (EU) General Product Safety Regulation (GPSR) is a set of rules that requires consumer products to be safe and our obligations to ensure this.

If you have any concerns about our products, you can contact us on ProductSafety@springernature.com

In case Publisher is established outside the EU, the EU authorized representative is:

Springer Nature Customer Service Center GmbH
Europaplatz 3
69115 Heidelberg, Germany

Batch number: 10732090

Printed by Printforce, the Netherlands